Basic Measurements in
Ophthalmology

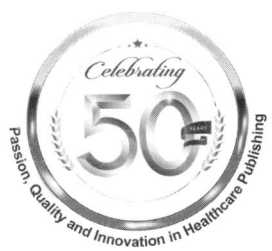

Basic Measurements in Ophthalmology

J Antony MS DO
Professor and Head
Department of Ophthalmology
Sree Gokulam Medical College and Research Foundation
Thiruvananthapuram, Kerala, India

Formerly, Professor
Regional Institute of Ophthalmology
Government Medical College
Thiruvananthapuram, Kerala, India

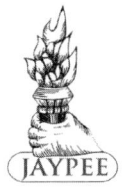

JAYPEE BROTHERS MEDICAL PUBLISHERS
The Health Sciences Publisher
New Delhi | London | Panama

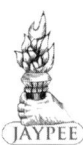 **Jaypee Brothers Medical Publishers (P) Ltd**

Headquarters

Jaypee Brothers Medical Publishers (P) Ltd
4838/24, Ansari Road, Daryaganj
New Delhi 110 002, India
Phone: +91-11-43574357
Fax: +91-11-43574314
Email: jaypee@jaypeebrothers.com

Overseas Offices

J.P. Medical Ltd
83 Victoria Street, London
SW1H 0HW (UK)
Phone: +44 20 3170 8910
Fax: +44 (0)20 3008 6180
Email: info@jpmedpub.com

Jaypee-Highlights Medical Publishers Inc
City of Knowledge, Bld. 235, 2nd Floor, Clayton
Panama City, Panama
Phone: +1 507-301-0496
Fax: +1 507-301-0499
Email: cservice@jphmedical.com

Jaypee Brothers Medical Publishers (P) Ltd
17/1-B Babar Road, Block-B, Shyamoli
Mohammadpur, Dhaka-1207
Bangladesh
Mobile: +08801912003485
Email: jaypeedhaka@gmail.com

Jaypee Brothers Medical Publishers (P) Ltd
Bhotahity, Kathmandu
Nepal
Phone: +977-9741283608
Email: kathmandu@jaypeebrothers.com

Website: www.jaypeebrothers.com
Website: www.jaypeedigital.com

© 2019, Jaypee Brothers Medical Publishers

The views and opinions expressed in this book are solely those of the original contributor(s)/author(s) and do not necessarily represent those of editor(s) of the book.

All rights reserved. No part of this publication may be reproduced, stored or transmitted in any form or by any means, electronic, mechanical, photocopying, recording or otherwise, without the prior permission in writing of the publishers.

All brand names and product names used in this book are trade names, service marks, trademarks or registered trademarks of their respective owners. The publisher is not associated with any product or vendor mentioned in this book.

Medical knowledge and practice change constantly. This book is designed to provide accurate, authoritative information about the subject matter in question. However, readers are advised to check the most current information available on procedures included and check information from the manufacturer of each product to be administered, to verify the recommended dose, formula, method and duration of administration, adverse effects and contraindications. It is the responsibility of the practitioner to take all appropriate safety precautions. Neither the publisher nor the author(s)/editor(s) assume any liability for any injury and/or damage to persons or property arising from or related to use of material in this book.

This book is sold on the understanding that the publisher is not engaged in providing professional medical services. If such advice or services are required, the services of a competent medical professional should be sought.

Every effort has been made where necessary to contact holders of copyright to obtain permission to reproduce copyright material. If any have been inadvertently overlooked, the publisher will be pleased to make the necessary arrangements at the first opportunity. The **CD/DVD-ROM** (if any) provided in the sealed envelope with this book is complimentary and free of cost. **Not meant for sale.**

Inquiries for bulk sales may be solicited at: jaypee@jaypeebrothers.com

Basic Measurements in Ophthalmology

First Edition: **2019**

ISBN: 978-93-5270-548-1

Printed at Rajkamal Electric Press, Kundli, Haryana.

Dedicated to

My beloved parents and my patients

Preface

Eyeball being a small mysterious globe of 24 mm diameter with its adnexa performing wonderful functions, it is important to know the measurements of various parts of eye for a better diagnosis of eye disorders and imparting skills in the medical and particularly in surgical management of various ophthalmic ailments.

An ophthalmic surgeon incising chalazion should know the thickness of tarsal plate (0.75–1 mm). To perform a good surgical correction of senile entropion, one should not only know the length of tarsal plate (about 25 mm) but also be aware of its width (upper tarsus 9–10 mm at its widest portion and lower tarsus 4–5 mm).

Though majority of measurements mentioned in this book are anatomical ones, many of them have been made bioluminescent by indicating their clinical usefulness. Proper location of measurements necessitated some amount of theoretical descriptions. Again, the measurements mentioned in this book are not strictly mathematical but biological and flexible and can be applied according to the clinical situations.

This book is thus an attempt to bring out some of the important measurements which are routinely used in ophthalmic practice with the hope that they might help all ophthalmologists as a reference tool for their learning and teaching purposes and also for their clinical practice.

J Antony

Acknowledgments

I am deeply indebted to Almighty God, my family members, teachers, colleagues and students who have helped me to shape the ideas to mold this book in this shape.

Again, I am extremely thankful to the artists Mr Arif (Sree Gokulam Medical College and Research Foundation, Thiruvananthapuram, Kerala, India) and Mr Rajasekharan (Government Medical College and Research Foundation, Thiruvananthapuram), who have drawn most of the diagrams. Mr NK Prasanth has performed the hard task of typing, setting, design work and layout of this book and he deserves great appreciation.

Finally, I express my sincere gratitude to Shri Jitendar P Vij (Group Chairman) and Mr Ankit Vij (Managing Director), Mr MS Mani (Group President), Ms Ritu Sharma (Director—Content Strategy), Ms Pooja Bhandari (Production Head), Ms Sunita Katla (Executive Assistant to Group Chairman and Publishing Manager), and staff of M/s Jaypee Brothers Medical Publishers (P) Ltd, New Delhi, India, for providing timely guidance and continued encouragement to me for the completion of this book.

Contents

1. **General Configuration and Gross Measurements of Eye**   1
   - Eyeball   1
   - Summary of general measurements of eyeball   4

2. **Measurements of Conjunctiva**   6
   - Structure   6
   - Portions of conjunctiva   7
   - Conjunctival sac   8
   - Attachments of bulbar conjunctiva   9
   - Fornix-based conjunctival flap   9
   - Goblet cells   10
   - Conjunctival impression cytology   11
   - Summary of measurements and dimensions of conjunctiva   12

3. **Measurements of Sclera**   14
   - Scleral dimensions   14
   - Structure of sclera   15
   - Insertion of extraocular muscles   16
   - Scleral apertures   16
   - Weak areas of sclera   20
   - Scleral rigidity   20
   - Ocular rigidity and applanation tonometry   24
   - Functions of sclera   24
   - Summary of measurements of sclera   24

4. **Measurements of Cornea**   26
   - Structure of cornea   26
   - Endothelium   30
   - Thickness of layers of cornea   32
   - Corneal innervation   32
   - Surface area of cornea   32
   - Corneal diameter   32
   - Microcornea   33
   - Megalocornea   33
   - Shape and curvature of cornea   35
   - Normal variations of corneal curvature   35
   - Measurement of corneal curvature and shape (Topography)   37
   - Computerized corneal topography (Videokeratography)   39
   - Refractive power   41
   - Refractive index   41
   - Corneal thickness   41
   - Summary of measurements of cornea   44

5. Measurements of Limbus — 46
- Limit (extend) of limbus 46
- Structure of limbus (layer by layer changes) 47
- Functions and importance of limbus 47
- Vulnerability limbus to diseases (medial limbus) 48
- Diseases particularly affecting limbus and adjacent regions 48
- Dimensions of limbus 49
- Landmarks of limbus 49
- Zones of limbus 50
- Surgical anatomy and dimensions of limbus 51
- Cyclodestructive procedures 55
- Cataract surgery and limbus 56
- Postlimbal—scleral incision 58

6. Measurements of Anterior Chamber — 62
- Boundaries of anterior chamber 62
- Dimensions of AC and its normal variations 63
- Summary of measurements of anterior chamber 63
- Angle of anterior chamber 63
- Trabecular meshwork 64
- Aqueous humor 67
- Intraocular pressure 69
- Glaucoma 70
- Tonometry 71
- Tonography 75

7. Measurements of Posterior Chamber — 81
- Parts of posterior chamber 81
- Boundaries of posterior chamber (summary) 83
- Functions of posterior chamber 83
- Dimensions of posterior chamber 84

8. Measurements of Uveal Tract — 85
- Iris 85
- Pupil 89
- Ciliary body 91
- Choroid 96

9. Measurements of Lens — 99
- Dimensions of lens 99
- Structure and surgical anatomy of lens 102
- Summary of dimensions of lens 107

10. Measurements of Zonules (of Zinn) — 109
- Dimensions and extent of zonules 109
- Parts of zonules 110
- Zonular bundles 110
- Functions of zonules 111
- Summary of dimensions and extent of zonules 111

11. Measurements of Vitreous Humor   112
- Structure of vitreous   112
- Primary, secondary and tertiary vitreous   113
- Vitreous topography   114
- Vitrectomy measurements   118

12. Measurements of Retina   126
- General structure (architecture) of retina   127
- Summary of measurement of retinal layers   131
- Gross measurements and general features of retina   132
- Clinical and functional differentiations and measurements of optic disk, macula and peripheral retina   135
- Methods of evaluation of different portions of retina particularly the retinal nerve fiber layer   146
- Summary of measurements of retina   151

13. Measurements of Optic Nerve   152
- Differences of optic nerve from other cranial nerves   152
- Structure and dimensions of various portions of optic nerve   153
- Variations in the arrangement of fibers in the distal and proximal portions of optic nerve   156
- In the proximal portion (chiasmal) of optic nerve   157
- Functions of optic nerve   158
- Summary of measurements of optic nerve   159

14. Measurements of Optic Chiasma   160
- Dimensions of optic chiasma   161
- Position of optic chiasma in the cranial cavity   161
- Relations of optic chiasma   162
- Measurements of sella   165
- Variations in the relationship of optic chiasma to sella turcica and pituitary gland   165
- Arrangement of fibers in optic chiasma   167
- Common lesions affecting optic chiasma   168
- Visual field defects in chiasmal lesions   168
- Clues for clinical suspicion of chiasmal lesions   171

15. Measurements of Eyebrows   172
- Dimensions of eyebrows   172
- Layers or structure of eyebrows   173
- Functions of eyebrows   174
- Clinical situations involving eyebrows   174

16. Measurements of Eyelids   178
- Gross measurements of upper lid   178
- Structure of upper lid   178
- Palpebral fissure   186
- Relative levels of medial and lateral canthi   187

- Measurements of ptosis   189
- Measurements of lower lid   191
- Functions of eyelids   195
- Measurement of upper lid (gross)   195
- Measurements of individual eyelid structures   195

17. Measurements of Lacrimal Apparatus   197
- Main lacrimal gland and its measurements   198
- Accessory lacrimal glands   199
- Lacrimal passages and their measurements   200
- Nasolacrimal duct   203
- Lacrimal sac surgery measurements   206

18. Measurements of Orbit   209
- Dimension of orbits   209
- Bones and walls of orbit   211
- Orbit-eyeball relationship—normal and abnormal   213
- Walls of orbit   215
- Lateral wall of orbit   217
- Floor of orbit   219
- Medial wall of orbit   222
- Orbital apex   223
- Communications of orbit   225
- Optic canal   225
- Superior orbital fissure   227
- Inferior orbital fissure   228
- General configuration and surface marking of recti muscle insertions   232
- Dimensions of extraocular muscles   235
- Angle or meridian of insertion of extraocular muscles   236
- Visual axis, optic axis, center of rotation of eyeball, orbital planes and orbital axis   236
- Center of rotation of eyeball   238
- General principles and measurements in surgical correction of squints   239

Suggested Readings   *243*

Index   *245*

PLATE 1

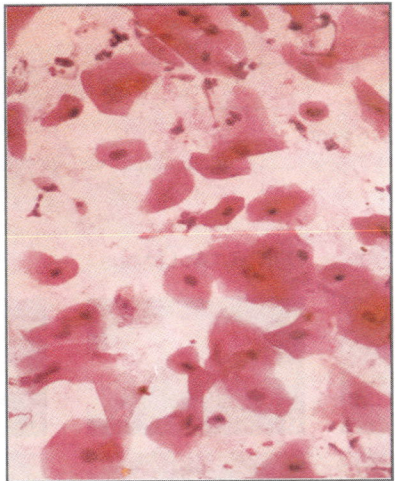

Fig. 2.7: Conjunctival impression cytology.

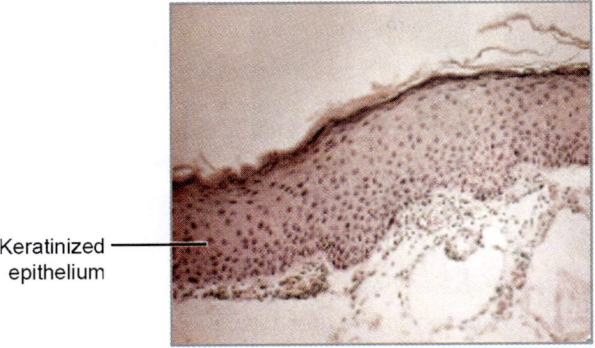

Keratinized epithelium

Fig. 2.9: Loss of goblet cells in conjunctival scarring.

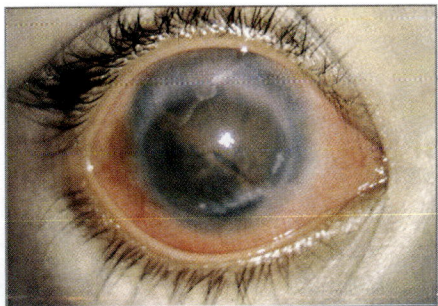

Fig. 4.12: Congenital glaucoma (buphthalmos) with enlarged corneal diameter and limbal stretching.

PLATE 2

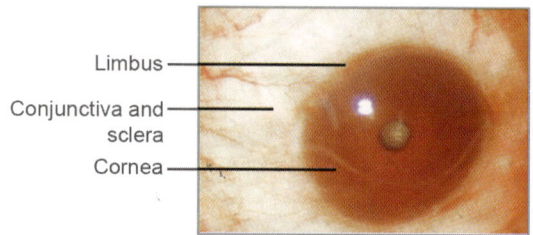

Fig. 5.1A: Limbus.

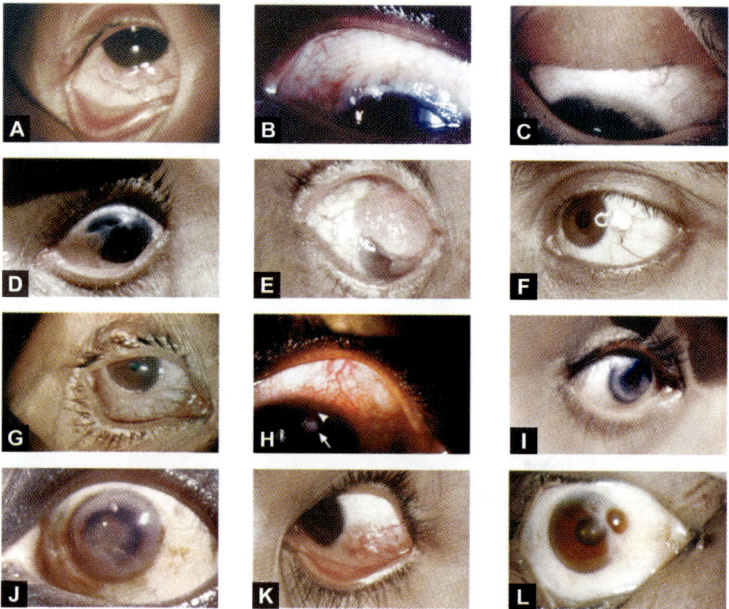

Figs. 5.3A to L: Diseases affecting limbus and adjacent regions: (A) Phlyctenular conjunctivitis; (B) Vernal conjunctivitis (limbal form); (C) Trachomatous pannus; (D) Pterygium; (E) Squamous cell carcinoma of conjunctiva; (F) Bitot's spot; (G) Marginal keratitis due to staphylococcal toxin; (H) Phlyctenular keratits; (I) Arcus juvenilis; (J) Kayser-Fleischer ring; (K) Episcleritis; (L) Peripheral corneal melting in rheumatoid arthritis.

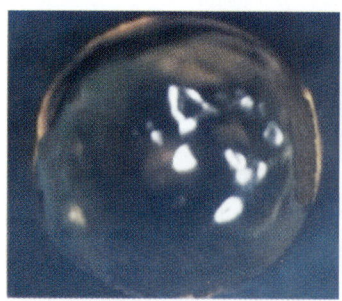

Fig. 9.1: Normal lens.

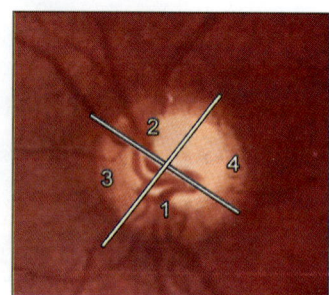

Fig. 12.8: Variations in thickness (breadth) of different regions of optic disk

PLATE 3

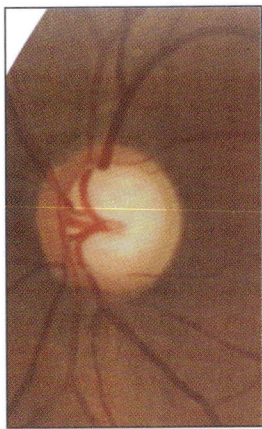

Enlarge vertically oval cup
cup-disk ratio >0.7

Fig. 12.9: Glaucomatous cupping.

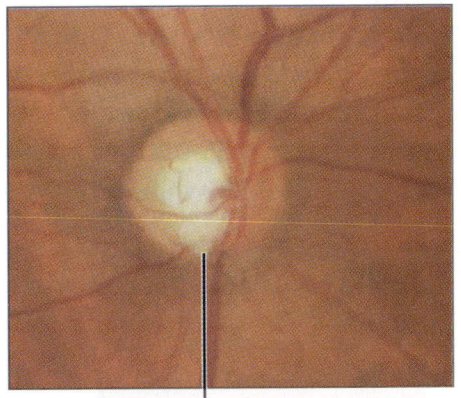

Inferior NRR

Fig. 12.10: Thinning of inferior neuroretinal rim (NRR) in glaucoma.

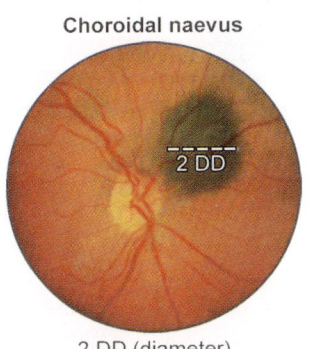

2 DD (diameter)

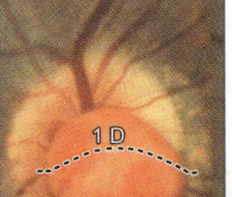

1 D (elevation)

Fig. 12.11: Disk diameter (DD) and diopter (D) elevation.

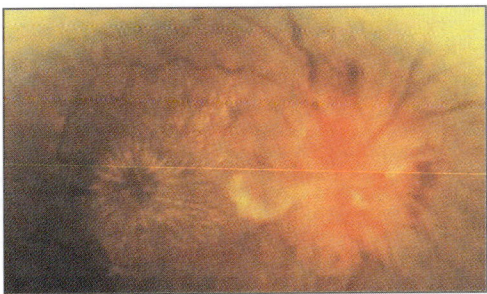

Fig. 12.12: Red swollen disk (papilledema).

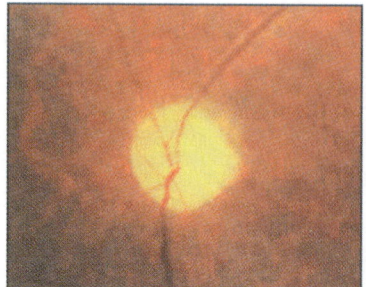

Fig. 12.13: Consecutive optic atrophy (yellowish waxy pale disk).

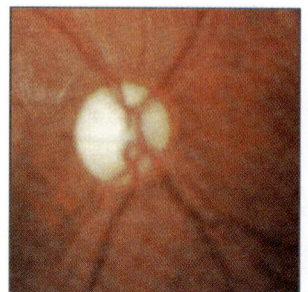

Fig. 12.14: Primary optic atrophy (papery white disk).

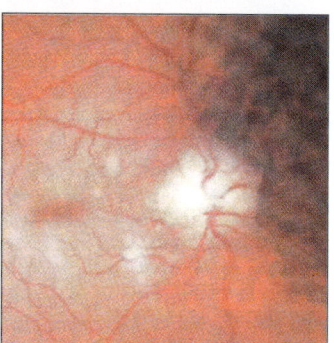

Fig. 12.15: Postneuritic (secondary) optic atrophy dirty gray color.

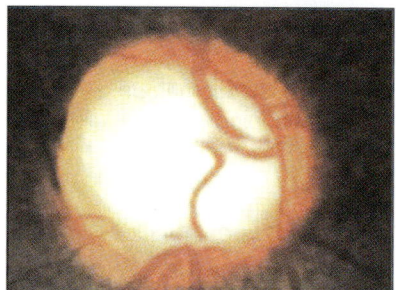

Fig. 12.16: Pale disk with deep wide (glaucomatous) cupping.

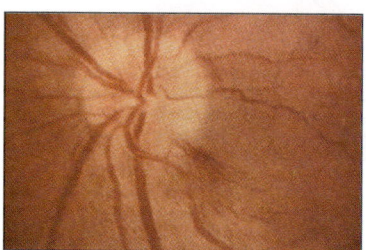

Fig. 12.17: Anterior ischemic optic neuropathy (pallid disk edema).

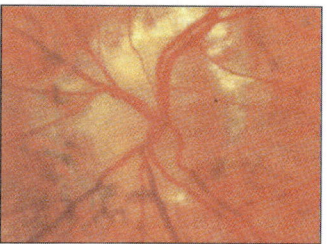

Fig. 12.18: Optic disk drusen (yellow swollen disk).

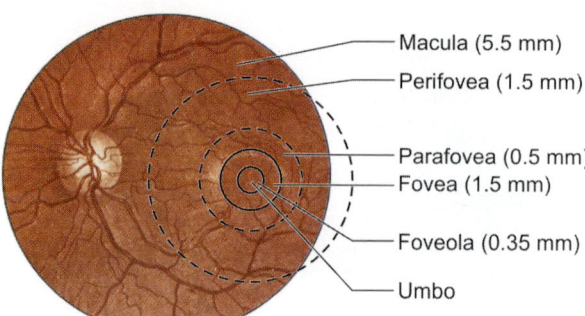

Fig. 12.20: Portions of macula.

PLATE 5

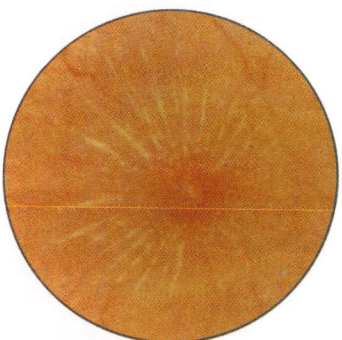

Fig. 12.23: Macular star.

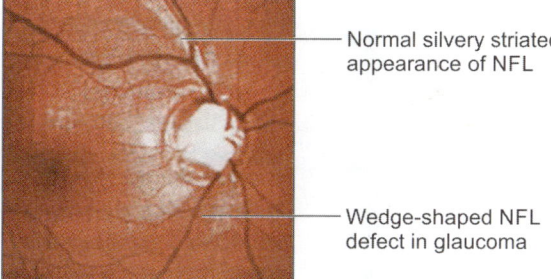

Fig. 12.25: Ophthalmoscopic appearance of normal and abnormal nerve fiber layer (NFL).

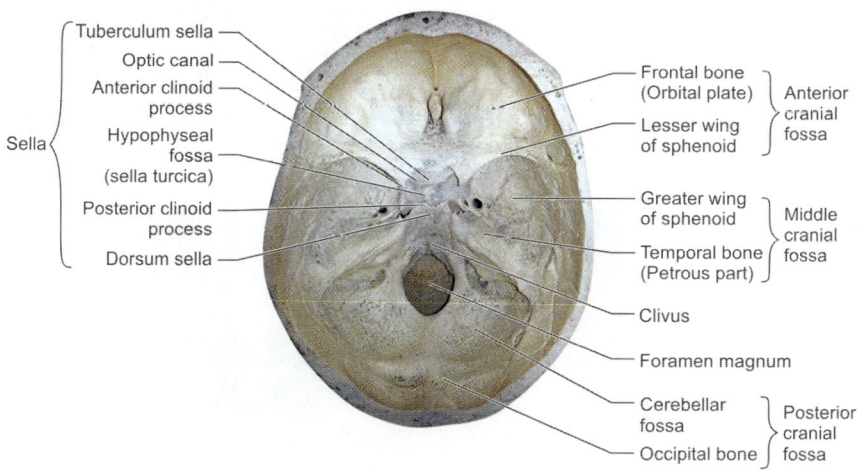

Fig. 14.6: Cranial fossae and sella.

PLATE 6

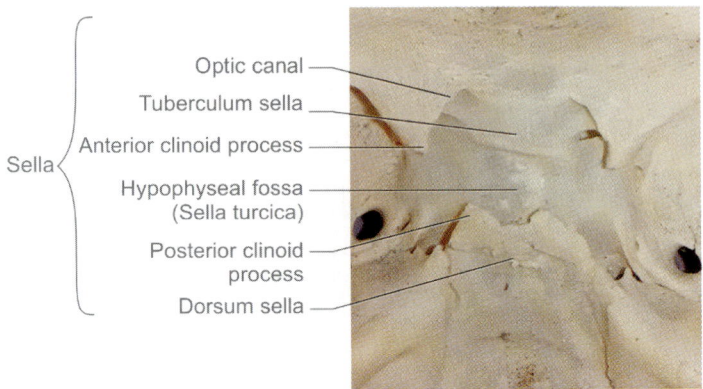

Fig. 14.7: Portions of sella.

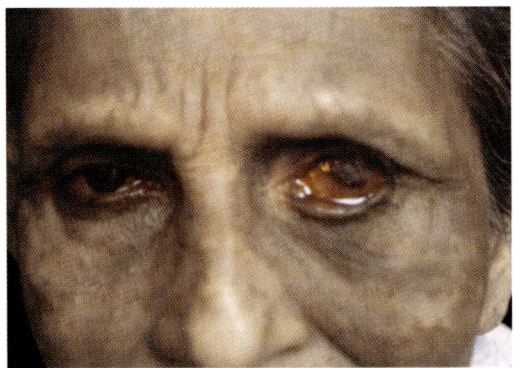

Fig. 15.3: Loss of eyebrow hairs in leprosy. (*For color version, see Plate 6*)

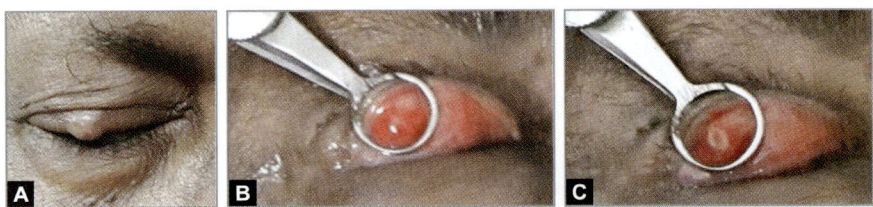

Figs. 16.20A to C: (A) Chalazion; (B) Lid everted with chalazion clamp to expose the granuloma; (C) Tarsal plate opened for removal of granuloma.

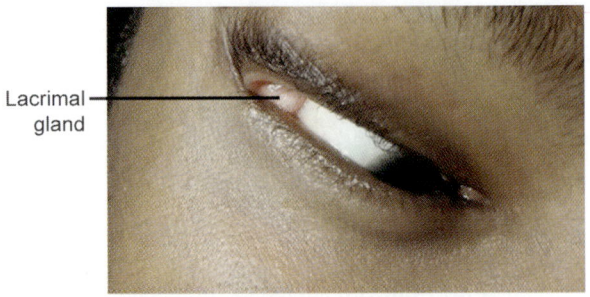

Fig. 17.3: Palpebral lobe of normal lacrimal gland visible in the upper and outer conjunctival fornix.

PLATE 7

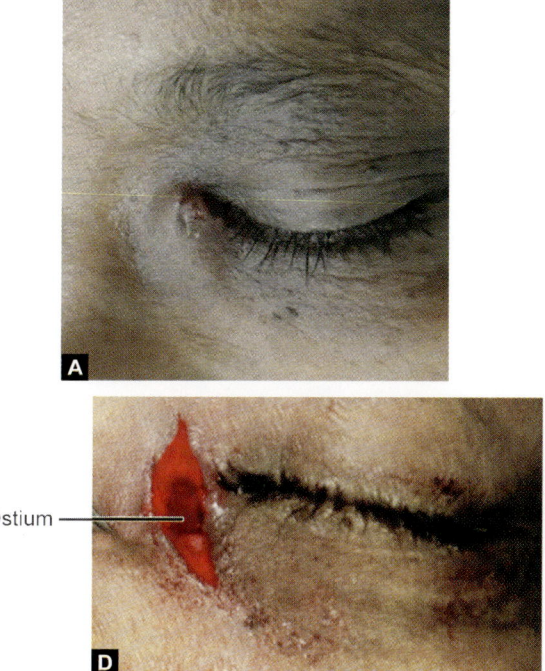

Ostium

Figs. 17.13A and D: DCR steps: (A) Dacryocystitis; (D) DCR incision closed.

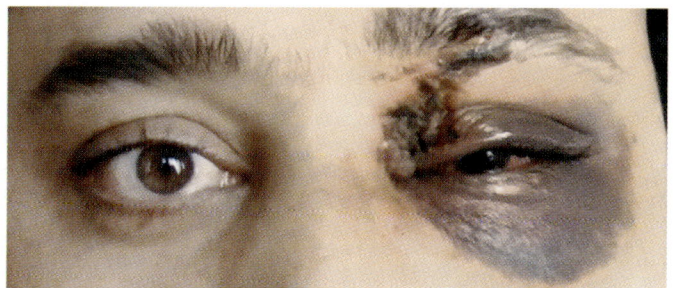

Fig. 18.17: Orbital floor injury (left).

CHAPTER 1

General Configuration and Gross Measurements of Eye

Eye consists mainly of Eyeball, Ocular adnexa (eyelids, lacrimal apparatus and orbit), their vascular connections and neurological pathways.

EYEBALL

Structure (Fig. 1)

Structurally the eyeball has three walls performing different visually vital functions, enclosing various intraocular structures like lens, vitreous cavity enclosing the vitreous and the anterior and posterior chambers filled with aqueous, arranged in order so that light comes to a focus on the retina resulting in image formation. The walls of the eye are as follows:

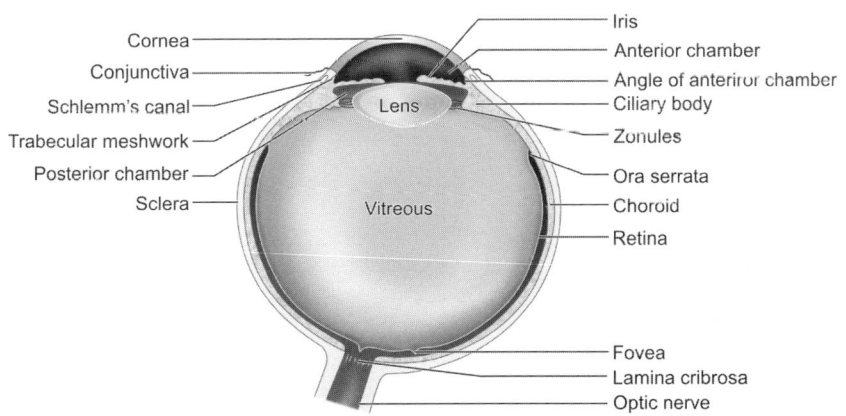

Fig. 1: General structure of eyeball.

- *Outer wall:* Is mainly protective in function and is made of cornea in front and sclera behind.
- *Middle wall:* Gives nutrition to many parts of eye and has three portions—iris, ciliary body and choroid.
- *Inner wall:* Performs predominantly neurological function—the retina.

General Dimensions

Eye ball is not a perfectly spherical globe, as its anterior and posterior segments have different curvatures.

Anterior 1/6th of outer wall, the cornea is more curved (steeper) than posterior 5/6th, the sclera which is less curved (flatter) with a transitional zone in between them (limbus)(Fig. 2).

Radius of Curvature of Globe

- *Radius of curvature of the anterior portion (cornea) is about 7.8 mm.*
- *Radius of curvature of the posterior portion (sclera) is about 12 mm.*

Summit of the curved anterior portion is the *anterior pole* and the apex of curved posterior portion is the *posterior pole* of the globe.

Diameter of Eyeball

Anteroposterior diameter (length) of eye ball is about 24 mm. Vertical diameter is 23.5 mm.

Equator of the Eyeball

- *External (Geometric) equator:* Externally the equator of the eye ball is a circular line drawn on the exterior surface of the ball equidistant from anterior and posterior pole. The circumference of equator is about 71 to 75 mm.
- *Anatomical equator:* Since the eye is slightly anatomically tilted backwards on temporal side for 1 to 1.5 mm and slightly nasally and sclera buldges

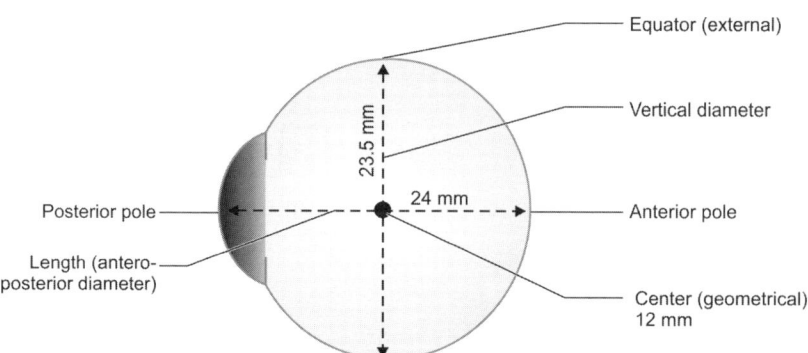

Fig. 2: Dimensions of eyeball.

slightly temporally, circle representing the anatomical equator may not be exactly in the middle of the globe.
- *Surgical equator:* Is the widest diameter of the globe in coronal plane.
- *Clinical equator:* Is an imaginary line drawn along the ampullae of vortex vein as seen on fundus examination (Fig. 3).

Center of (geometrical) eyeball: Center of eye ball is about 12 mm behind the anterior pole of globe.

Center of rotation of eyeball: Center of rotation of eyeball is slightly behind the center of the eyeball and is about 13 mm behind the anterior pole.

Nodal point of the eyeball: Different points of visual field are connected to the retinal points by visual planes, each of them passing through the nodal point of eye. This point is situated in the posterior pole of the lens and is about 7.2 mm behind the apex of cornea (Fig. 4).

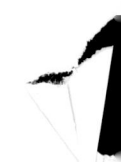

Visual Axis

Visual axis is an imaginary line connecting object of fixation, nodal point of the eye and fovea.

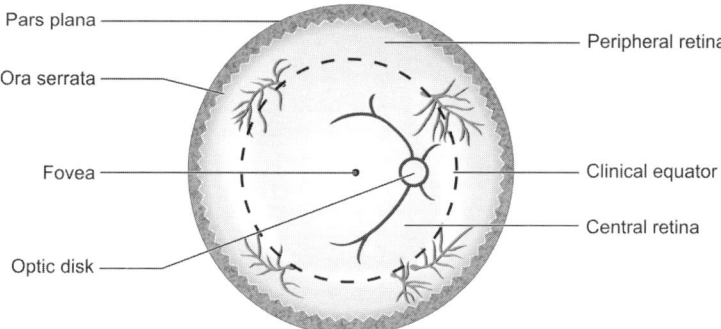

Fig. 3: Internal (clinical) equator.

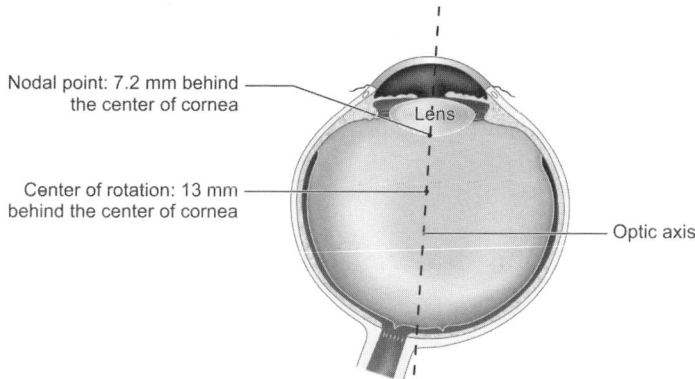

Fig. 4: Optic axis, nodal point and center of rotation of eyeball.

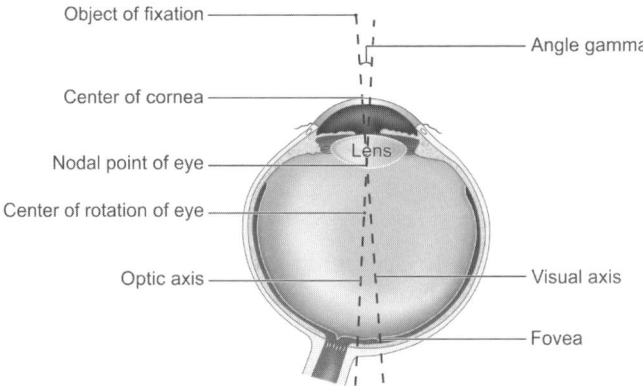

Fig. 5: Optic axis, visual axis and angle gamma.

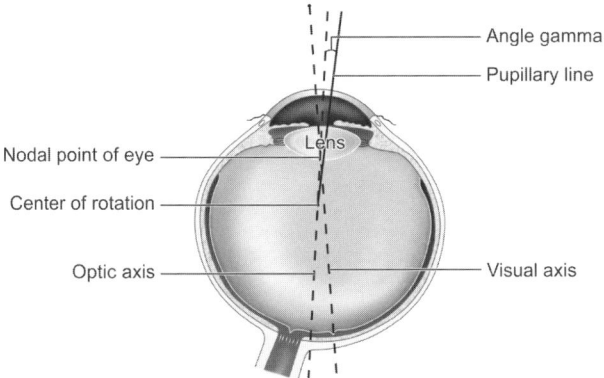

Fig. 6: Optic axis, visual axis, pupillary line and angle kappa.

Optic Axis

Optic axis passes from a point 0.25 mm nasal to the center of cornea, lens, center of rotation of eyeball and approximately through the center of pupil intersecting visual axis at nodal point and extent more nasally posteriorly. Pupillary line passes through center of cornea and center of pupil almost near the optic axis.

The angle between visual axis and optic axis is called angle gamma. This angle is assessed clinically at the pupillary plane (not very accurate) and is called angle Kappa also (Figs. 5 and 6).

SUMMARY OF GENERAL MEASUREMENTS OF EYEBALL (FIG. 7)

- Radius of curvature anterior
  1/6th of eyeball (cornea)   : 8 mm
- Radius of curvature of posterior
  5/6th of eyeball (sclera)   : 12 mm

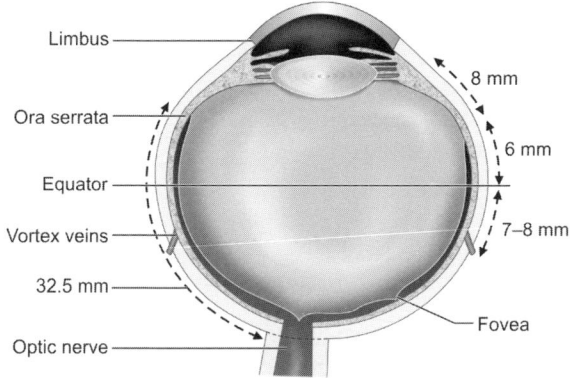

Fig. 7: Approximate distance of ora serrata, equator and vortex veins in mm from limbus as marked on surface of sclera.

- Length (anteroposterior diameter) of eyeball : 24 mm
- Vertical diameter of eyeball : 23 mm
- Horizontal diameter of eyeball : 23.5 mm
- Center of eyeball (geometrical) : 12 mm behind apex of cornea
- Nodal point of eyeball : 7.2 mm behind apex of cornea
- Center of rotation of eyeball : 13 mm behind anterior pole
- Distance of limbus to ora serrata : 8 mm
- Distance of ora serrata to equator : 6 mm
- Distance of limbus to equator : 14 mm
- Weight of eyeball : 7.15 grams in adult and 3 grams in infant
- Surface area : 22.86 cm^2
- Specific gravity : 1.077
- Volume : 7.2 mL

CHAPTER 2

Measurements of Conjunctiva

Conjunctiva is a thin membrane which extends between eyelids and eyeball connecting them. It is a continuous, translucent, mucous membrane lining the posterior surface of eyelid and anterior portion of sclera.

STRUCTURE (FIG. 1)

Structurally conjunctiva has three layers from surface to depth.
- *Non-keratinized stratified epithelium:* It is two layered in palpebral conjunctiva and many layered in fornices and limbal portions. Superficial layers carry goblet cells which secrete mucus.
- *Adenoid layer:* Under epithelium is the adenoid layer made of loose connective tissue containing few leukocytes. In inflammatory and irritative conditions of conjunctiva, they proliferate and elevate the epithelium to form follicles.

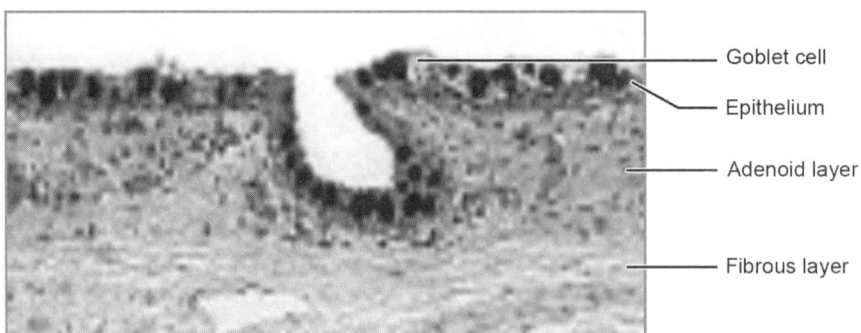

Fig. 1: Structure of conjunctiva.

Fibrous layer: Under the adenoid layer is dense fibrous tissue layer which merges with underlying tissue of lid or eyeball.

PORTIONS OF CONJUNCTIVA

Conjunctiva has following portions (Figs. 2 to 4):
- *Marginal portion:* Lining the posterior portion of lid margins. It starts in the middle of lid margin posterior to the opening of meibomian glands and extends up to the sharp posterior margin of lid.
- *Tarsal conjunctiva:* Conjunctiva is then continued from posterior lid margin to the posterior surface of eyelid and is closely adherent to tarsal plate. About 2 mm above the posterior margin of upper eyelid margin there is a shallow groove on the back of eyelid—sulcus subtarsalis. This sulcus tends to trap small foreign bodies which get into the conjunctival sac, and is clinically important. Unlike the upper tarsal conjunctiva, the lower is adherent for only to upper half of the lower tarsal width.
- *Orbital conjunctiva:* Is that portion of conjunctiva between upper border of tarsal plate and upper fornix in upper lid and lower border of tarsal plate and fornix in lower lid. It is loosely attached to subjacent Muller's muscle and is important in ptosis surgery.
- *Conjunctival fornix:* Conjunctiva then bends acutely to form a continuous annular recess, the conjunctival fornix and then gets reflected over the sclera. The conjunctival fornix has different portions with different dimensions.
    - *Superior fornix*—reaches about almost 13 mm from upper lid margin and 8-10 mm from limbus.

      Ducts from the lacrimal gland and accessory glands of Krause open into upper fornix. Upper fornix has important attachments to:
        - Portion of levator palpebrae superioris
        - Some fibers of superior rectus muscle
        - Muller's unstriped muscle and
        - Orbital septum.
    - Inferior fornix extends down only about 9 mm from lower lid margin and 8 to 10 mm down from the limbus.

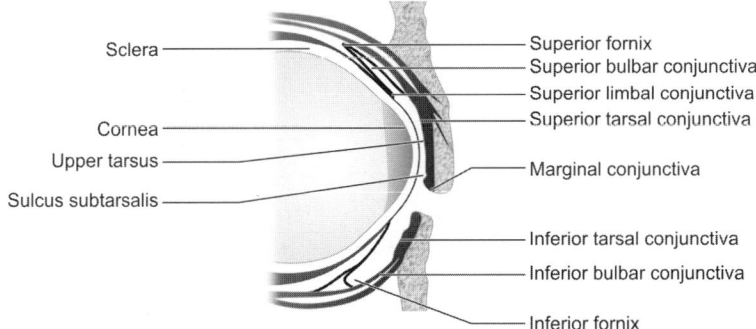

Fig. 2: Portions of conjunctiva.

- Lateral fornix extents about 5 mm from lateral margin of lid and 14 mm from the limbus, reaching just posterior to equator.
- Medial fornix—is the shallowest, comprising medial ends of superior and inferior fornices. Extends to about 7 mm from limbus.
- *Bulbar conjunctiva:* Fornicial conjunctiva gets reflected on to the anterior part of eyeball (sclera) to form bulbar conjunctiva and stops at the limbus. Conjunctival epithelium alone continues as the corneal epithelium.

CONJUNCTIVAL SAC

All the above five parts of conjunctiva particularly the fornices together form a conjunctival sac which open at the palpebral fissure. Ointments and drops are instilled into this region especially lower fornix.

Conjunctival sac normally contains about 7 microliter of tear fluid but can accommodate even up to 30 microliter. If eye drops are instilled in excess of this volume are either drained into lacrimal sac or overflow the lids.

In the intertendinous intervals behind the fornices, the conjunctiva adjoins orbital fat. So a hemorrhage due to a fracture of base of skull can advance under conjunctiva to the limbus.

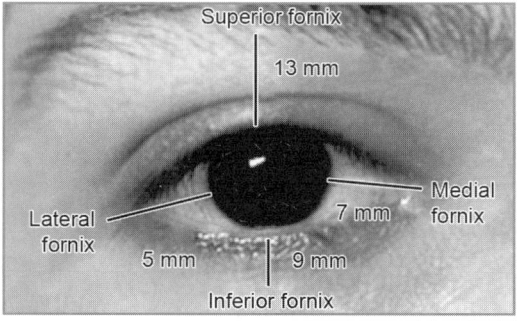

Fig. 3: Level of dimension of conjunctival sac in mm from lid margin.

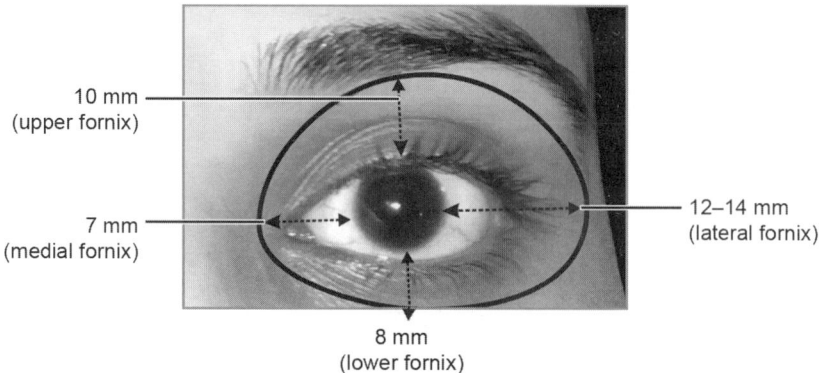

Fig. 4: Extent (distance) of fornices from limbus.

Incisions at the superior fornix enter areolar tissue between levator and superior rectus.

At the inferior fornix incisions enter between the inferior palpebral and inferior rectus muscles and the expansions from inferior ocular muscles.

ATTACHMENTS OF BULBAR CONJUNCTIVA

Bulbar conjunctiva is tied down to Tenon's facia (fascia bulbi) by areolar tissue and is mobile. Fascia bulbi (capsule of Tenon) is a thin fibrous sheath which envelops the globe from behind the limbus to the level of optic nerve.) Anteriorly Tenon's facia is under bulbar conjunctiva and for about 3 mm behind limbus it is separated from bulbar conjunctiva by loose connective tissue (containing subconjunctival vessels) and can be distinguished from it during surgery.

At about 2 or 3 mm posteriorly from limbus—conjunctiva, fascia bulbi (Tenon's capsule) and sclera are firmly adherent. Because the conjunctiva is less mobile here, a firmer hold of globe can be obtained with forceps during surgery. At this union conjunctiva form a slight ridge, obvious in infections.

Behind this, conjunctiva is in contact with the tenon capsule coverings of extraocular muscle tendons (fascia bulbi), both have to be divided to expose the tendons of muscles during squint surgery.

Bulbar conjunctiva, except around limbus, is lax and mobile. It contains a good amount of elastic tissue. It is maximum loose in the fornices and the periphery of bulbar conjunctiva. The amount of conjunctiva available for conjunctival grafting is more on the temporal side of bulbar conjunctiva and then nasal and in the upper fornix than in the lower fornix. So conjunctival flaps are usually made and mobilized from above and temporal side.

FORNIX-BASED CONJUNCTIVAL FLAP

Fornix-based conjunctival flaps (Fig. 5) are preferred in most of the surgeries of eyeball, like cataract surgery (SICS), antiglaucoma surgeries, retinal detachment surgeries (scleral indentation), etc.

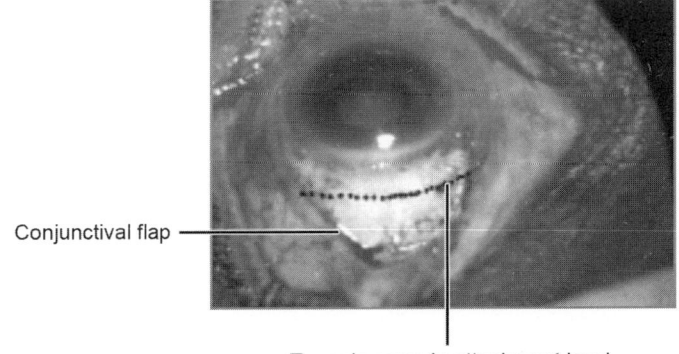

Fig. 5: Fornix-based conjunctival flap.

In cataract surgery, generally a fornix-based conjunctival flap of varying length 2-6 mm consisting of bulbar conjunctiva and Tenon's capsule is made according to technique of the surgery. Conjunctiva with Tenon's capsule is held with fine forceps (holding perpendicular to the ocular surface), behind the limbus, is buttonholed and undermined with spring scissors, cut and separated from limbal attachment to desired extend. *The firm attachment of bulbar conjunctiva to the tenon's capsule at about 3 mm behind has to be released to expose sufficient clear scleral bed to fecilitate good scleral tunnel incision.*

GOBLET CELLS

Goblet cells are the main source of mucin—which is an essential portion of precorneal tear film, making ocular surface hydrophilic. These glands are intracellular glands present in most of the portions of conjunctival epithelium. Goblet cells are modified conjunctival epithelial cells which get enlarged due to accumulation of mucus shifting the nucleus to the base of cells. Goblet cells develop from basal layer of epithelium. *Goblet cells are round or oval in shape, 10 to 20 micrometer wide with flat basal nuclei. The cells become larger (25 µ × 26 µ) and more* oval as they approach the surface where they develop a stoma and discharge their mucin content. They are finally shed into conjunctival sac. Goblet cell openings are 1 to 3 micrometer in size on the tarsal conjunctiva and 2 to 5 micrometer elsewhere (Fig. 6).

They make about 15% of superficial epithelial cell population and 8% of basal epithelial cell population in children. Their mean linear density is about 10 cells/mm.

Though goblet cells occur throughout conjunctiva, singly or along epithelial crypts, goblet cell population is maximum in the nasal portion of the conjunctiva especially in plica semilunaris. Goblet cell density decreases in the temporal portion especially in the upper temporal fornix and almost absent at the limbus and mucocutaneous junctions of eyelid margin.

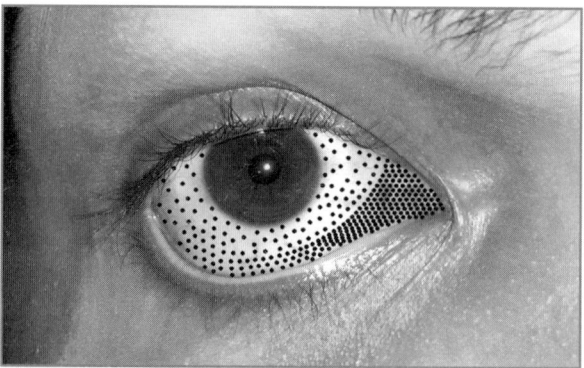

Fig. 6: General density of goblet cells in conjunctiva.

CONJUNCTIVAL IMPRESSION CYTOLOGY (FIG. 7)

Conjunctival impression cytology (CIC) is a noninvasive simple technique of studying the histological changes in the conjunctival epithelium—introduced by Egbert et al.

After anesthetizing the conjunctiva using topical proparacaine 0.5% or lignocaine 4% eye drops, cellulose acetate paper (HAWP 01300) cut into small pieces of 5×5 mm^2. Size are applied to the upper bulbar conjunctiva, about 2 mm above the limbus, one on 11 O'clock and another on 1 O'clock position with forceps and gentle pressure is applied for 3 to 5 seconds. Then filter papers are removed.

One of them is fixed in a combined solution of 70% ethyl alcohol, 37% formaldehyde and glacial acetic acid (mixed in a ratio 20:1:1) for 10 minutes. This filter paper piece is stained with PAS and hematoxylin stain.

Other piece of filter paper is fixed in 95% ethyl alcohol and stained with Papanicolaou stain.

Both the pieces are cleared in xylene and examined under light microscope for cytological changes.
- Goblet cell density and loss
- Epithelial changes
- Any abnormality in nuclear chromatin, etc.

Natadisastra et al. have suggested a staging from 0 to 5 for cytological changes noted in conjunctival epithelium on microscopic examination in normal and various conjunctival disorders (Figs. 8 and 9).
- Stage 0 : Normal epithelium with abundant goblet cells and mucin spots.
- Stage 1 : Small epithelial cells, few goblets cells and mucin spots.
- Stage 2 : Enlargement of epithelium cells and loss of goblet cells and mucin spots.
- Stage 3 : Enlargement and separation of epithelial cells.

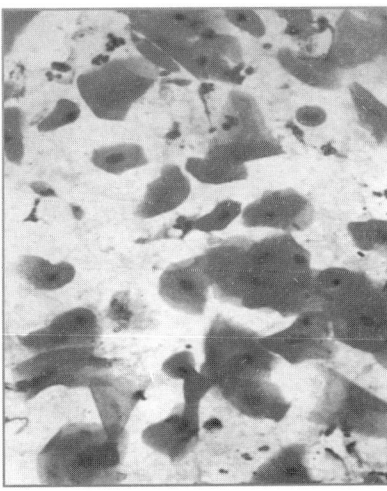

Fig. 7: Conjunctival impression cytology. (*For color version, see Plate 1*)

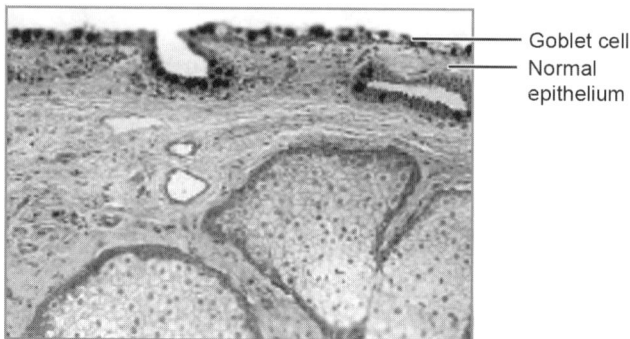

Fig. 8: Goblet cells in conjunctival epithelium.

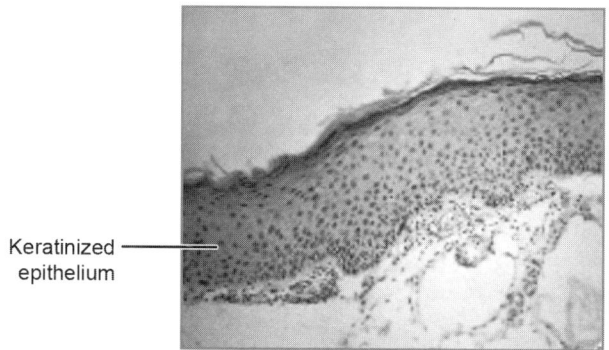

Fig. 9: Loss of goblet cells in conjunctival scarring.
(*For color version, see Plate 1*)

- Stage 4 : Large epithelial cells with scattered keratinization.
- Stage 5 : Large keratinized epithelial cells with nuclear loss.

The number of goblet cells increases in chronic inflammation. Their numbers decrease in keratinzation as in vitamin A deficiency and scarring—(Trachoma and burns of conjunctiva). Pemphigus, Steven Johnson syndrome, etc. leading to dry eye.

SUMMARY OF MEASUREMENTS AND DIMENSIONS OF CONJUNCTIVA

Level of Conjunctival Sac

1. Superior fornix : 13 mm from upper lid margin and 8 mm from limbus (almost up to the level of upper orbital margin)
2. Inferior fornix : 9 mm from lower lid margin and from limbus (to a few mm from inferior orbital margin)

3. Lateral fornix : 5 mm from lateral margin of lid and 14 mm from limbus (reaching just posterior to equator)

4. Medial fornix : 7 mm from limbus to medial canthus (just posterior to equator)

   – Volume of conjuctival sac : It can accommodate 30 microliters of tear fluid but normally contain only 7 microliters
   – Adherence of Tenon's capsule to conjunctiva : 3 mm behind limbus
   – Sulcus subtarsalis : 2 mm above lid margin
   – Mean goblet cell density : 10 cells per mm

CHAPTER 3

Measurements of Sclera

Sclera *forms the posterior five sixths of outer coat of eyeball,* is opaque and mainly performs protective function. Though the sclera is not a visually vital structure, scleral diseases can affect the visual function a lot, due to loss of protection to intraocular structures. Anteriorly sclera is continuous with the cornea and the line of union is known as corneoscleral junction or limbus. Posteriorly sclera is perforated by the optic nerve.

SCLERAL DIMENSIONS

Average *coronal diameter of scleral coat is between 22 to 24 mm.* In males diameter is 0.5 mm larger than females. At birth *anteroposterior diameter* is 16 to 17 mm increasing to **22.5 mm** by age of 3 years and reaching about 24 mm by age 13 years (Fig. 1).

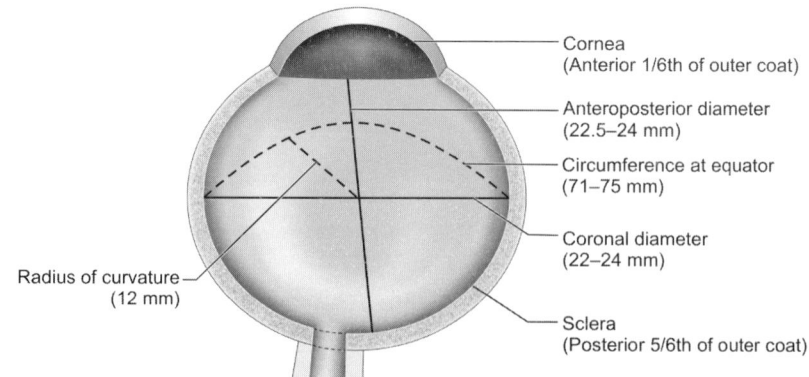

Fig. 1: Dimension of sclera.

The anterior portion of sclera is visible clinically (beneath transparent conjunctiva) as ***white of eye*** and has a dull white color in adults. In children it has a bluish tinge. Sclera may develop a yellowish color variation due to fatty deposits in elderly.

Following scleral inflammations, injuries, osteogenisis imperfecta, Ehlers-Danlos syndrome and other collagen diseases that produce a defect in collagen synthesis, sclera becomes abnormally thin and is *blue in color*—due to the underlying choroidal pigment showing through thin sclera.

STRUCTURE OF SCLERA

Sclera has Three Layers

- *Episclera*—is outermost layer and is made of loose connective tissue. It is connected to the Tenon's capsule over it by fine strands of tissue. Episclera slowly merges with the underlying scleral stroma. Anterior portion of episclera has blood supply from anterior ciliary vessels arising from the muscular branches of extraocular muscles. They form a plexus around sclerolimbal junction which will become conspicuous in inflammations of uveal tract and sclera—circumciliary congestion ("ciliary flush").
- *Scleral stroma*—The main mass of sclera is made of dense fibrous tissue intermingled with fine elastic fibers. Unlike cornea, the individual *collagen fibrils vary in diameter from 28 to 280 nanometer with periodicities of 8 and 11 micrometer.* The bundles of fibrils run in *whorls, loops and arches random forming a felt like matting of the bundles.* Few fibroblasts and melanocytes are found between collagen bundles.
- *Lamina fusca*—is the innermost layer of sclera, which is brown in color due to the presence of melanocytes. This layer has many grooves, caused by the passage of ciliary vessels and nerves. It is separated from the underlying choroid by the perichoroidal space but fine collagen fibers produce a weak connection between sclera and choroid.

Thickness of Sclera—Varies in its Different Parts

- Anterior portion (near the corneolimbal junction) : *0.8 mm*
- Posterior portion near optic nerve is (the thickest) : *1 mm*
- Equator : *0.6 mm*
- At the insertion of extraocular muscles (along with tendons) : *0.66 mm*
- Beneath the insertions : *0.33 mm*
- Behind tendinous insertion (subrectus) (Thinnest) : *0.3 mm*

In strabismus surgery *(recession and resection) which involves extraocular muscles and sclera, it is important to remember that sclera is very thin at and behind the insertions (about 0.3 mm). When tendons and muscles are sutured to sclera at these regions the suture needle passes through half of this thickness of sclera without perforating it.*

In high myopia the sclera is thinner than emmetropes and hypermetropia. These facts have to be kept in mind while performing, squint and retinal detachment surgeries. Temporal sclera is more prone to develop dehiscences and staphyloma than nasal.

INSERTION OF EXTRAOCULAR MUSCLES

Sclera acts as a rigid support or base for the insertion of extrinsic muscles of eyeball, facilitating eyeball rotation in all directions.
- Superior rectus inserts on the sclera about : *7.7 mm behind the limbus*
- Inferior rectus : *6.5 mm behind the limbus*
- Medial rectus : *5.5 mm behind the limbus*
- Lateral rectus : *6.9 mm behind the limbus*
- Superior oblique : *is inserted behind the equator on the sclera above the posterior pole*
- Inferior oblique : *is inserted on sclera behind equator below posterior pole*

SCLERAL APERTURES (FIG. 2)

Sclera has three groups of foramina through which important structures pass in and out of eyeball—anterior, middle and posterior groups.

Anterior Group of Foramina

- *Anterior scleral foramen:* It is at the junction where sclera and cornea meet. The outer and inner margins of the scleral portion of this foramen extend more anteriorly than the main body of sclera (Fig. 2).
  - *External scleral margin of anterior scleral foramen is oval. It is diameter is 11.7 mm horizontally and 10.6 mm vertically.* This is responsible for the difference in the width of limbus horizontally and vertically.

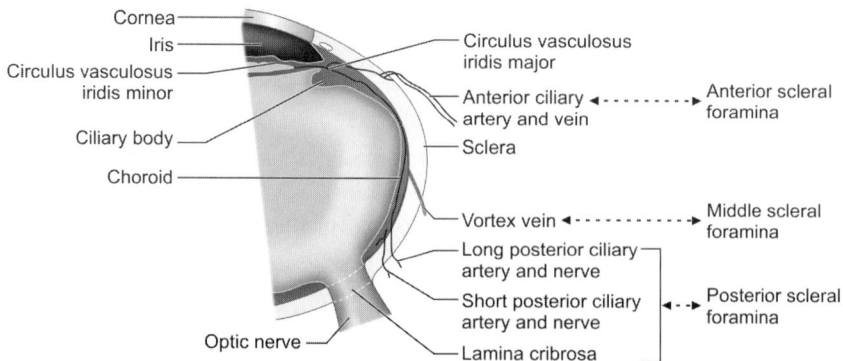

Fig. 2: Scleral foramina and structures passing through them.

These produce a shallow groove externally just posterior to the corneoscleral junction called external scleral sulcus or sulcus sclerae. It is not very clear in living eye as it is occupied by conjunctival tissue and blood vessels.
- *Internal scleral margin:* The above extension produces a concave circumferential groove internally called the internal scleral sulcus. This sulcus is occupied by canal of Shlemm and the trabecular meshwork. *Internal margin of anterior scleral foramen is circular, 11.7 mm in diameter and so corresponds with internal diameter of the cornea.*
- *Foramina for anterior ciliary vessels:* Anterior ciliary arteries arise from the muscular branches ophthalmic artery. After supplying recti muscles, two anterior ciliary arteries arise from each recti (with the exception of lateral rectus which has only one). After coming out of recti they run forward and *pierce the sclera obliquely about 5 to 6 mm from corneoscleral junction.* The largest of these vessels enters the ciliary body and form part of major arterial circle. These do not produce a capillary bed in sclera but small branches bend anteriorly and along with subconjunctival vessels to form the episcleral plexus—*gets congested in anterior uveitis—circumcorneal congestion.*

Each anterior ciliary artery has two accompanying anterior ciliary veins emerging from ciliary body—share a common channel with a branch of posterior ciliary nerve, which passes almost to the surface before looping back to enter ciliary body—nerve loop of Axenfeld, present in 12% of eyes. In living eye, they appear as a smooth, glistening gray dome-shaped appearance.

Middle Group Foramina

Vortex Veins (Fig. 3)

Vortex veins exit through middle group of scleral foramina. They drain blood from choroid and exit through the middle group of scleral foramina (small percentage of blood from choroid is drained through anterior ciliary veins also). Each quadrant of choroid is drained by one vortex vein. *Small afferent veins from each quadrant of choroid converge to a wide ampulla (1.5 to 2 mm wide and 5 mm long) which then narrows to form the main vortex vein. This vein passes through an oblique channel of sclera, which is about 4 mm long and situated 2.5 to 3.5 mm behind the equator (14 to 25 mm from limbus) and joins the superior ophthalmic vein.* Thus each eye has **four vortex veins** mainly. They are:
- Superior temporal vortex vein
- Superior nasal vortex vein
- Inferior temporal vortex vein
- Inferior nasal vortex vein

  Some eyes may have two or more accessory vertex veins, making a total of seven.

Basic Measurements in Ophthalmology

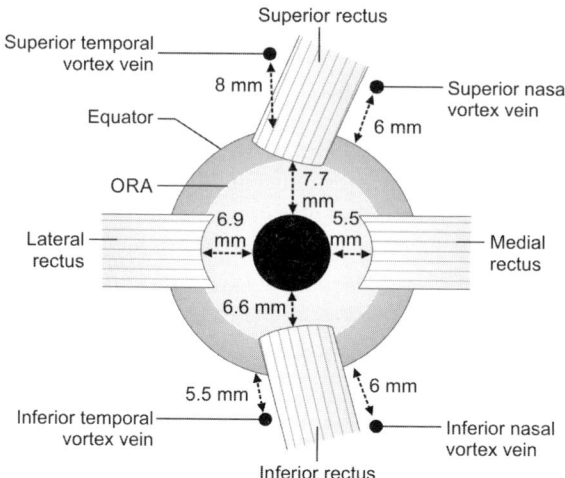

Fig. 3: Approximate distance of vortex vein exit through sclera in mms from equator and limbus.

The site of exit of accessory vortex veins is searched within 1 to 2 mm from those of the main veins.

Positions of Vortex Veins

A good awareness of the distance of ora serrata, equator and optic nerve from limbus (Fig. 4) and their relative positions of vortex veins in relation to them is important when performing retinal detachment, scleral and orbital surgeries. Damage of vortex veins during surgical procedures can lead to severe ocular disturbance.

- *The usual distance from limbus to ora serrata is about 8 mm on temporal side and 7 mm on nasal side.*
- *The average distance of ora serrata to equator is 6.8 mm.*
- *Distance of ora serrata to optic nerve is around 32.5 mm on temporal side and 27 mm on nasal side and on superior and inferior aspect about 31 mm.*
- *Distance of equator to macula is 18 to 20 mm.*
- *The average point of emergence of vortex veins varies from 14 to 24 mm (about 20 mm from limbus).*
  Superior vortex veins come out of sclera near the lateral and medial margins of superior rectus muscle.
- *Superior temporal vortex vein leaves the sclera about 8 mm behind equator.*
- *Superior nasal vortex vein exit sclera about 6 mm behind equator.*
  Inferior vortex veins lie on *either side of inferior rectus muscle*.
- *Inferior temporal vortex vein is placed 5.5 mm behind the equator.*
- *Inferior nasal vortex vein exit sclera about 6 mm behind equator.*
  Upper temporal vortex vein is sometimes hidden under superior oblique muscle tendon.

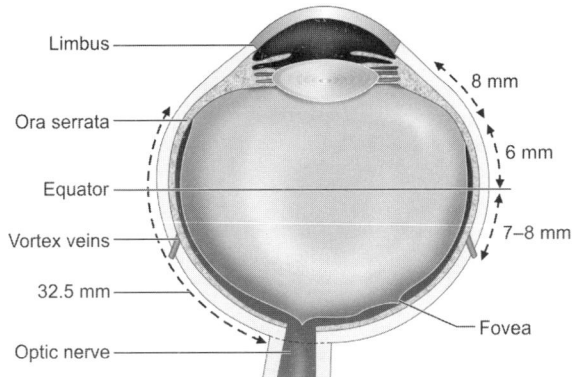

Fig. 4: Approximate distance of ora serrata, equator and vortex veins in mm from limbus as marked on surface of sclera.

Posterior Foramina (Fig. 5)

1. **Posterior scleral foramen:** It is the canal *for the exit of optic nerve from globe.* This short scleral canal has the shape of a *truncated cone and about 1 mm long. The internal opening of cone is about 1.5 to 2 mm and external is about 3.5 mm in diameter.*
   Canal is situated 3 mm medial to midline and 1 mm below horizontal meridian.
   In the posterior scleral foramen (not like the anterior) scleral fibers extend across leaving only openings for exit of optic nerve fibers. This network of bands of scleral fibers is called **lamina cribrosa**. It is concave on the intraocular aspect. It provides support and anchorage for the optic nerve fibers passing through it. But a sustained increase of intraocular pressure and ischemia of optic nerve can lead to a posterior displacement of lamina cribrosa leading to deepening of optic cup (Glaucoma).
   The fibers from outer 2/3rd of sclera do not traverse the foramen, but turn a right angle and run outwards to blend with the dural covering of optic nerve.
2. **Foramina for posterior ciliary arteries and nerves:** Posterior ciliary arteries arise below optic nerve from ophthalmic artery as two trunks and divide into:
   - **Long posterior ciliary arteries**—two in number—one on the nasal and other on the temporal side of globe in the horizontal meridian. They *pierce the sclera about 3 to 4 mm anterior to the optic nerve, traverse the sclera very obliquely forwards for 3 to 5 mm to suprachroidal space* and supply ciliary body anastomosing with anterior ciliary arteries to form arteriosus iridis major, supplying the iris.
   - **Short posterior ciliary arteries** *about 20 in number* pierce the sclera around optic nerve and supply posterior sclera and choroid.

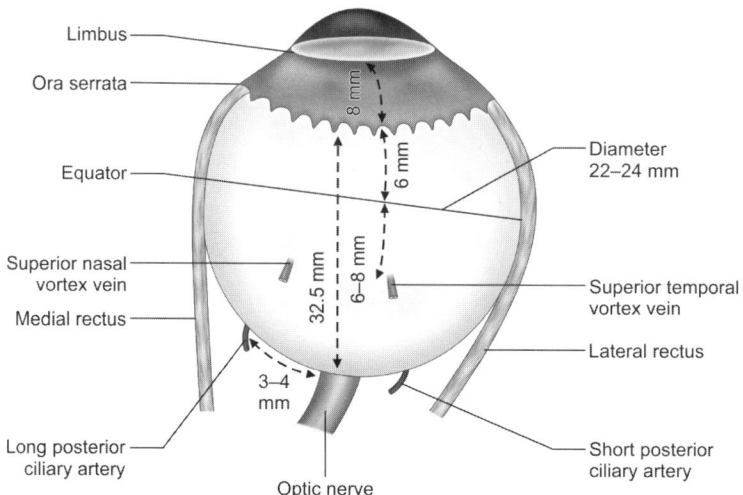

Fig. 5: Approximate distance of ora serrata, equator, vortex veins and optic nerve in mm from limbus as marked on dorsal surface of sclera.

- **Long ciliary nerves** are branches of nasociliary nerve. With the short ciliary nerves they pierce the sclera around optic nerve, pass between sclera and choroid and *supply sensory fibres to iris, cornea and ciliary body and sympathetic fibers to dilator pupillae.*
- **Short ciliary nerves** are branches from ciliary ganglion, *6 to 10 in number contain sensory, parasympathetic and sympathetic fibers.* They accompany short ciliary arteries above and below optic nerve, connect with each other and long ciliary nerves, and supply branches to optic nerve and ophthalmic artery, pierce the sclera around optic nerve run forwards between sclera and choroid and supply ciliary body, iris and cornea.

WEAK AREAS OF SCLERA (FIG. 6)

Sclera may rupture due to a blow to eyeball, mostly at the limbus or sites of muscle insertion. Weak areas of sclera are:
- Limbus: Collagen fibrils run a circular course at limbus which is the weakest portion of corneoscleral envelope.
- Sclera is thinnest just behind muscle insertion (subrectus).
- Equator: Sclera is thinner than other areas in equator.

SCLERAL RIGIDITY

Scleral rigidity is the resistance of sclera to distension. Theoretically most people associate the term rigidity with resistance to bending than to stretching.

Rise of intraocular pressure can cause slight stretching of sclera especially when it is thin and weak.

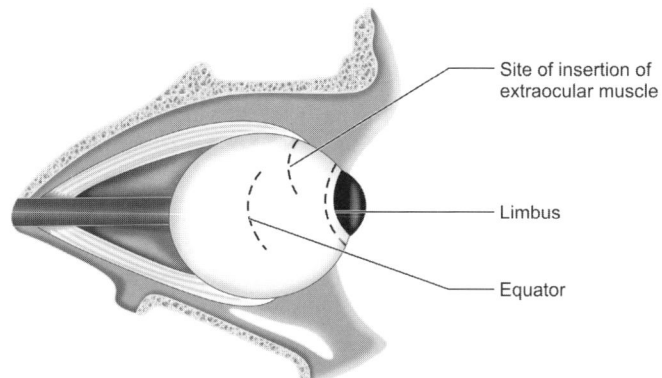

Fig. 6: Weak areas of sclera.

In children a rise of intraocular pressure (infantile glaucoma) leads to a slow stretching of sclera and limbus producing a buphthalmic globe. As the age increases this proportionate stretching of sclera in response to rise of intraocular pressure does not occur.

Though controversial, the clinical phenomenon of scleral rigidity exists. Friedenwald studied this rigidity factor in Cadaveric eye and calculated average value of coefficient of scleral rigidity (E) as 0.0215.

Lowered scleral rigidity occur in following situations:
- Myopia
- During water drinking test (Provocative test)
- Application of strong miotics (Cholinesterase inhibitors)
- Following diffuse scleritis
- Cystoid cicatrix
- Following retinal detachment surgery and intravitreal injection of compressible gases, etc.

In the above condition of lowered scleral rigidity, a falsely low intraocular pressure estimation (less than actual) can occur especially when IOP measurements are done with indentation tonometer (Schiotz).

Increased ocular rigidity can occur in:
- Hypermetropia
- Nanophthalmos (Dwarf cyc)

An ocular rigidity coefficient higher than normal can lead to an erroneously high estimation of IOP by indentation tonometry.

Ocular Rigidity Variation and Indentation Tonometry

When the indentation (Schiotz) tonometer is applied (16.5 g) on eye, the weight of tonometer (indentation) on cornea displaces some amount of aqueous through AC angle. The aqueous cannot flow out at once, and so eye gets distended, the ***resistance of sclera against this distension is ocular rigidity***. Rigidity may differ in different eyes.

The calibration of Schiotz tonometry (Table 1) refers to an average rigidity and when there is considerable deviation of readings from average, the indentation tonometer readings can be misleading.

If both measurements correspond to the same value in mmHg in calibration table and the rigidity is normal, probably IOP measurement is correct.

If the rigidity is lower, that is when the eye is more distensible than normal, the intraocular pressure recorded is lower than actual in patients with raised IOP. Then we have to evaluate and make adjustment for abnormal scleral rigidity to bring out correct IOP measurement. The error is more with higher weight.

For example, 10 g weight will show a much lower value in calibration table than 5.5 g weight; indicating a lower rigidity. The real intraocular pressure is even higher than the value indicated by the measurement with 5.5 g weight.

A **nomogram** can be used to find out the actual intraocular pressure. The scale readings with 5.5 and 10 g weight are noted (on the curves in the center of the nomogram), and the two points should be joined by a straight line. The inter section of this line with perpendicular indicates the true intraocular pressure. The intersection of a parallel to this line through zero (the intersection of abscissa and ordinate) will indicate on the arc in the left lower field the value K for rigidity (Fig. 7).

There are three slanting curves showing scale reading with 5.5, 7.5 and 10 g weights. The ordinate (left margin) of nomogram shows the IOP in mm of Hg. The abscissa (lower margin) of nomogram shows the value of indentation in cu mm. The semicircular scale in the lower left hand corner shows coefficient of ocular rigidity (Fig. 8).

To use Friendwall normogram, plot the results of differential tonometry on the nomogram. In the Figure 8 the point A represents the scale reading with 5.5 and B with 10 g weight during differential tonometry. The line joining A and B if extended to left intersects the ordinate at the point C which shows the actual value of IOP (Po). Draw another line DE extended through lower left

TABLE 1: Scale readings corresponding to the intraocular pressure of 20.5 mm Hg in cases of abnormal rigidity (Leydecker)

		Weight		
	Rigidity	*5.5 g*	*7.5 g*	*10.0 g*
Low	0.0050	8.0	12.0	16.0
	0.0100	6.25	10.00	12.0
	0.0150	5.25	8.0	10.5
High	0.0250	3.5	6.0	8.0
	0.0300	3.0	5.25	7.5
	0.0350	2.75	4.75	6.75
Normal	0.0215	4.0	6.5	8.75

Measurements of Sclera

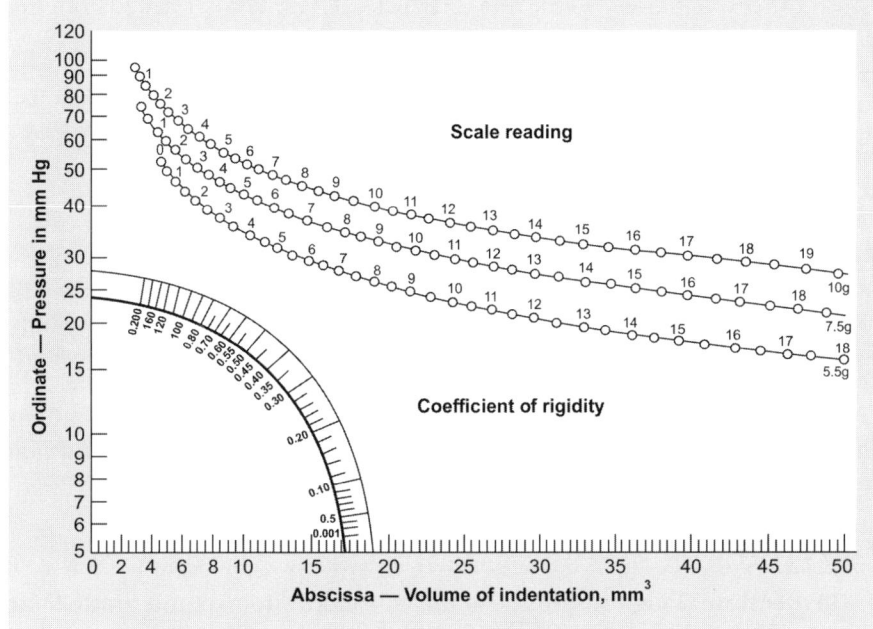

Fig. 7: Friedenwald nomogram—for calculation of scleral rigidity (Leydecker—glaucoma).

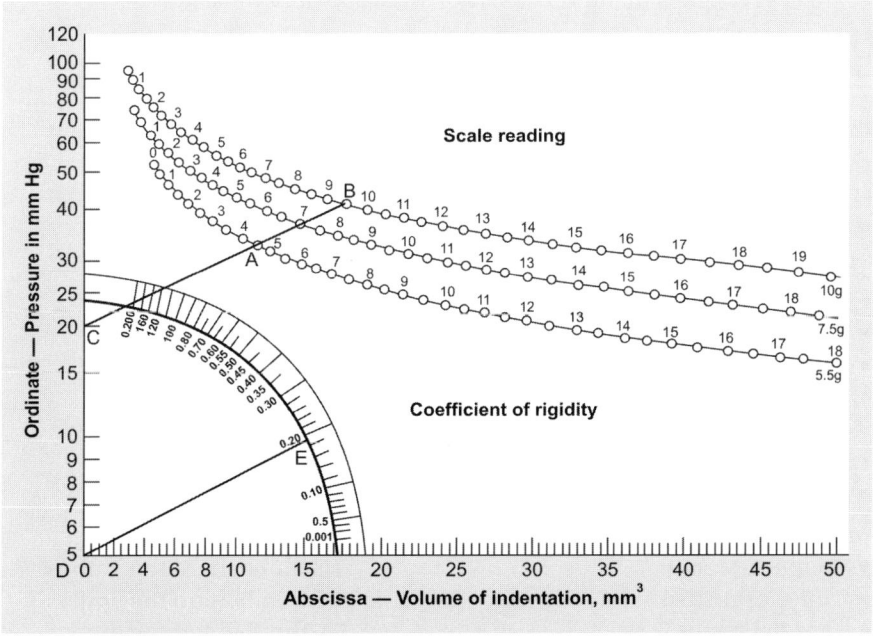

Fig. 8: Friedenwald nomogram—for calculation of scleral rigidity (Leydecker—glaucoma).

hand corner and parallel to the line CAB. Scleral rigidity can be read from the point where the line DE crosses semicircular scale.

So, Schiotz tonometry though a useful procedure, is carried out as far as only in situations where an applanation tonometer is not available for intraocular pressure measurement.

OCULAR RIGIDITY AND APPLANATION TONOMETRY

Fairly accurate measurement of IOP is possible only if the changes in the quantity of aqueous displaced at angle of AC and change in the volume of aqueous are least during applanation tomometry. This can be achieved only by using applanation tonometer. *This tonometer displaces only small amount (0.5 mL) of aqueous during tonometry compared to indentation tonometer and is independent of basal intraocular pressure which is negligibly altered. Thus the factor of ocular rigidity is eliminated and so the factor of scleral rigidity will not come to play during applanation tonometry.*

FUNCTIONS OF SCLERA

- **Protection:** Tough fibrous structure of sclera protects the intraocular contents from trauma and mechanical displacements.
- **Preserves shape of eyeball:** Firmness and strength of sclera together with intraocular presure contributes to the shape of eyeball.
- *Maintains exact position of different parts of optical system.*
- Acts as a *rigid wall* for the insertion of extraocular muscles.

SUMMARY OF MEASUREMENTS OF SCLERA

Sclera forms posterior 5/6th of the outer coat of eye ball.

Diameter
- Coronal diameter : 22–24 mm
- Anteroposterior diameter : 22.5 mm

Thickness
- Near the limbus : 0.8 mm
- Near optic nerve : 1 mm (thickest)
- Equator : 0.6 mm
- At the insertion of extraocular muslces (along with tendons) : 0.66 mm
- Beneath the insertion : 0.33 mm
- Behind insertion (subrectus) : 0.3 mm (thinnest)

Insertion of extraocular muscles
- Superior rectus : 7.7 mm behind the limbus
- Inferior rectus : 6.5 mm behind the limbus
- Medial rectus : 5.5 mm behind the limbus
- Lateral rectus : 6.9 mm behind the limbus

- Superior oblique : Behind equator above posterior pole
- Inferior oblique : Behind equator belowposterior pole

Scleral foramina
- Anterior scleral foramina : 11 mm in diameter
- Foramina for anterior ciliary vesseles junction : 5-6 mm behind corneoscleral
- Foramina for vortex veins (average) : Situated 20 mm behind limbus

Posterior foramina
- Posterior scleral foramina for exit of optic nerve : Average 2 mm in diameter and 32 mm behind ora serrata
- Long ciliary arteries : 3-4 mm in front of optic nerve
- Long ciliary nerves
- Short ciliary nerves and anterior pierce sclera : Around exit of optic nerve
- Diameter of collagen fibers of sclera : 28-280 nanometer
- Water content of sclera : 68%

CHAPTER 4

Measurements of Cornea

Cornea constitutes the anterior 1/6th of outer ocular wall. It is the only transparent window through which light enters the eye. Cornea is a visually vital structure as it transmits about 99% of incident light and contributes about 65% (+40 Diopters) of refractive power (Total + 6OD) to the eye. The average diameter cornea is about 11–12 mm, thickness is 0.5–1 mm, radius of curvature is 6.5–8 mm and surface area is 1.3 cm² (Fig. 1).

STRUCTURE OF CORNEA (FIG. 2)

Cornea has a precise architectural structural arrangement of following layers culminating in its unique function of transparency and light transmission.

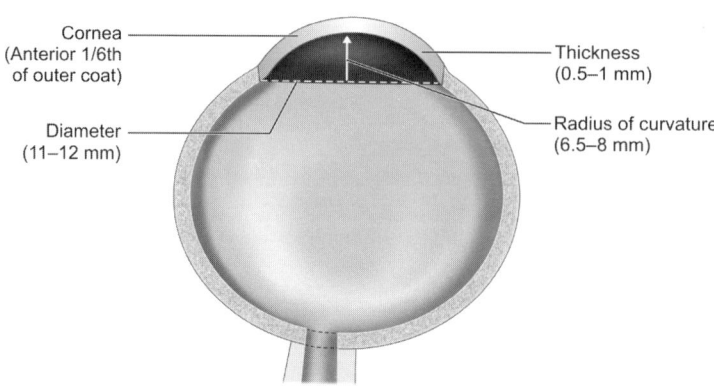

Fig. 1: Dimensions of cornea.

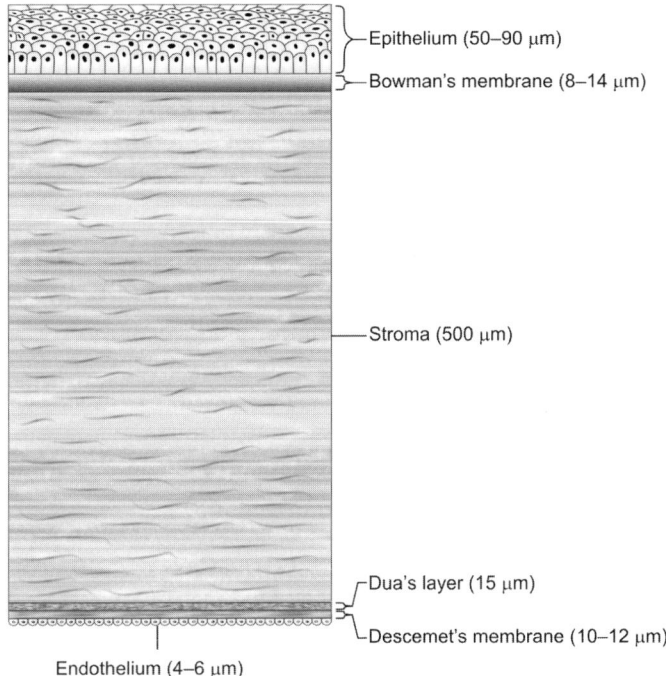

Fig. 2: Structure (layers) of cornea.

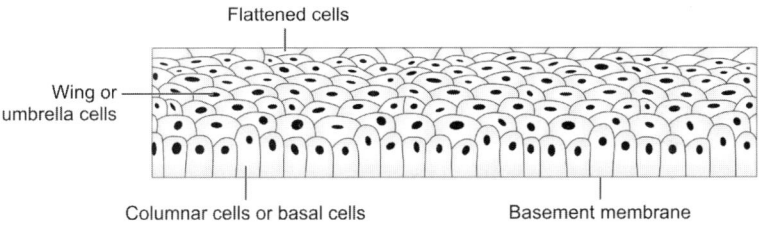

Fig. 3: Corneal epithelium.

Epithelium (Fig. 3)

Epithelium, the anterior layer of cornea is a *50–90 μm thick stratified, non-keratinized non-secretory squamous epithelium. It makes about 5% (0.05 mm) of total thickness of cornea.* It is made of 3 types of cells—flattened cells, wing or umbrella cells and columnar or basal cells arranged in *five to seven layers.* The lower most single layer of basal cells have mitosis and adheres to a basement membrane. The primary **function** of epithelium is:
- It forms a very *strong refractive surface*
- The extraordinary *dense sensory nerve* plexus induces rapid response to touch and injuries
- It form a *barrier to invasion of eye by pathogens*
- Prevent the uptake of excess of *fluid* by stroma.

Basement Membrane or Basal Lamina

Basement membrane or basal lamina of epithelium is 40 to 60 nm thick, contains type IV collagen, laminin proteoglycan and fibrin. Epithelium attaches to this basement membrane and Bowman' layer by hemidesmosomes and type VII collagen fibrils called anchoring fibrils. The anchoring fibrils penetrate as deeply as 2 μm into stroma ending in structures called anchoring plaques. This adhesion is complete and is destroyed in photorefractive keratectomy and must be reassembled during the healing process. *Following corneal injury (abrasion), though, epithelialization and hemidesmosome formation can occur as early as 18 hours, anchoring fibrils form only after many days and full structural integrity is achieved only after many months. This may be the reason for recurrent erosions following injury of cornea by sharp objects.*

Bowman's Membrane

Bowman's membrane is an acellular narrow *homogenous 8-14 μm thick membrane* underlying the epithelium. It consists of a felted meshwork of fine collagen fibrils of uniform size lying in a ground substance. *The diameter of fibrils is about 24-27 nm and it less than that of corneal stroma.* The compact arrangement of collagen fibers confers great strength to this zone. Thus, it is relatively resistant to trauma (mechanical) and infection. Once destroyed it is not reformed but is replaced by scar tissue. It is perforated in many places by unmyelinated nerves proceeding to epithelium. It is considered as condensation and barrier of superficial stroma.

Function of Bowman's membrane are:
- It may be functioning as a smooth, rigid base for maintaining epithelial uniformity for refraction.
- It prevents the close contact between stromal and epithelial cells which might induce stromal activation.

Stroma (Substantia Propria) (Fig. 4)

Stroma is 500 μm thick. The stromal portion of cornea mainly contributes to the structure and optical properties of cornea and *makes up to 90% of its thickness.* Stroma is made of regularly arranged *bundles of fibers of 200-300 numbers centrally and 500 peripherally.* These vary in width between 9 and 260 nm and 1.5 and 2 nm in height. Lamellae are arranged in layers parallel with each other and with corneal surfaces. They stretch from limbus to limbus. *At limbus they*

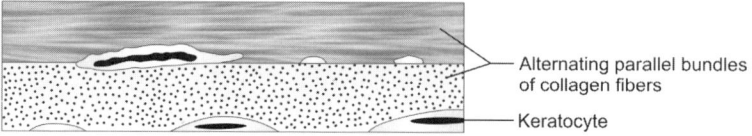

Fig. 4: Parallel arrangement of bundles of fibers in alternating lamellae in corneal stroma.

run circumferentially forming an annulus of 1.5–2 mm wide around the cornea. It is this annulus that maintains the curvature of cornea.

Union between neighboring bands slightly hinders separation of cornea into lamellae, anteriorly than posteriorly. *So, lamellar separation is readily achieved* by blunt dissection and is the basis for lamellar corneal grafting.

In deeper stroma, the lamellae form strap like ribbons which run approximately at right angles to those in consecutive layers. *Functions of stroma are:*
- Maintains transparency and allows passage of light into eye
- It forms part of the rigid framework of eyeball and helps in maintaining intraocular pressure
- It contributes to alignment of optic pathway.

Dua's Layer

Dua's layer was hypothesized in 2013 by Dr Harminder Singh Dua and his colleagues at University of Nottingham as the fourth layer of cornea located between corneal stroma and Descemet's membrane. *It is about 15 micrometers (0.00059 inch) thick.* Though very thin it is strong enough to withstand a bursting pressure of 70 mm–900 mm Hg and is impervious to air.

Dua's layer is made of 5–8 thin compact lamellae of type I, IV and VI collagen fibers which traverse in longitudinal and oblique direction. Keratocytes are lacking in this layer.

This layer was first observed during deep lamellar keratoplasty (DALK) procedures and related research on donated eyes. The cleavage of this layer from stroma could be accomplished for about 8.5–9 mm diameter area from center of cornea and there after it is firmly adherent to stromal bed to periphery but not up to Schwalbe line.

More studies about this layer in future will help in understanding more about the diseases of cornea like keratoconus, descemetocele, pre-Descemet's dystrophies, etc. and will improve the outcome of lamellar keratoplasties.

Descemet's Membrane (Fig. 5)

Descemet's membrane (DM), the basal lamina of endothelium is *about 10–12 µm thick in adult and binds to stroma posteriorly and is the plane of separation usually used in lamellar keratoplasty.* Though appear homogenous, it has a laminated structure, *anterior 1/3rd having a vertically banded pattern and posterior 2/3rd appearing amorphous and granular.* Termination of Descemet's membrane at the corneal periphery (internal landmark of corneal limbus) appears Gonioscopically as a glistening line called Schwalbe's line to which the apex of trabecular meshwork is attached. It is prominent in 15–20% of individuals and hypertrophied in congenital anomalies; then it may appear as a visible shelf on gonioscopy—posterior embryotoxon.

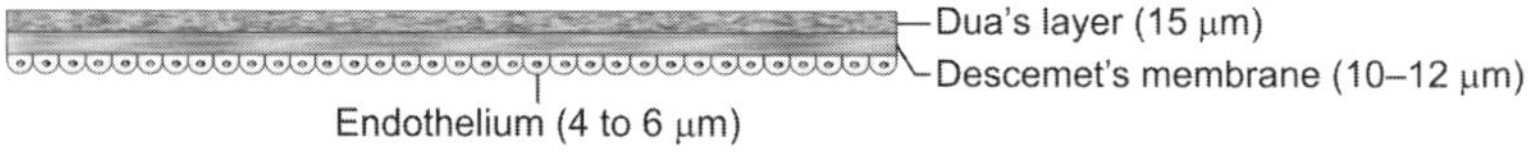

Dua's layer (15 μm)
Descemet's membrane (10–12 μm)
Endothelium (4 to 6 μm)

Fig. 5: Dua's layer, Descemet's membrane and endothelium.

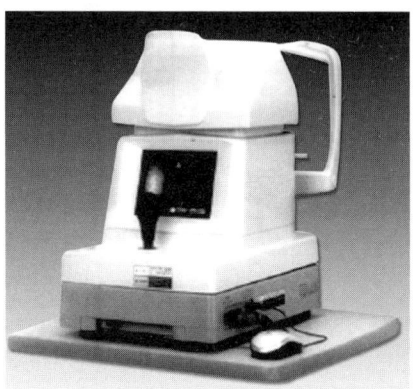

Fig. 6: Specular microscope.

ENDOTHELIUM

Endothelium is a *monolayer of about 500000 hexagonal cuboid cells attached to the posterior surface of Descemet's membrane.*

The corneal endothelium can be studied on the slit lamp by specular reflection under high magnification and also by specular microscopy (Fig. 6). Normal endothelial cells are approximately *20 μm in diameter and 4-6 μm thick*. These cells contain numerous mitochondria, prominent cytoplasmic reticulum and Golgi apparatus. The endothelial cells are metabolically active in *transport, synthesis and secretory activities.* Endothelial cells are interconnected by tight junctions and gap junctions (macula occludens). This makes the endothelium a "leaky barrier" by permitting paracellular diffusion of aqueous humor into cornea but preventing bulk fluid flow between aqueous humor and stroma. *Endothelium plays a major role in maintaining corneal transparency by regulating corneal hydration.*

Specular microscopic studies show that average endothelial cells population is around 2500-5000 cells/mm^2 in adult (Fig. 7).

At birth the endothelial cell density is about 6000/mm^2 and falls by about 26% in first year. A further 26% is lost over the next 11 years but rate of loss possibly stabilizes around middle age. At birth cells are 10 mm in height, but become extremely flat (3-5 mm) with age.

Normally, there is a 0.6% decrease in cell density per year in typical patients with no history of corneal disease or surgery.

Minimum level of endothelial cell density required for maintenance of normal corneal function and transparency is about 400-700 cells per mm^2.

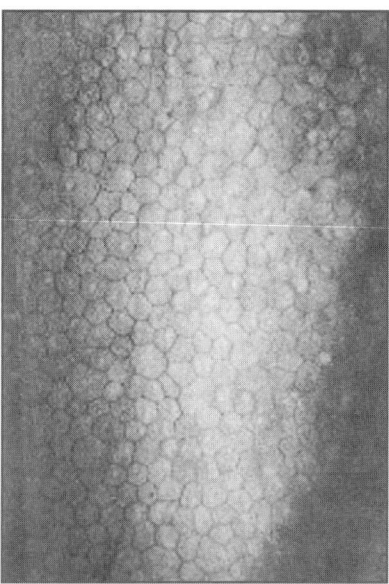

Fig. 7: Specular micrograph of endothelium.

The *degree of uniformity of cell* size is determined by measuring the areas the apical membranes of a population of cells and calculating the *coefficient of variation (CV) of cell size (standard deviation (SD) of mean cell area/mean cell area)*. The normal endothelium has a CV of about 0.25. An increase in this value indicates a variation of cell size, known as polymegathism. This may be *indicative of a stressed or unstable endothelium in which cell volume is not adequately regulated.*

Endothelial cell density and size variations in various clinical conditions.

- **Contact lens wear:** Polymegathism of corneal endothelial cells have been reported following long-term use of rigid PMMA *contact lenses* and daily wear extended wear CLs. Contact lens induced hypoxia may be the cause.
- **Glaucoma:** In glaucoma patients with elevated IOP, there is a *significant decrease* in *endothelial* cell density.
- **Diabetes mellitus:** In type 2 diabetes patients (more than 10 years duration) *CV is increased and the percentage of hexagonal cells decreases to 50%.* These changes are related to changes in cell metabolism.
- **Keratoconus:** Keratoconus patients have normal cell density but *percentage of hexagonal cells drops from normal to 50% showing stress.*
- **Keratoplasty:** Penetrating keratoplasty (PK)patients showed endothelial cell loss rate of *7.8% per year from 3-5 years after PK,* on long-term follow-up of clear grafts.
- **Cataract surgery:** Endothelial cell loss following *phacoemulsification* with 10 L implantation using peribulbar block was *about 8.5% after 12 months.* Using intracameral 1% preservative free lidocaine for anesthesia, the mean

decrease in cell density was 5.5% after 1 month. CV increased 12.5% and hexagonality decreased 4.7%.
- **LASIK:** Following LASIK for correction of 2.25 to 14.5D of myopia, there was *no significant effect* on endothelial cell density or the percentage of hexagonal cells 3 years after surgery. A residual corneal thickness of 200 µm of stroma above corneal endothelium after refractive should be left unablated to protect the corneal endothelial structure and barrier function.

THICKNESS OF LAYERS OF CORNEA

1. Epithelium : 50–90 µm
2. Bowman's membrane : 8–14 µm
3. Stroma : 500 µm
4. Dua's layer : 15 µm
5. Descemet's membrane : 10–12 µm
6. Endothelium : 4–6 µm

CORNEAL INNERVATION

Cornea is one of the *most densely innervated of all tissues* of body. Corneal epithelium is almost highly innervated of all epithelia with approximately 300–400 *more nerve endings per unit area than epidermis.* Sensitivity of cornea is 100 times *more than conjunctiva.* The nerves supplying the cornea are mostly sensory nerve fibers from *long ciliary* nerves arising from ophthalmic division of trigeminal nerve. The long ciliary nerve enters the cornea from perichoroidal space a short distance posterior to limbus. Here they form an annular plexus. About 1mm outside limbus they lose their perineurium and myelin sheaths (which contribute to corneal transparency). Branches then pass forwards in a radial fashion to enter stroma.

After crossing Bowman's membrane and epithelial basement membrane (maintaining Schwann cell sheath) the bundles again turn 90° and run parallel to the base of epithelium. These bundles are called leashes.

At this point of crossing the epithelial basement membrane, Schwann sheath is lost. Beaded nerves of leashes pass between epithelial cells terminating in outer squamous cells to form an intraepithelial plexus. There is no specialized nerve endings and axons are naked and devoid of Schwann sheath.

SURFACE AREA OF CORNEA

The area of anterior surface of cornea is about 1.3 cm^2 (one-sixth of surface area of globe).

CORNEAL DIAMETER (FIGS. 8 AND 9)

Anterior surface of cornea appear slightly oval horizontally because of the greater overlap of sclera and conjunctiva above and below than laterally. *Thus, the*

Measurements of Cornea

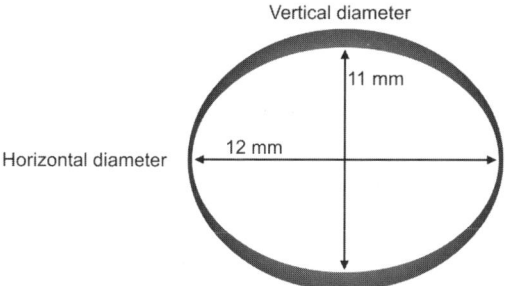

Fig. 8: Diameter of anterior surface of cornea.

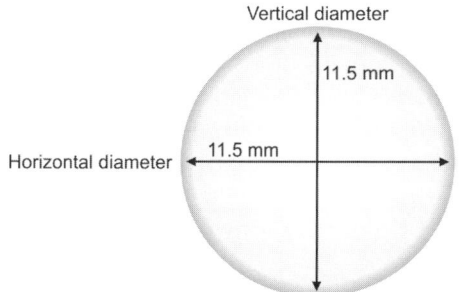

Fig. 9: Diameter of posterior surface of cornea.

diameter of anterior surface of normal adult cornea is about 11 mm vertically and 12.6 mm horizontally.

Posterior surface of cornea is circular. So, the vertical and horizontal diameter of posterior surface are 11.5 mm. Cornea is 1 mm wider in males than females.

Measurement of corneal diameter with a caliper is important in the diagnosis and management of conditions like buphthalmos, microcornea and megalocornea, etc. Cornea reaches its adult size by 2 years of age.

MICROCORNEA (FIG. 10)

In microcornea *adult horizontal diameter is less than 11mm.* It can occur as a true (isolated) condition (rest of globe normal) or associated with other ocular anomalies as in Ehlers-Danlos syndrome, intrauterine rubella, toxoplasmosis and trisomy 13, etc.

MEGALOCORNEA

Megalocornea is primarily an *enlarged diameter of cornea more than 13 mm in horizontal diameter in absence of increased intraocular pressure.* This is a rare condition caused by bilaterally symmetric corneal enlargement.

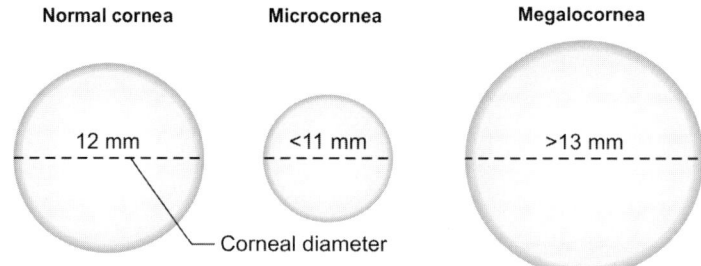

Fig. 10: Corneal diameter variation of microcornea and megalocornea from normal.

Normal horizontal diameter of cornea of newborn is about 10 mm. If the diameter is 12 mm or more in a neonate or 13 mm or more in adult megalocornea is present. Megalocornea can occur as:
- **Simple megalocornea**, not associated with any other ocular anomalies
- **In megalocornea of megalophthalmos** (X-linked) there are iris and angle anomalies and also early subluxation and cataract formation of lens.

Keratoglobus and Corneal Diameter

In keratoglobus there is generalized thinning of stroma resulting in a spherical protuberance but corneal diameter is normal.

Corneal Diameter and Intraocular Pressure

At birth the normal horizontal corneal diameter is between 9.5 to 10.5 mm. It enlarges about 0.5 mm in first year of life. Distension of the globe in response to increased IOP (Buphthalmos) leads to enlargement of cornea especially near the corneoscleral junction. *Thus corneal diameter larger than 12 mm in first year is suspicious. When the corneal diameter becomes 13 mm or more it strongly suggests abnormalities, like childhood glaucoma or buphthalmos.* (Figs. 11 and 12). Corneal diameter may be a more reliable guide than axial length in assessment of congenital glaucoma. A surgical interference in buphthalmos earlier than 13.5 mm corneal diameter can give good visual results (Table 1).

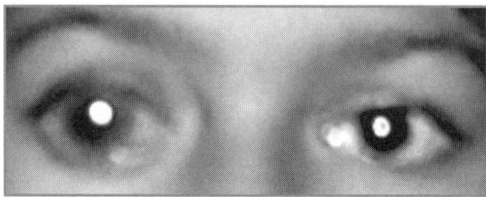

Fig. 11: Enlarged corneal diameter in buphthalmic right eye.

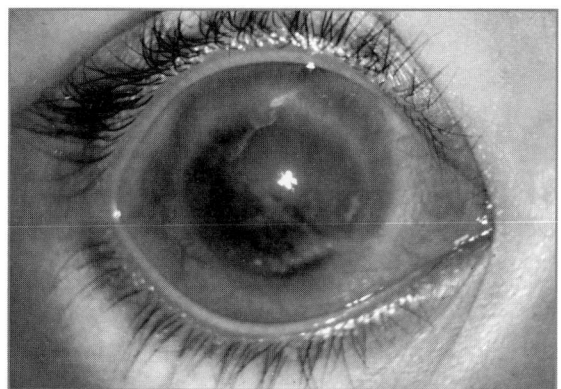

Fig. 12: Congenital glaucoma (buphthalmos) with enlarged corneal diameter and limbal stretching. (*For color version, see Plate 1*)

TABLE 1: Horizontal corneal diameter (in mm) in normal and buphthalmic eyes.

Age	Normal	Possible glaucoma
Birth to 6 months	9.5–11.5	>12 mm
1–2 years	10–12	> 12.5 mm
Older child	≤12	>13 mm

SHAPE AND CURVATURE OF CORNEA

A study of curvature and shape of cornea using keratometer, keratoscope or corneal topographer is an essential step in diagnosis and management of corneal ectasias and conditions of corneal irregularities. They are also important in contact lens fitting, pre and postoperative assessment of cataract surgery, keratoplasty and refractive surgeries.

Average radius of curvature of anterior surface of cornea ranges from 7.2 mm to 8.4 mm (mean 7.8 mm) and radius of curvature of posterior surface is 6.5 mm in adult male (Fig. 13).

NORMAL VARIATIONS OF CORNEAL CURVATURE

Cornea is flatter (radius of curvature more) in infants. Cornea slightly flattens on convergence.

Anterior Corneal Astigmatism

Though normal cornea appears spherical, having same radius of curvature from limbus to limbus on slit lamp examination, *in reality it is a spherical and has different curvatures in different parts and meridians.*

Cornea is normally more curved in vertical meridian than horizontal meridian for about 0.25 D. This is direct astigmatism or astigmatism with rule (Fig. 14A).

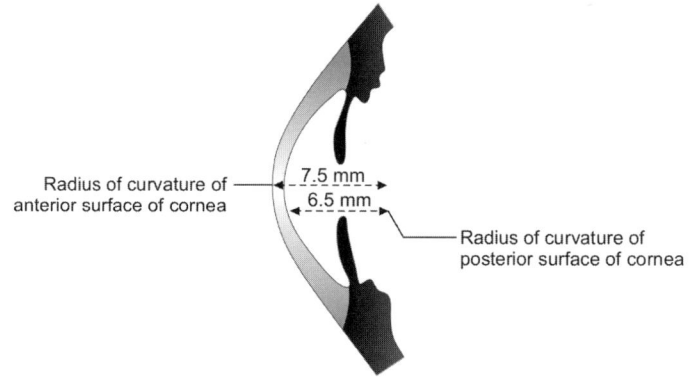

Fig. 13: Radius of curvature.

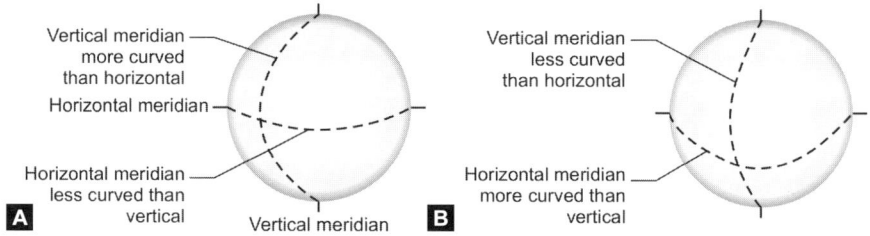

Figs. 14A and B: (A) Astigmatism with-the-rule; (B) Astigmatism against-the-rule.

As age advances or surgical or other types of scarring in upper or lower part of cornea, direct astigmatism tends to disappear or even reverses itself into an *inverse astigmatism or astigmatism against rule, with vertical curve less than horizontal (Fig. 14B)*.

Posterior Corneal Astigmatism

Posterior surface of cornea also has an irregularity in its curvature ranging from 0.25 to 0.75 D with the rule (WTR) or against the rule (ATR). Posterior corneal astigmatism can be measured separately from anterior corneal astigmatism using Barrett's (more accurate) or Bayer's calculators and the measurements are useful in calculating the power and the meridian of toric intraocular lens (IOL) in cataract surgery.

Corneal Topographic Zones

Normally, the central third of cornea (2–4 mm area) is more curved than periphery—the corneal cap. This area is decentered upwards and outwards relative to visual axis but correctly centered for papillary aperture (which is less 0.4 mm temporally).

Cornea flattens peripherally, greater flattening nasal than temporal, above than below (Fig. 15).

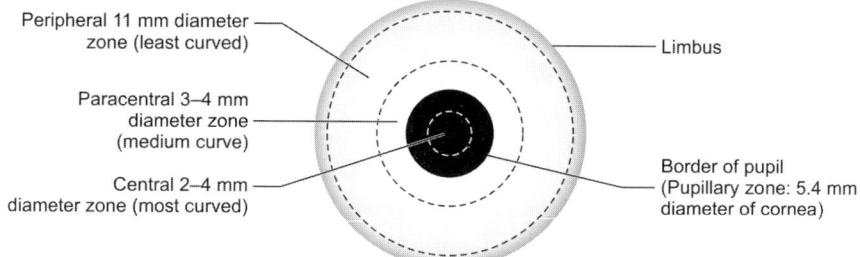

Fig. 15: Corneal topographic zones.

Clinically cornea is a spherical and has three zones with different curvatures.
- **Central zone:** Central zone is 1–2 mm which is almost spherical and steepest.
- **Paracentral zone:** A progressively flattening adjacent 3–4 mm portion with an outer diameter of 7–8 mm.
  Central and paracentral zone mainly provide the refractive power of cornea and the optical zone of cornea overlying the pupil is the central 5 mm diameter area.
- **Peripheral zone:** Adjacent to paracentral zone of 11 mm diameter has maximum flattening and asphericity. Rest of the portion near the limbus cornea steepens further before joining the sclera.
  Conventional keratometry measure the shape of central 3 mm of cornea and the videokeratoscopy measure the mid peripheral and central zones (central 7–8 mm area) of cornea.

MEASUREMENT OF CORNEAL CURVATURE AND SHAPE (TOPOGRAPHY)

An accurate measurement of corneal shape is important in preoperative assessment of refractive surgery, diagnosis of corneal irregularities (ectasias, dystrophies, etc.) unexplained visual loss, etc. Topography can be obtained mainly by three methods.

Keratometry

Keratometry measures the corneal curvature and the corneal element of astigmatism. It *studies the curvature of central part of anterior surface of cornea at four points*. Keratometry is based on the physical principle; anterior surface of cornea acts as a convex mirror so that size of image reflected by it, varies with curvature. *The steeper the cornea (more curved) smaller the image and flatter (less curved) larger the image.* Four keratometric images (mires) are reflected from points of about 1.5 mm either side of corneal apex by a device which double the image by a double refracting prism, is used.

The average radius of curvature of cornea measured by a keratometer ranges from 7.2 to 8.4 mm. The shorter the radius of curvature, steeper the cornea and the more refracting power it has.

Basic Measurements in Ophthalmology

Most clinicians consider the dioptric power of cornea than corneal curvature in mm in practice. Thus, most keratometers give reading in diopters by converting curvature into diopter assuming refractive index of cornea as 1.3200. This gives the reading of total corneal power, anterior surface minus posterior surface rather than anterior surface alone. Baush and Lomb keratometer gives both refractive power and radius of curvature of cornea and has the advantage that both horizontal and vertical meridians can be measured simultaneously (Fig. 16).

Keratoscopy

Keratoscopy measures the shape of whole cornea and can study distortion of large areas of cornea. A keratoscope (an illuminated placidos disk) is used to project *a series of concentric rings into corneal surface*. The principle of corneal contour mapping is employed. Closer the lines together steeper the curvature. A loss of *sharpness the outline of image denotes a loss of normal polish of corneal surface, while irregularities in the rings reflect irregularities of corneal surface* (Figs. 17A and B). An instant camera photographs the ring pattern and its

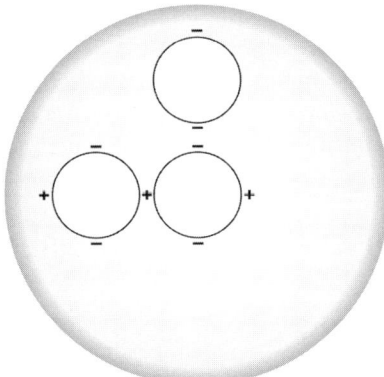

Fig. 16: Keratometric mires (Bausch and Lomb).

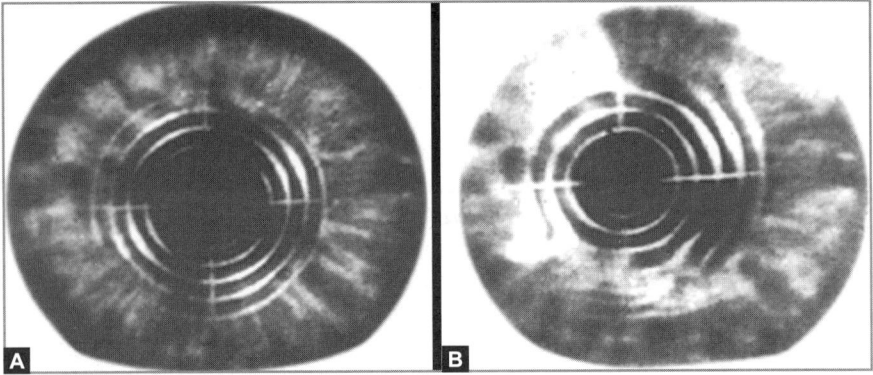

Figs. 17A and B: Keratoscopic corneal reflex. (A) Normal; (B) Distorted.

analysis made by a corneoscope can be used for comparison with standard corneal curvature measurements.

This technique is not effective in studying larger irregularities that occur keratoplasties, keratoconus and trauma, etc.

COMPUTERIZED CORNEAL TOPOGRAPHY (VIDEOKERATOGRAPHY)

This can analyze corneal topography more accurately even in corneal disorders producing symptoms such as halos, glare, reduced contrast, etc. and we can obtain a more complete assessment of corneal surface contour than can be obtained with keratometry.

The equipment is a combination of keratoscope and a video camera. A series of concentric illuminated rings are projected into the cornea, and the image is enlarged and photographed. The data thus obtained are analyzed using a computer program, that evaluates the geometric properties of the ring pattern and converts the coordinates into linear data. Calculation of the geometric average data for every 2 degrees of arc enables the keratoscopic analysis pattern to derive a three-dimensional representation of cornea.

Color-Coded Contour Map (Fig. 18)

We can collect the topographic information through color association and pattern recognition—color-coded contour map. *Power near normal power appear as green, lower powers (flatter) as cool colors (blue) and higher than normal powers (steep) as warm colors (red).* Only a few common colors are selected for assessing the corneal powers so that specific power intervals can be identified easily. *This allows the recognition of severe astigmatic patterns of corneal topography as a bow tie pattern for keratoconus (local area of steepening), pellucid marginal degeneration, (inferior arcuate steepening), characteristic patterns associated with refractive surgeries, etc.*

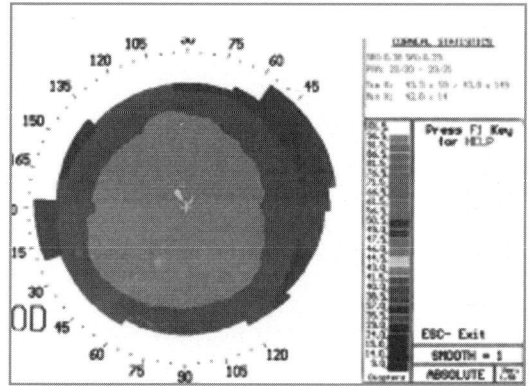

Fig. 18: Topography of a cornea with low asphericity.

Standard Scales

Since even normal cornea can exhibit a variety of topographies—round, oval and irregular patterns—a fixed universal scale is essential to allow only features of clinical significance to be displayed. *Scale ranging from 28 to 65.5D at uniform 1.5D intervals is a practical scale—as sufficient for clinical use, in high resolution topographers.*

Recent developments in corneal topography is its association with *wave front analysis.*

Orbscan: Utilizes slip scanning technology to image the cornea. In addition to corneal topography it also images posterior surface of cornea, AC and lens. It uses both placido mires and dual slip scanning technique to image the cornea. So it is a hybrid system. Orbscan takes more time to scan the cornea, so it does not image a common point and is affected by eye movement.

Pentacam (Fig. 19): Manufactured by Ocular Inc. is a still more advanced diagnostic tool which image the entire anterior segment of eye from anterior surface of cornea to posterior surface of lens. It employees Scheimpflug principles and provide wide depth focus and generates color-coded topographic maps (Fig. 20) of cornea revealing its elevations and curvature.

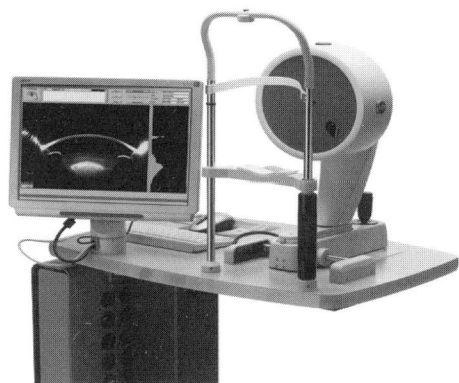

Fig. 19: Pentacam.

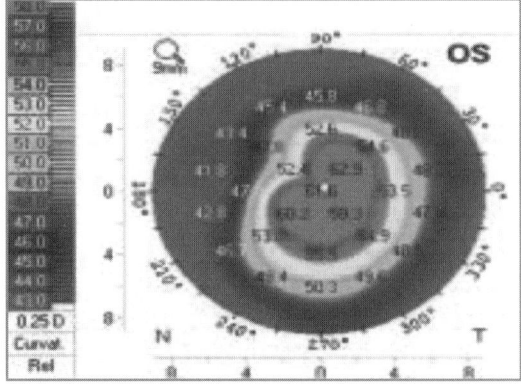

Fig. 20: Kerataconus (Pentacam, front tangential curve map).

Pentacam maintains a fixed reference point on cornea compensating for eye movement and allows examinations of a specific area. Again, when placidio based system do not detect the lesions of corneal periphery, pentacam images cornea from limbus to limbus revealing corneal periphery disorders also.

General Principles of the Effect of Incision and Suturing on the Shape and Curvature of Cornea

Incisions on cornea can change its shape depending on their direction, depth, location, and number.

To produce a good therapeutic response incision may be made up to 85–90% depth of cornea to allow intact posterior lamellae and maximum anterior bowing of lamellae.

1. All incisions cause local flattening of cornea.
2. Radial incisions flatten the adjacent cornea and cornea 90° away.
3. Tangential incisions (arcuate and linear) lead to flattening in meridian of incision and steepening in the meridian 90° away that may be equal to or less than the magnitude of decrease in primary meridian.
4. Tissue removal produce flattening over the area of removal.
5. Full thickness tissue addition produces steepening over the site of tissue addition and flattens adjacent cornea.
6. Tight sutures in the limbal area tightens cornea adjacent to it leading to steepening.
7. Cornea flattens adjacent to loose suture.

REFRACTIVE POWER

Cornea contributes about *65% of the total refractive power of eye*. The refractive power of *anterior surface of cornea is about +40 Diopters*. Refractive power of *posterior surface is -5D. Thus, the net refractive power is +43D.*

REFRACTIVE INDEX

Refractive index of cornea is 1.376. But refractive index of 1.3375 is used in calibrating the keratometer on account of the combined optical power of the anterior and posterior curvatures of cornea.

CORNEAL THICKNESS (FIG. 21)

The thickness of cornea is about 0.52 mm in its center, 1 mm in the periphery and 0.75 mm in between. In myopia, the thickness is less and varies between 0.46 and 0.67 mm. There is no age or sex difference. Thickness of cornea may vary in different quadrants (Fig. 22). *Superior nasal quadrant is the thickest. Inferior nasal quadrant is thinner than superior nasal quadrant. Upper temporal quadrant is next in thickness. Inferior temporal quadrant is the thinnest.* Thin corneas are diagnostic of keratoconus and other ectatic conditions and

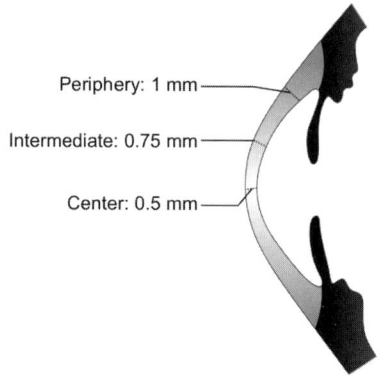

Fig. 21: Thickness of cornea in various portions.

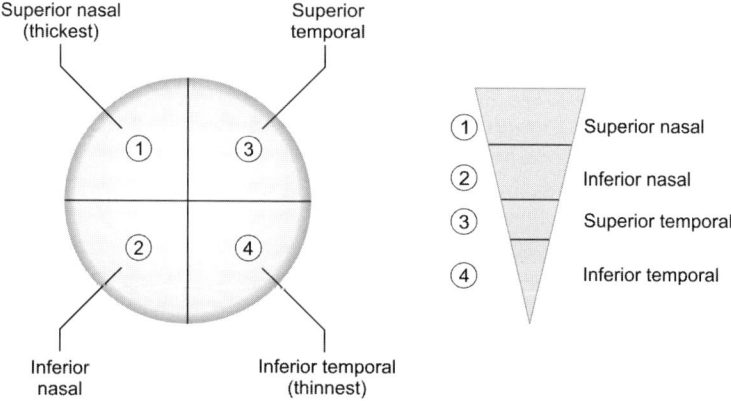

Fig. 22: Normal variations in thickness of different quadrants of cornea.

thick corneas indicate increase in tissue in normal cornea and endothelial dysfunction.

Measurement of Corneal thickness (Pachymetry)

Accurate measurement of corneal thickness is necessary for:
- Evaluation of glaucoma
- Refractive surgeries
- Assessment of various disease conditions.

Pachymeters

Corneal thickness can be *measured by pachymeters.*
- **Optical pachymetry** can be performed by using a device attached to the slit lamp; but this device is not accurate (Fig. 23).

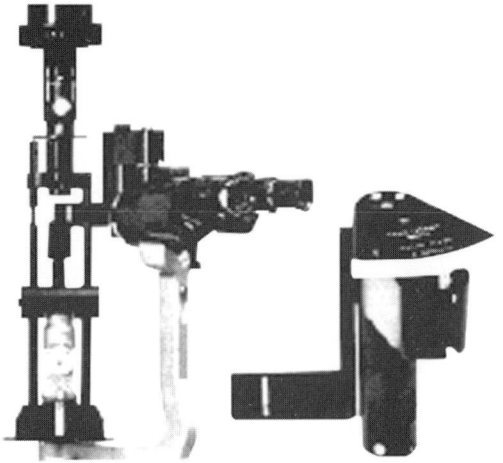

Fig. 23: Pachymeter (optical).

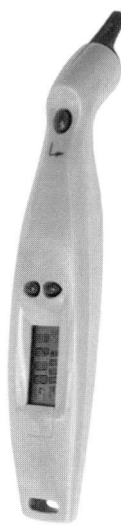

Fig. 24: Handheld pachymeter.

- **Ultrasonic pachymetry** is more easier and accurate. It is based on the speed of sound in normal cornea (1640 m/sec). Applanating tip must be perpendicular to cornea to avoid error (Fig. 24).
- **Orbscan** can produce maps of outer corneal thickness.
- Laser interferometer allows mapping corneal thickness precisely.
- **Optical coherence tomography** can be used to image curvature and thickness of cornea.
- Pentacam—provides very accurate measurement of corneal thickness from limbus to limbus in color-codded maps. Since mapping can be repeated

Corneal Thickness and Intraocular Pressure Measurement

Variation in corneal thickness can produce intraocular pressure measurement differences up to *4 mm of Hg in 20% of patients. Thicker corneas due to increase in tissue cause an overestimation IOP; conversely thinner corneas lead to an under estimation of IOP.*

Goldmann applanation tonometer (GAT) is designed with the assumption that, the central corneal thickness (Central 2 to 3 mm) is about 0.52 mm. *In corneas thicker than normal, GAT records an artificially high measure of IOP since they require a greater flattening force. In eyes with thinner than normal corneas a lower estimate of IOP than normal occurs since these corneas are more easily flattened. Thus, central corneal thickness above or below the normal standard 0.52 mm can lead to erroneous IOP measurements. Correction formulas like Ehlers or Dresden are useful to rule out increased IOP due to corneal thickness.*

Ocular hypertensive persons have significantly thicker CCT ranging from 0.57 to 0.60 mm. But patients with normal tension glaucoma have thinner than average CCT from 0.51 to 0.52 mm. Every 0.04 mm of central corneal thinning can have a two of fold increased risk in persons with ocular HT of developing POAG over 5 years.

Thus, corneal pachymetry is useful in IOP evaluation and assessment of the risk of visual loss and to find out a target IOP.

So, it is ideal to perform pachymetry in all glaucoma patients. But the value of pachymetry should be utilized in the diagnosis of glaucoma only in the following situations.
- When clinical diagnosis of glaucoma is mainly based on IOP level.
- When disk and field status cannot be easily correlated.
- In normal tension glaucoma and ocular HT patients (when disk and field changes are inconsistent with IOP).
- Following refractive surgery.

Thus, thin CCT in glaucoma patients can lead to advanced glaucoma due to under estimation of IOP and inadequate treatment. Thick CCT particularly in aphakic and pseudophakic patients with high IOP may be misled to have unnecessary treatment.

SUMMARY OF MEASUREMENTS OF CORNEA

Cornea forms the anterior 1/6th of the outer coat of eyeball.
Diameter
- Anterior surface—oval
    - Horizontal diameter : 12.6 mm
    - Vertical diameter : 11 mm
- Posterior surface—round
    - Diameter : 11.7 mm

- Microcornea—Diameter : Less than 11 mm
- Megalocornea—Diameter : More than 13 mm
- Corneal diameter of an infant is 10–11 mm
- Enlargement of diameter more than 12–13 mm with other evidence of glaucoma in a child suggests in buphthalmos.

Curvature
- Anterior surface (average) : 7.8 mm
- Posterior surface (average) : 6.5 mm

Refractive power
- Anterior surface : +40 diopters
- Posterior surface : –5 diopters

Refractive index : 1.376

Thickness
- Center : 0.52 mm
- Periphery : 1 mm
- In-between center and periphery : 0.75 mm

CHAPTER 5

Measurements of Limbus

The limbus is an 1 to 2 mm wide about 1 mm thick translucent zone of transition between transparent cornea on one side and opaque sclera and conjunctiva on other side (Figs. 1A and B). This blue-grey zone is of great medical and surgical importance to ophthalmologist. Since anatomically tissues on either side are continuous, disease of conjunctiva can readily spread into corneal epithelium, those of sclera to corneal stroma and those of uveal tract to corneal endothelium through limbus.

LIMIT (EXTEND) OF LIMBUS

Anterior limit: Anatomically (histologically also) the anterior extend of the limbus is superficially at the level of peripheral end of Bowman's membrane and deeply at the level of termination of Descemet's membrane. Level of these terminations is not in the same vertical plane, but slightly inclined posteriorly.

Posterior limit of limbus is about 1.5 mm behind the anterior limit, in the sclera and is in a vertical plane (perpendicular) to the surface of globe.

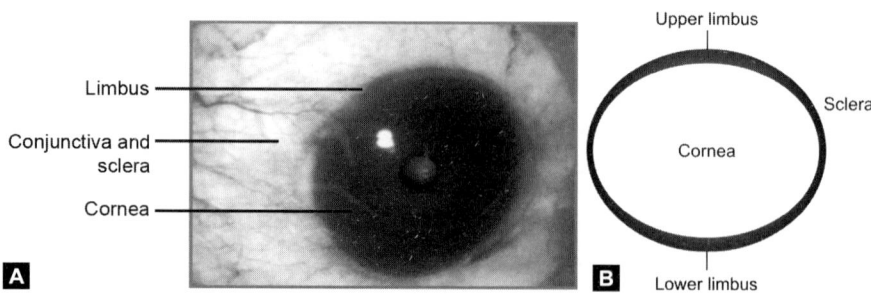

Figs. 1A and B: Limbus. (*For color version, see Plate 2*)

Important structures carrying out the drainage of aqueous like trabecular meshwork, canal of Schlemm and most of the draining vessels are situated mainly in this scleral portion of the limbus.

STRUCTURE OF LIMBUS (LAYER BY LAYER CHANGES)

Several morphological and structural changes occur in layers of limbus when cornea transforms to sclera through limbus (Fig. 2).

- When the corneal epithelium becomes bulbar conjunctival epithelium, in limbus, the latter is thrown into folds by subepithelial connective tissue which runs radially into cornea to form the palisades of Vogt. These folds greatly increase the surface area of basal cells which is important for regeneration purposes. The connective tissue within the folds contains blood vessels and lymphatics.
- Bowman's membrane of cornea becomes continuous with lamina propria of conjunctiva and Tenon's capsule in the limbus.
- Substantia propria of cornea gradually loses its uniform orderly pattern in limbus and become sclera. The fibril diameter increases (broad) and becomes coarse and collagen fibers run a circular course at limbus, which is the weakest region in sclerocorneal envelope.
- Descemet's membrane ends abruptly as Schwalb's line at the beginning of limbus to which apex of trabecular meshwork is attached.
- Endothelium of cornea becomes continuous laterally through similar endothelial lining of trabecular meshwork and anterior surface of iris.

FUNCTIONS AND IMPORTANCE OF LIMBUS

- Limbus carries many portions of aqueous outflow pathway mechanisms
- Contains adult stem cell population.

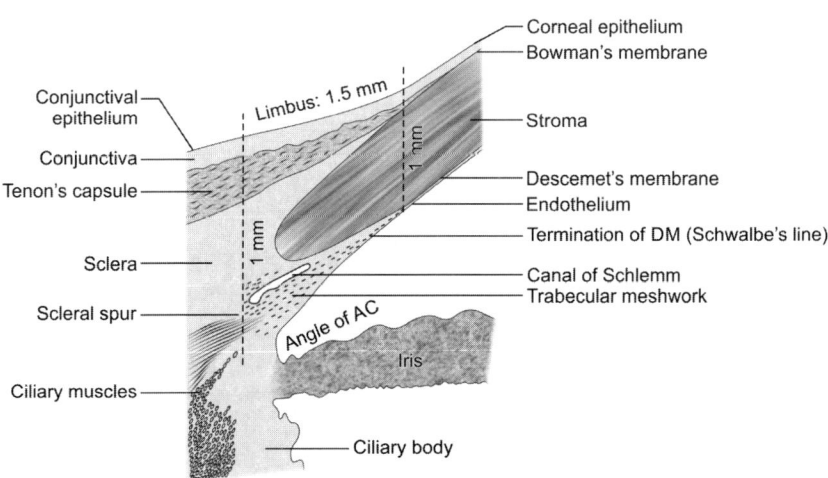

Fig. 2: Structure of limbus.

- Limbus is a major surgical and anatomical reference point for many intraocular and extraocular surgeries.
- Limbus is often assume the principal site of many toxic, immunologic and degenerative disorders.

VULNERABILITY LIMBUS TO DISEASES (MEDICAL LIMBUS)

The word limbus has two literal meanings:
- "Edge of organs or body parts"
- "Borders of hell or prison".

The first meaning is more applicable anatomically. The second interpretation is more appropriate clinically as the limbus and its adjacent peripheral cornea and conjunctiva (**medical limbus**) and to a certain extend in adjacent sclera, are prone to a host of diseases. Following *factors* may be contributing to this:
- Diseases of conjunctiva and sclera can directly spread to peripheral cornea due to the anatomical continuity.
- Limbus being a transitional, vascularized zone is prone to endogenous and exogenous allergens.
- Toxins liberated in bulbar conjunctiva can diffuse into limbus and involve peripheral cornea.
- Limbus is more vulnerable to metabolic and metastatic disorders due to almost the same reasons.

DISEASES PARTICULARLY AFFECTING LIMBUS AND ADJACENT REGIONS (FIGS. 3 A TO L)

- Superior limbic keratitis
- Marginal corneal ulcers caused by staphylococcal toxins and catarrhal ulcer caused by *Moraxella lacunata*.
- Ring ulcer or abscess of cornea caused by *Pseudomonas, Proteus*, etc.
- Superior limbus pannus caused by trachoma and molluscum contagiosum.
- Phlyctenular disease
- Vernal disease
- Pinguecula and pterygium
- Arcus senilis and juvenilis
- Bitot's spots
- Copper deposit—Kayser-Fleischer ring
- Iron deposit—at the base of glaucoma filtering bleb (Ferry line) and at advancing edge of pterygium (Stocker line).
- Pellucid marginal degeneration
- Terrien's marginal degeneration
- Limbal manifestation of collagen vascular disorders
- Dellen
- Benign dyskeratosis
- Intraepithelial epithelioma
- Squamous cell carcinoma

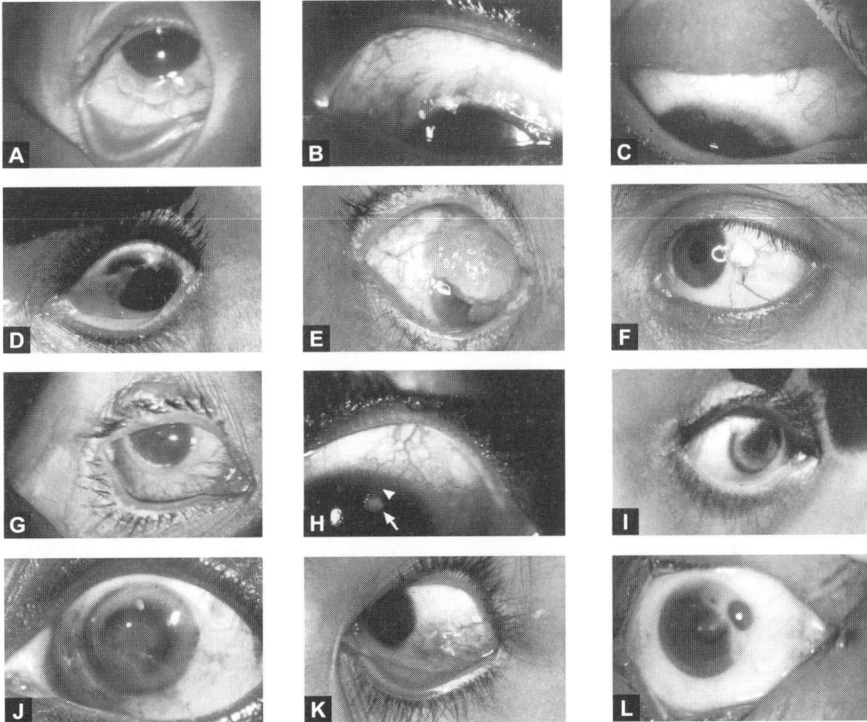

Figs. 3A to L: Diseases affecting limbus and adjacent regions: (A) Phlyctenular conjunctivitis; (B) Vernal conjunctivitis (limbal form); (C) Trachomatous pannus; (D) Pterygium; (E) Squamous cell carcinoma of conjunctiva; (F) Bitot's spot; (G) Marginal keratitis due to staphylococcal toxin; (H) Phlyctenular keratits; (I) Arcus juvenilis; (J) Kayser-Fleischer ring; (K) Episcleritis; (L) Peripheral corneal melting in rheumatoid arthritis. (*For color version, see Plate 2*)

- Conjunctival episcleritis of gout
- Deep pigmentation of limbus and peripheral sclera in alkaptonuria (Ochronosis), etc.

DIMENSIONS OF LIMBUS (FIG. 4)

- **Externally** conjunctiva inserts more anteriorly in the superior and inferior quadrants of limbus. Consequently, limbus is wider in these quadrants. Limbus is *approximately 2 mm wide in the upper quadrant, 1.5 mm in the lower quadrant and about 1mm in temporal and nasal quadrants.*
- **Internally** limbus is only about *1mm wide.*

LANDMARKS OF LIMBUS

A good awareness of the external landmarks and the corresponding internal structures of limbus and how to relate them each other is key to the success of various surgical procedures performed at and near limbus (Fig. 5).

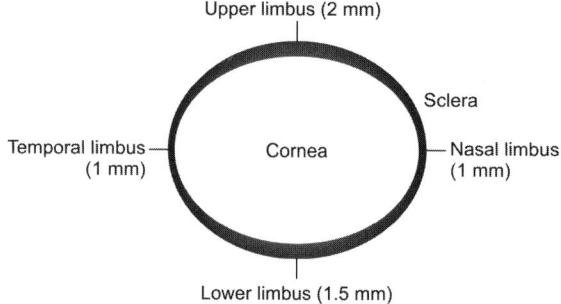

Fig. 4: Dimensions of limbus.

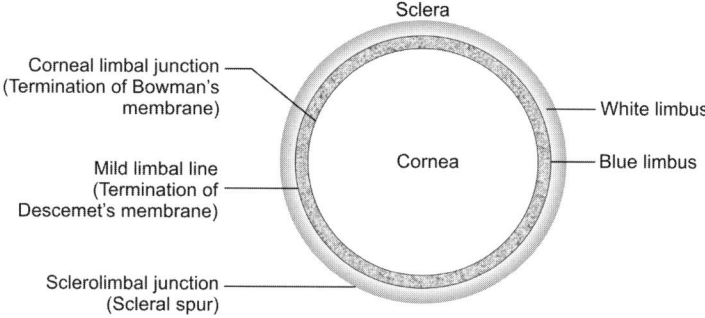

Fig. 5: Landmarks of limbus.

External Landmarks

- **Anterior limbal border or corneolimbal junction:** It is the anterior boundary of limbus externally. It overlies the *termination of Bowman's membrane* of cornea. This is identified on slit lamp by the *internal limit of marginal arcade of corneal vessels at the limbus*. This is 0.5 mm anterior to the insertion of conjunctiva and Tenon's capsule.
- **Posterior limbal border or sclerolimbal junction**—*overlies scleral spur* deeply under sclera and so less clearly defined externally.
- **Mid limbal line:** An (imaginary) line between anterior limbal border and posterior limbal border which probably *overlies Schwalbe's line* internally.

Internal Landmarks

- **Anteriorly:** The Schwalb's line which is the termination of Descemet's membrane.
- **Posteriorly:** Scleral spur to which the base of trabecular meshwork and ciliary muscles are attached.

ZONES OF LIMBUS (FIG. 6)

Thus externally the limbus has two zones.
- **Blue limbus:** Blue limbus is an *1 mm anterior blue portion of limbus* starting from corneolimbal junction corresponding to *termination of Bowman's*

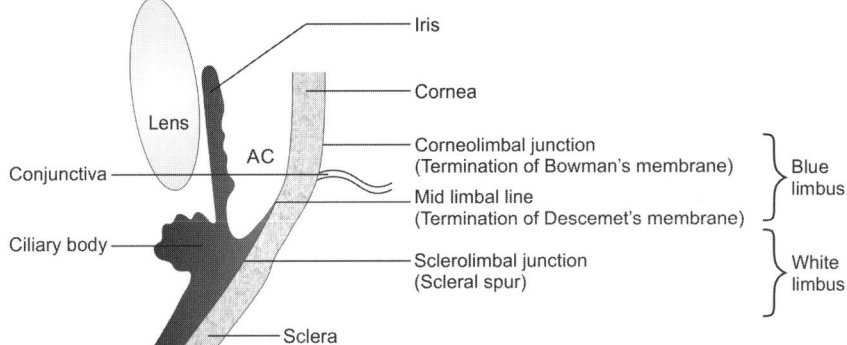

Fig. 6: Zones of limbus.

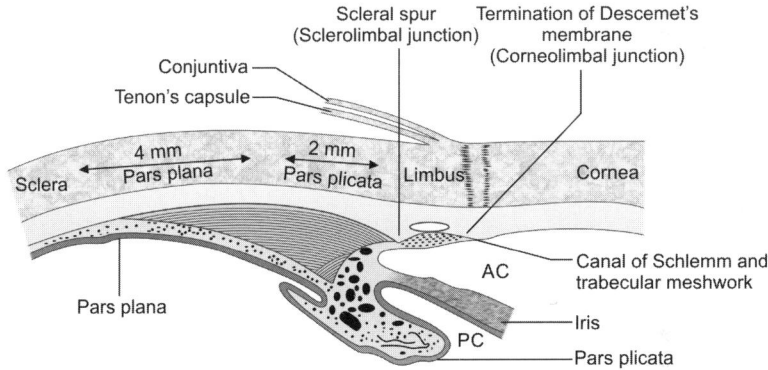

Fig. 7: Surgical anatomy and dimensions of limbus.

membrane (at the level of the marginal arcades of corneal vessels) to the middle of limbus (imaginary)—which corresponds to *termination of Descemet's membrane* (Schwalbe's line – Gonioscopically).

- **White limbus:** Continuous with the anterior 1 mm blue limbus is the zone of *1 mm white limbus* which stops at the posterior limbal border (corresponds to scleral spur internally) and less clearly visible externally.

SURGICAL ANATOMY AND DIMENSIONS OF LIMBUS (FIG. 7)

Kasener compares the constitution of limbus as, *1 mm wide blue limbus and 1 mm wide white limbus with an imaginary midlimbal line in between them to a tennis court.* Midlimbal line represents the net of court with blue limbus anterior and white limbus posterior portions of the court on either side of it.

Blue limbus probably overlies between the termination of Bowman's membrane and Descemet's membrane (Fig. 8).

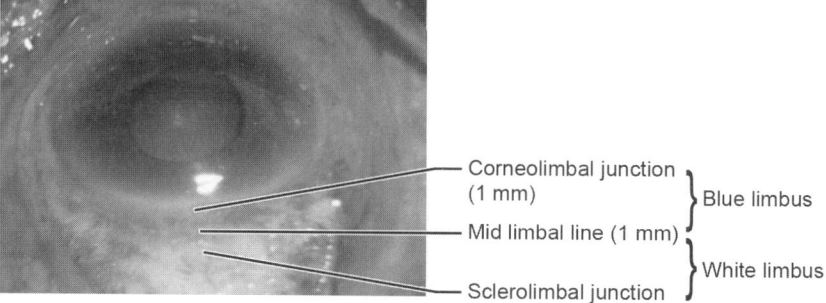

Fig. 8: Zones of limbus (landmarks of limbus).

White limbus probably overlies scleral spur, iris root and approximately canal of Schlemm and trabecular meshwork.

The sclerolimbal junction is also called **surgical limbus** or posterior limbus. It is a more useful landmark than corneolimbal junction in intraocular surgeries. It helps to identify the location of deep internal structures of angle of anterior chamber so that surgeon will be confident about the exact position and quantity of tissue to be incised or excised in surgery particularly in antiglaucoma and other surgeries, avoiding complications and culminating in a successful outcome.

When conjunctiva and Tenon' fascia are reflected from limbus, *surgical limbus* becomes visible *at the junction of bluish-grey limbus anteriorly and opaque white sclera posteriorly.*

The scleral spur is located just posterior to the sclerolimbal junction and Schlemm's canal would be just anterior to this landmark.

This landmarks become more clear, when we take a superficial lamellar (1/2 to 2/3rd thickness) scleral flap, for antiglaucoma surgeries.

As the dissection is carried out anteriorly, till the blue grey barrier is crossed, *where the white opaque sclera with its crisscrossing fibers merging to the grey band of parallel fibers—overlies the scleral spur. The junction of posterior border of blue-grey zone is trabecular band.*

The Schlemm's canal is usually situated just anterior to the circumferential fibers of the scleral spur, sometimes it is found behind it.

Trabeculectomy (Figs. 9A to L)

In trabeculectomy, after a conjunctival flap, a superficial half thickness 4 × 4 mm scleral flap is made. Then a deep scleral flap of 2 × 1 mm is marked at the area of sclerolimbal junction, probably containing trabecular meshwork canal of Schlemm. After entering AC, this deep scleral flap is excised. A peripheral iridectomy is done. The superficial flap is also replaced over deep scleral trabeculectomy ostium and sutured. Conjunctival flap is replaced over the superficial scleral flap and sutured meticulously over it. Aqueous from PC, passes through iridectomy into angle of AC, then drain into the cut ends of

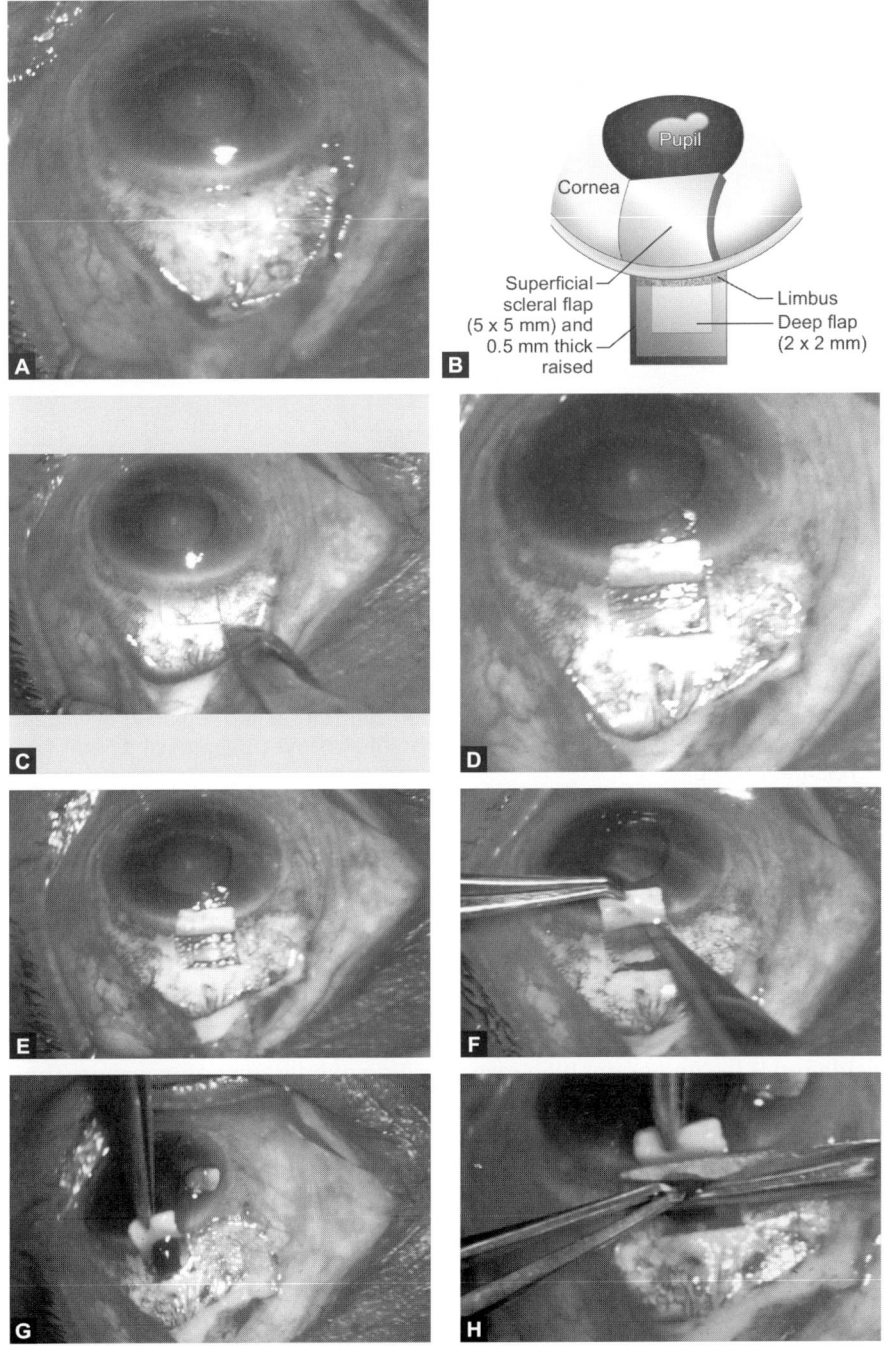

Figs. 9A to H

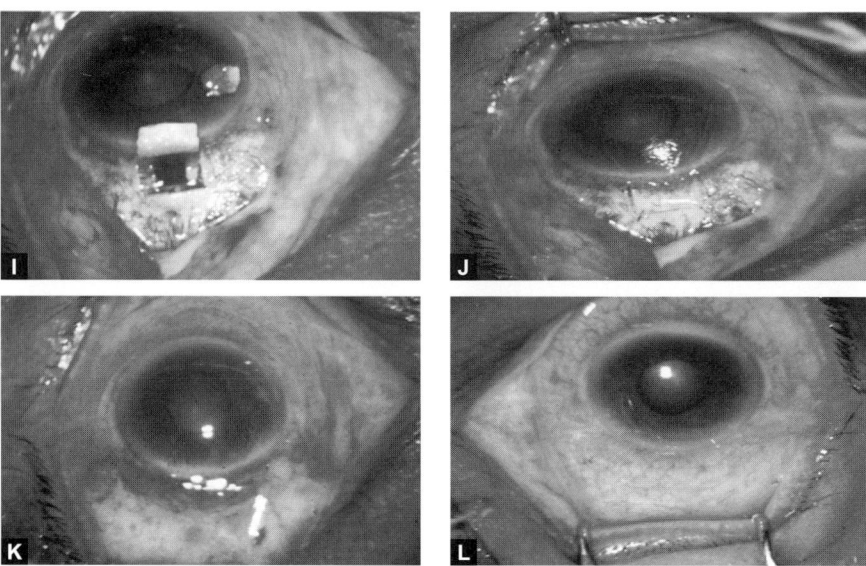

Figs. 9A to L: Trabeculectomy steps: (A) Fornix-based conjunctival flap (9 mm); (B) Size and thickness of scleral flaps; (C) 5 x 5 mm superficial half-thickness lamellar scleral flap marked; (D) Lamellar scleral flap raised up to clear cornea; (E) 2 x 2 mm deep scleral flap made; (F) Anterior chamber entered; (G) 2 x 1 mm trabecular tissue block excised; (H) Peripheral iridectomy; (I) Trabeculectomy ostium after removal of trabecular tissue block; (J) Superficial scleral flap replaced over deep and sutured in place; (K) Conjunctival flap sutured over superficial scleral flap; (L) Surgery completed.

trabecular meshwork and, canal of Schlemm then under superficial scleral flap at the subconjunctival level producing a filtering bleb.

Trabeculotomy

Trabeculectomy is done for congenital or infantile glaucoma with hazy cornea. Under a small flap of conjunctiva and partial thickness scleral flap, the canal of Schlemm is located under high magnification of operating microscope. Then Schlemm's canal is exposed and opened by making a small radial incision across the sclerolimbal junction (posterior part of grey zone). The long prong of Harms Trabeculotomy Probe is passed along Schlemm's canal to the right, the upper prong being used as guide and rotated into AC as so cut the miner wall of AC. This is repeated on left side also.

Viscocanalostomy

Viscocanalostomy is a nonpenetrating surgical procedure for treatment of uncontrolled primary open angle glaucoma with good success rate and less complications than penetrating filtering surgeries. It can relieve outflow obstruction by creating a Trabecular-Descemet's window, that removes the inner wall of canal of Schlemm and juxtacanalicular trabecular meshwork tissue.

After creating a fornix-based conjunctival flap (8 mm chord length), a limbal-based half thickness superficed scleral flap (5 × 5 mm) extending 1.5 mm forward into clear cornea is made. A deep smaller scleral flap (4 × 4 mm) is also prepared beneath the superficial flap. This flap extends to Descemet's membrane and perforation into AC should be avoided. Under high magnification, then carefully look for landmarks on surgical limbus, locate canal of Schlemm. It is unroofed, any fibrotic tissue removed from canal. The dissection is continued into clear cornea using methyl cellulose sponge exposing anterior trabecular meshwork and DM, creating a trabecular Descemet's window. Then high viscosity sodium hyaluronate (Healon GV) is injected into the cut ends of canal of Schlemm on both sides using Grieshaber viscocanalostomy cannula relieving obstruction. In successful surgery one will be able to see viscoelastic leaving AC and flowing through emissary vessels in to sclera.

Then the deep scleral flap is excised and superficial flap is sutured over it using four or five separate 10 zero nylon sutures. Healon GV is injected under the flap and conjunctival flap sutured with two 10-nylon sutures.

If the incisions and the subsequent steps for above surgeries are done incorrectly and more posteriorly than usual can injure ciliary body and can lead to sudden and severe bleeding. Again if the fistula is made more posterior can get blocked by the uveal tissue leading to non-drainage and failure of surgery.

CYCLODESTRUCTIVE PROCEDURES

Cyclodestructive procedures are done on the area of pars plicata of ciliary body which cannot be visualized externally. Here again we have to depend on external landmarks (Fig. 10).

- **In cyclocryotherapy:** The cryoprobe for destruction of CB tissue, should be *placed 2–3 mm behind the corneolimbal junction* (length of plicata is 2 mm from the level of corneolimbal junction) to produce desired of IOP lowering effect (aqueous is formed mainly from pars plicata). When we perform surgery involving different portions of ciliary body (e.g. cyclocryotherapy, parsplana incision, etc.) one should remember that *these structures are slightly more posterior in relation to apparent limbus in superior and inferior quadrants.*
- **Transscleral laser cyclophotocoagulation:** Laser beam must be placed *1.5 mm behind the corneolimbal junction superiorly and inferiorly* and 1mm temporally and nasally to reach pars plicata.

Pars Plana Surgery

Pars plana surgery may be required to relieve malignant glaucoma, drainage of fluid collection in choroidal detachment and hemorrhage, vitrectomy, etc.

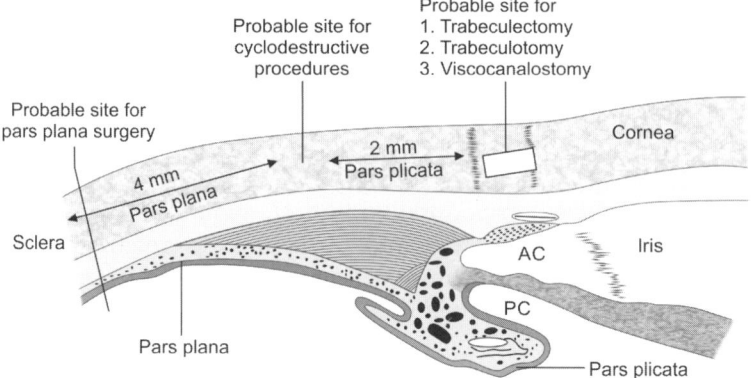

Fig. 10: Measurement and sites for antiglaucoma surgeries and pars plana surgeries.

The pars plana incision (posterior sclerotomy) *for these procedures should be made 3 mm (in aphakic and pseudophakic eyes) and 4 mm (in phakic eyes) behind corneolimbal junction* (The length of pars plana is 4.5 mm).

Limbus and Surgical Entry into Anterior Chamber

Anterior chamber is surgically opened for a variety of procedures like paracentesis, peripheral iridectomy, cataract surgery, antiglaucoma filtration surgeries, etc. The site of entry at or near the limbus into AC can be slightly different for different techniques and different surgeries for successful, least traumatic outcome. Many of these have already been described.

CATARACT SURGERY AND LIMBUS

Conventionally AC entry for cataract surgery can be made through either of the following incision sites (Fig. 11).
- Corneal incision
- Limbal incision
- Scleral incision.

Corneal incision

A clear corneal incision is done just anterior to the insertion of conjunctiva to limbus, just ahead of the limbal vascular arcade. This is not an ideal incision for cataract surgery and is mainly reserved for rare situations like:
- Eyes which have undergone filtering surgeries
- Eyes with bleeding disorders
- Scleral thinning
- Large volume camp surgeries

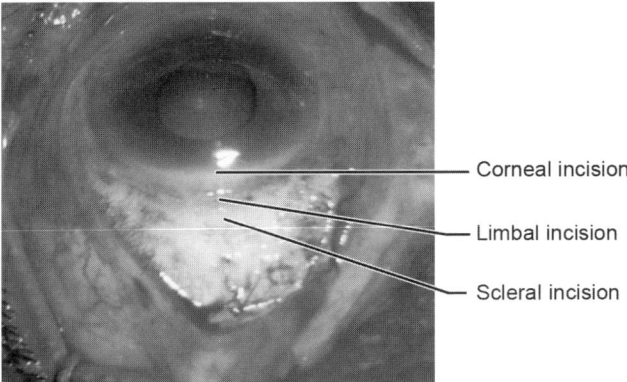

Fig. 11: AC entry level for (cataract) surgeries.

Disadvantages

- High postoperative astigmatism
- More corneal trauma like DM stripping
- May require suturing
- High incidence of postoperative endophthalmitis.

Limbal Incision

Limbal incision may be done on blue limbus, white limbus or in between them (mid limbus). A limbal incision is more easier to perform (especially for beginners), produces less astigmatism, minimum bleeding and least visual disturbance from scarring. This incision is the preferred one for intracapsular and conventional extracapsular cataract extraction.

Limbal incision may be done at 3 levels.
- **Blue limbal incision**—is done in the blue limbal zone.
- **Mid limbal incision**—is done in an area between blue and white limbus externally.
- **White limbal incision**—is done near the sclerolimbal junction. Though postoperative astigmation is less, this incision can cause damage to the underlying trabecular meshwork and also produce excessive bleeding.

Chord length of incisions in various techniques of cataract surgeries vary in different techniques cataract surgery and the nucleus management (Figs. 12A to G).
- Intracapsular cataract extraction: 10–12 mm
- Conventional extracapsular extraction: 7–8 mm
- Manual small incision cataract surgery: 5–6 mm
- Phacoemulsification with rigid IOL implantation: 3–3.5 mm
- Phacoemulsification with foldable IOL implantation: 2 mm
- Microincision cataract surgery: 1mm
- Coaxial microincision cataract surgeries: Less than 1mm

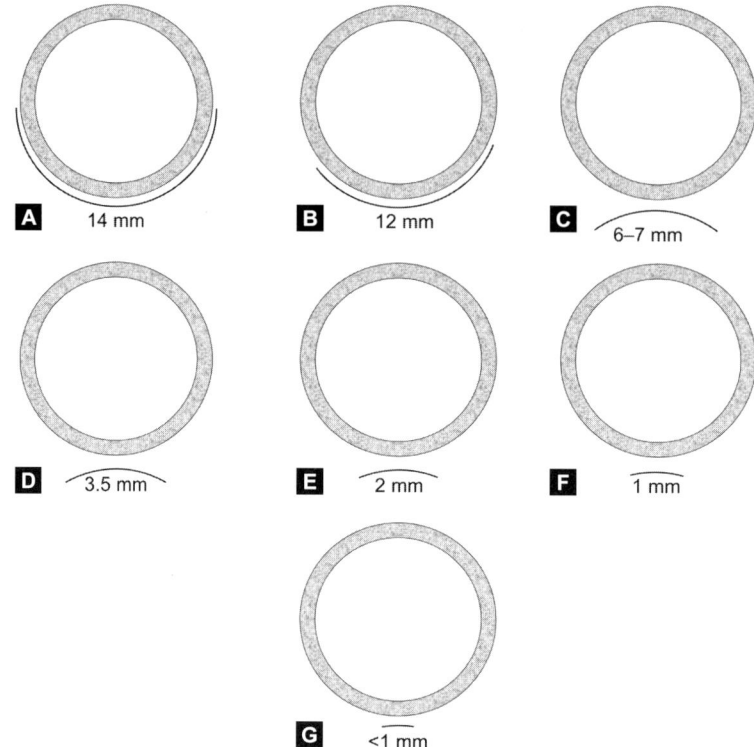

Figs. 12A to G: Chord length of incisions in various techniques of cataract surgery. (A) Intracapsular cataract extraction; (B) Conventional extracapsular cataract extraction; (C) Manual small incision cataract surgery; (D) Phacoemulsification with rigid IOL implantation; (E) Phacoemulsification with foldable IOL Implantation; (F) Microincision cataract surgery; (G) Coaxial microincision cataract surgery.

POSTLIMBAL—SCLERAL INCISION

Are done slightly behind the limbus.

Scleral Tunnel or Scleral Pocket Incision

This is the most ideal and versatile incision practised currently for cataract surgery procedures and is done on sclera posterior to limbus.

Classical scleral tunnel incision consists of an external incision on sclera, 1.5–2 mm posterior to limbus, a scleral tunnel (internal incision) and a corneal valve.

Advantages
- Better wound stability
- The surface area of opposed wound edges is increased which can enhance an earlier wound healing.

- Reduction of induced astigmatism and stability of refraction
- Greater patient comfort and early visual rehabilitation
- Lesser chance of AC collapse during surgery
- Dreaded complications like expulsive hemorrhage can be avoided
- Suture related complications can also be avoided
- Fewer postoperative follow-up visits.

Dr Richard Kratz (1980) designed and carried out this incision for first time away (posterior) from limbus on sclera as the initial step for AC entry. He believed that (it is true also!). Scleral tunnel is an astigmatically neutral way of entering anterior chamber.

Mathematical Principle

This design of scleral tunnel incision is based on a flexible rule—the postoperative astigmatism is directly proportional to the cube of the length of incision and inversely proportional to the distance of incision from limbus.

Incisional Funnel (Fig. 13)

The relationship between incision length, its distance from limbus and the induced postoperative astigmatism can be projected on the scleral surface, producing the so called incisional funnel. *It consists of an imaginary pair of curved lines representing the outer limits of scleral incision that produce same amount of astigmatism.* These lines diverge outwards from limbus as separating the distance from limbus increases. *Incisions made within the funnel will for all practical purposes be astigmatically neutral. Accordingly short incisions made closer to the limbus, and longer ones away will have equivalent effect on corneal curvature.*

Architecture of Scleral Tunnel Incision

The conventional scleral tunnel incision has a square (shape) incisional geometry (Fig. 14); length of the tunnel is equal or exceed width of tunnel which will be self-sealing.

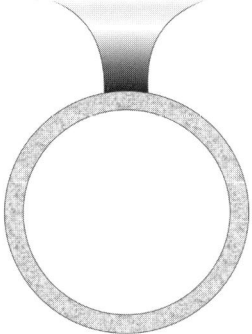

Fig. 13: Incisional funnel (Paul Kosh).

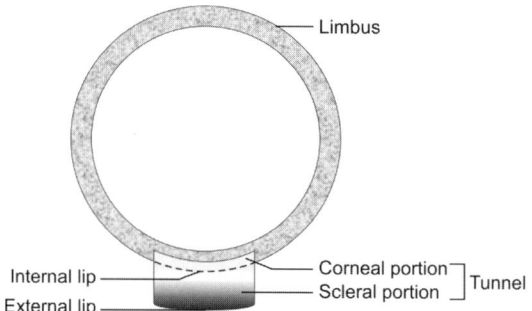

Fig. 14: Conventional square-shaped corneoscleral tunnel incision.

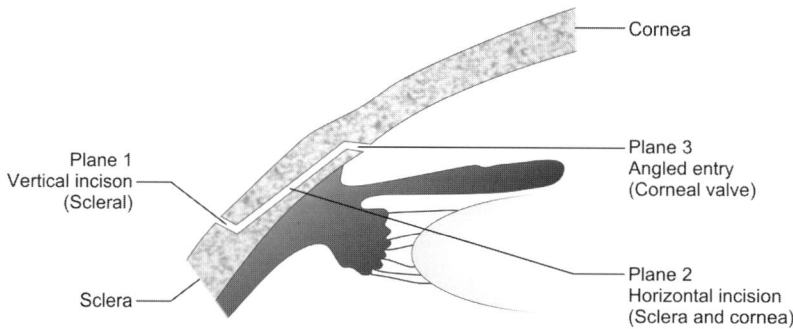

Fig. 15: Scleral tunnel corneal valve incision.

The *internal corneal lip* of tunnel incision was popularized by Paul Ernest. This has a corneal valve which prevents fluid escape from AC and hyphemas from scleral tunnel.

It is a *three step incision*, shaped like 'Z' and has 3 planes or steps (Fig. 15).
- **Plane (Step) 1:** Is a vertical incision on sclera involving 1/3rd or half of its thickness.
- **Plane (Step) 2:** Is a horizontal incision through sclera and cornea (the tunnel itself).
- **Plane (Step) 3:** AC entry portion is an angled, beleveled incision through cornea, producing a corneal valve. The corneal valve involves stroma (DM and endothelium of cornea and seals the internal lip of tunnel on itself (self-sealing) when IOP returns to normal level postoperatively.

Dimensions or Limits of Scleral Tunnel (Fig. 16)
- **Location of incision from limbus:** The ideal distance of vertical limb of incision from limbus is *1–2 mm*. As the distance of this incision on sclera increases from limbus, the induced astigmatism less, but the tunnel making and the maneuverability of instruments into the AC become more difficult.
- **Depth of incision** is about 1/3rd or 1/2th thickness of sclera. Deeper incision (roof of tunnel thick) can lead to inadvertent entry into AC. Thinner

Measurements of Limbus

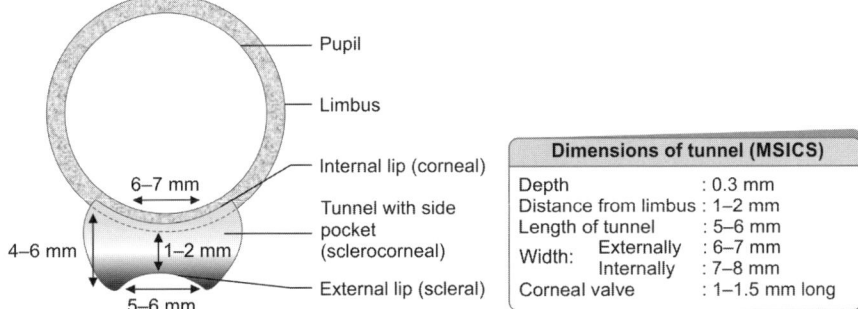

Fig. 16: Shape and dimensions of corneoscleral tunnel (funnel-shaped) for manual small incision cataract surgery (SICS).

roof of tunnel result in its button-holing or tearing of the scleral roof of the tunnel.
- **Length of incision:** The distance between two ends of incision and varies according to technique (refer chord length) and is about 5–6 mm for cortical cataract and 7 to 8 mm for nuclear cataract in manual SICS.
- **Length of tunnel:** The distance from vertical scleral incision to the site of angled entry into AC. The length will be usually equal or slightly exceed width.
- **Angled entry** into AC producing a corneal valve.

In a funnel-shaped tunnel made for manual SICS, creating side pockets for easier nuclear delivery, *the dimensions of internal lip of tunnel has to be larger than outer lip; the inner lip will have a width of about 6.5–8 mm and outer lip around 5–6 mm.*

CHAPTER 6

Measurements of Anterior Chamber

Anterior chamber (AC) is the space in the anterior segment of eye between cornea (in front) and iris (behind) filled with aqueous humor.

BOUNDARIES OF ANTERIOR CHAMBER

Anteriorly: Anterior chamber is bordered by:
- Cornea
- A small anterior portion of sclera.

Posteriorly: The boundaries from center towards periphery are:
- The part of lens exposed through pupil
- Anterior surface of iris
- A small portion of anterior face of ciliary body (Fig. 1).

Anterior chamber communicates with the extracellular spaces of the iris, ciliary body, trabecular meshwork and through pupillary aperture to the posterior chamber of eye.

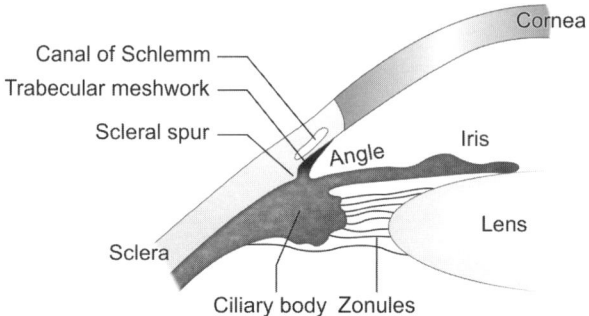

Fig. 1: Boundaries of anterior chamber.

DIMENSIONS OF AC AND ITS NORMAL VARIATIONS (FIG. 2)

The average depth of AC is about 3.1 mm in the center in normal adult but can vary from 2.5 mm to 4.5 mm. It is shallower in very young children and in old people. Hypermetropic eye has a shallower AC and myopic patient has a deeper AC than emmetrope. *An increase in depth of AC due to any cause for about 0.06 mm induce myopia of 1D.*

AC depth decreases by about 0.01 mm per year of life. AC depth is diminished slightly in accommodation, partly due to the increased anterior lens curvature and partly by the forward translocation of lens.

The depth of anterior chamber becomes less and less towards the periphery.

SUMMARY OF MEASUREMENTS OF ANTERIOR CHAMBER

- **AC depth:** 2.5–4.5 mm in the center in normal adults
- **Volume of AC:** It is about 250 µL
- **Diameter of AC:** It is varies from 11.3 to 12.4 mm.
- **Surface area:** It is 323 mm^2.

ANGLE OF ANTERIOR CHAMBER

At the periphery of anterior chamber where its anterior and posterior boundaries meet, it becomes progressively shallow and form a recess called angle of anterior chamber (Fig. 3). The *boundaries* of this angle are:

Anteriorly

Peripheral portion of cornea and adjacent small anterior portion of sclera.

Posteriorly

- The peripheral portion (root) of iris anteriorly
- A portion of anteromedial surface of ciliary body (pars plicata) above iris root attachment.

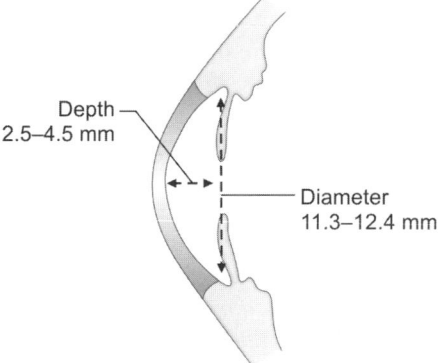

Fig. 2: Dimensions of anterior chamber.

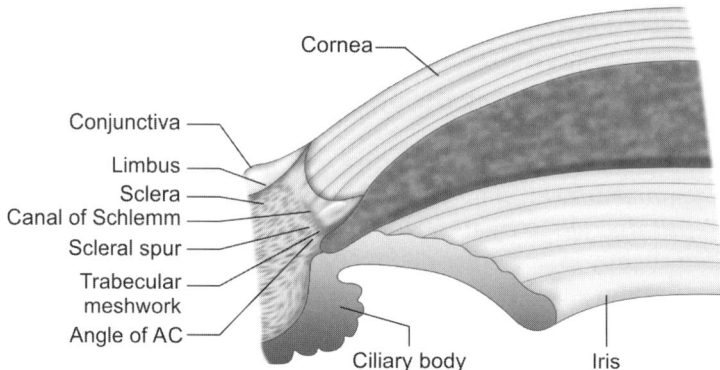

Fig. 3: Anterior chamber.

The anterior boundary accommadates the *aqueous drainage system of eye*.
- Canal of Schlemm: A circular venous channel occupying the inner layers of sclera which form the anterior boundary of AC angle.
- Trabecular meshwork: A triangular meshwork of tissues (carrying fine channels) situated between canal of Schlemm and extreme periphery of AC angle.

TRABECULAR MESHWORK

At the periphery of angle between canal of Schlemm and the recess of angle of AC, a loosely constructed meshwork of tissue is situated called trabecular meshwork. It is a sponge work of connective tissue beams arranged as superimposed perforated sheets. These beams are diposed circularly in AC angle. Trabecular meshwork is triangular in shape in meridional section. Its apex of the beam is directed anteriorly and arise from (1) the termination of Descemet's membrane (Shwalbe ring) and (2) subjacent fibers of corneal stroma. Base is directed posteriorly and gets attached to (1) scleral spur and (2) junction of iris and ciliary body.

Trabecular meshwork has 3 portions:
1. **Uveal (portion) meshwork:** The inner layers which border the anterior chamber. The individual sheet has a *diameter of 4–6 µm and intratrabecular spaces arrange in size from 20–75 µm*.
2. **Corneoscleral (portion) meshwork:** It is the next layer. Sheets are *about 5–12 µm in thickness and separated from each other by space of 5 to 20 µm*.
3. **Juxtacanalicular portion** is between corneoscleral portion and inner endothelial wall of Schlemm's canal. It has a *thickness of 2–20 µm and consists of 2–5 layers of loosely arranged cells*.

   The spaces of trabecular meshwork decrease in size progressively from within outwards. The meridional width of trabecular meshwork posteriorly near the scleral spur is 120–180 µm. The dimensions are wider in myopic than hypermetropic eye.

With advancing age the thickness of trabecular sheets increases and the open spaces of meshwork reduce due to accumulation of curly collagen. A number of structural changes are observed in the drainage angle with advancing age that may contribute to resistance of aqueous outflow. An exaggeration of this leads to *primary open angle glaucoma*.

Scleral Spur

Scleral spur is a wedge shaped circular ridge projecting from the inner aspect of anterior sclera. *The scleral spur is triangular in shape with apex pointing anteriorly and inward and base posteriorly.* Base of trabecular meshwork is attached to the apex of scleral spur. The longitudinal portion of ciliary muscles gets attached to its base. It consists of mainly collagen type I and III and elastic tissue (5%) oriented in a circumferential fashion. It contains collagen and elastic fibers. *The collagen fibers vary in diameter from 35 to 80 nanometers and widens towards sclera.* Structures attached to scleral spur are:
1. Inferomedial portion (base) forms the posterior margin of scleral sulcus and receives the posterior attachment of trabecular meshwork.
2. The anterior tendons of longitudinal ciliary muscles are also attached on its inner aspect.

Contraction of the ciliary muscle pulls the spur posteriorly and opens the spaces of trabecular meshwork which is attached to scleral spur. This is a likely mode of action of mitotics, e.g. pilocarpine, thereby by increasing the facility of outflow of aqueous in treatment of open angle glaucoma and lowering of intraocular pressure (IOP).

Schlemm's Canal

Schlemm's canal is a vascular venous channel which occupies a sulcus on the inner surface of corneoscleral limbus called internal sulcus (a circular groove extending from termination of Descemet's membrane anteriorly and scleral spur posteriorly). The sulcus completely accommodates canal of Schlemm externally and corneoscleral portion of trabecular meshwork internally. Thus, the canal is surrounded by sclera, trabecular meshwork and scleral spur.

This canal is a narrow circular vascular sinus of some 36 μm in circumference extending around entire globe and is lined by endothelium. Shape of the canal varies. The lumen is *elongated and oval or sometimes triangular in cross-section.* It is *about 200–400 μm long in its meridional axis and 10–25 μm in its shorter axis.*

The size or diameter of the lumen varies according to IOP, the space can be absent in high IOP and very large in low intraocular pressures.

Schlemm's canal is lined by single layer of spindle shaped endothelial cells, oriented parallel to the circumference. In the inner wall they are 40 to 120 μm long, 4 to 12 μm wide and 0.2 μm thick.

Canal Schlemm conducts aqueous humor from trabecular region to the episcleral venous network via collector channels (Fig. 4).

About 25–30 collector channels arise at irregular intervals in from outer wall of canal of Schlemm and pass through three interconnecting venous plexuses of sclera before reaching anterior ciliary veins.

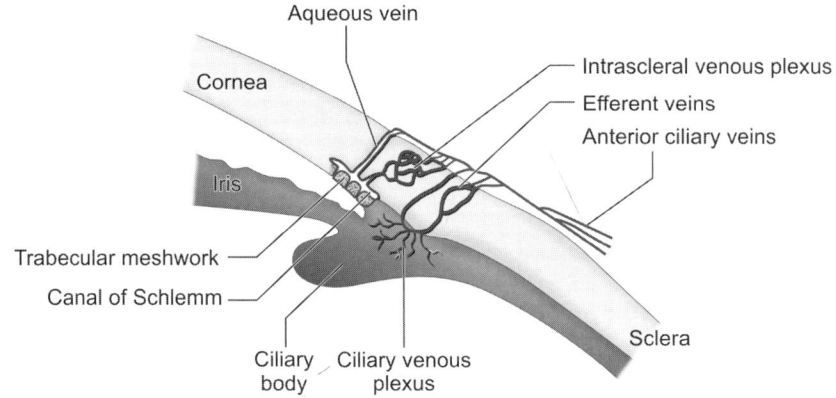

Fig. 4: Aqueous humor channels.

Of the above 32 collector channels, some 8 channels bypass the deep scleral venous plexus and pass directly through sclera from canal of Schlemm into episcleral veins. These channels are known as the aqueous veins, because they contain mostly clear aqueous.

With slit lamp they may be seen subconjunctivally, either as clear vessels or showing a bilaminar flow pattern representing the presence of blood and aqueous. *They are found about 2 mm behind limbus, most often inferiorly and often commencing in a hook shaped bend where they emerge from sclera. They may run a course of 1–10 mm before joining episcleral vein.*

Pathways of Aqueous From Anterior Chamber to Systemic Circulation

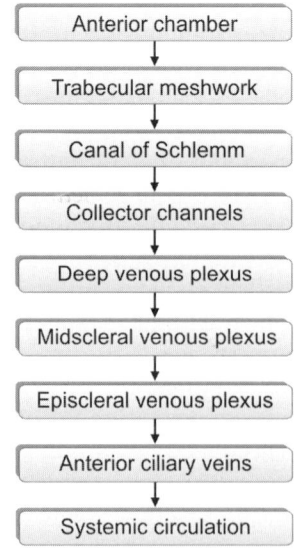

Summary of Measurements of Drainage angle

- Circumference : 35.5–38 mm
- Trabecular width : 0.8 mm (anterior posterior)
- Diameter of Schlemm's canal : 200–400 μm long axis
  10–25 μm short axis
- Number of collector veins : 25–35
- Width of collector veins at origin : 20–90 mm
- Number of aqueous veins : 2–8

AQUEOUS HUMOR

Aqueous humor is a clear fluid formed from the blood vessels and epithelium of ciliary processes by ultrafiltration, diffusion and secretion into posterior chamber, and then passes through pupil into anterior chamber and its angle. Aqueous humor returns from angle of AC to venous system (systemic circulation) through following pathways.

- Canalicular (Conventional) pathway: Here aqueous exits through the canals of angle of AC—trabecular meshwork, canal of Schlemm, the lumen of which directly communicates with episcleral veins and aqueous veins, completing the circulatory pathway of aqueous return to heart. *About 83–96% (average 90%) of aqueous drains through this pathway.*
- Uveoscleral (unconventional) pathway: This is also known as extracanalicular or uveovortex flow. A smaller amount of aqueous drains out of eye through this route consisting of ciliary muscle and iris into supraciliary and suprachoroidal space either by diffusion or spaces around the nerves and blood vessels which pass through sclera and absorbed into the uveal vascular system including vortex veins (uveovortex outflow). This pathway accounts for *about 5–15% of aqueous exit (average 10%) of total aquous outflow. Outflow via uveoscleral pathway is 0.3 mL/minute.*

  Ciliary muscle tone determines the rate of uveoscleral outflow. Factors which produce contraction of ciliary muscle (like pilocarpine) lower the uveoscleral outflow and those relax ciliary muscle (as atropine) increase uveoscleral outflow.

  Uveoscleral outflow is significantly increased by prostaglandin analogues and they are among the potent topical IOP lowering drugs available. In cyclodialysis surgery, a portion of ciliary body is surgically detached from its attachment to scleralspur thereby increase uveoscleral outflow and helping to lower intraocular pressure.

- Subsidiary pathways are:
  - Exchange across the anterior vitreous face
  - Exchange across the iris vessels.
  - Exchange across corneal endothelium.

The role of these unconventional pathways is not very significant in normal situations but in pathological situations accessory drainage routes attain importance and help in drainage of aqueous humor.

Aqueous Humor—Measurements

Total volume	:	0.4 mL
Formation rate	:	0.25 mL/min
Refractive index	:	1.3333
Viscosity	:	1.025–1.040
Total outflow facility	:	0.25 mL/min/mm Hg around age of 20–30 years.

Drainage

Conventional pathway	:	83–96% (average 90%)
Unconventional pathway	:	5–15% (10%)

Composition of Aqueous Humor

The composition of aqueous humor differs in many respects from blood plasma (from which it is formed) due to the existence of blood aqueous barrier and the active transport of various organic substances by ciliary epithelium. Some of the important differences of aqueous humor from plasma are:

- *Low protein content*: Through the protein content of plasma is about 6–8 g%, the protein content of aqueous is only 5–15 mg% due to the ultrafiltration occurring in the ciliary region.
  When the protein content of aqueous rises above 20 mg/100 mL due to a disturbance of blood aqueous barrier, the resultant light scattering makes the slit lamp beam visible as it traverses the anterior chamber. This is phenomenon of "***aqueous flare***"—is one of the early signs of uveitis especially acute exudative iridocyclitis (Fig. 5).
- *High ascorbate concentration*: Ascorbate content of aqueous is about 20 times greater than plasma. Ascorbate functions as an antioxidant, regulates the sol-gel balance of mucopolysaccharides in the trabecular meshwork and partially absorbs ultraviolet radiation.
- *Lactate* is also normally excess than in plasma probably as a result of glycolytic activity of lens, cornea and other ocular structures.
- *Chloride ions* and certain amino acids are in excess relative to plasma.

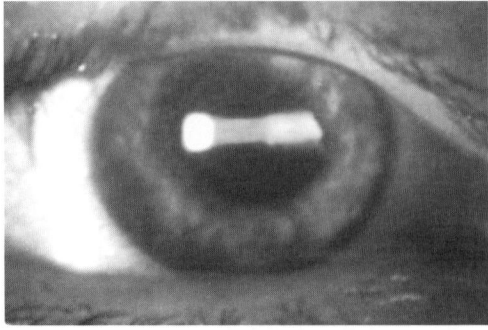

Fig. 5: Aqueous flare.

- *Glucose, urea and nonprotein nitrogen* concentrations are slightly less than plasma. Smaller water-soluble molecules like creatinine, sucrose and urea are not restricted by capillaries of ciliary body. Lipid soluble molecules readily pass through nonpigmented epithelium of the ciliary body.
- *Oxygen concentration* of aqueous is between 13 to 80 mm of Hg.

Diseases, drugs, trauma, etc. breakdown blood aqueous barrier leading to movement of plasma into aqueous humor and aqueous become 'plasmoid'.

Peculiarities of the Chemical Composition of Aqueous Humor Compared to Plasma

		Plasma	Aqueous humor
1.	pH	7.40	7.21
2.	Protein	7%	0.02% (200 times less than plasma)
3.	Ascorbate	0.06 nano Molecule/kg H_2O	0.92 nano Molecule/kg H_2O (20 times greater than plasma)
4.	Sodium ions	176 nano Molecule/kg H_2O	163 nano Molecule/kg H_2O
5.	Chloride ions	117 nano Molecule/kg H_2O	126 nano Molecule/kg H_2O
6.	Bicarbonate ions	26 nano Molecule/kg H_2O	22 nano Molecule/kg H_2O
7.	Lactate in aqueous is excess than plasma		
8.	Glucose, urea and nonprotein concentration of aqueous is less than plasma		
9.	Oxygen concentration of aqueous is between 13 and 80 mm Hg		

Functions of Aqueous Humor

1. Carries nutrients and oxygen to avascular structures of eye—lens, cornea, trabecular meshwork, etc.
2. Removes toxic products of metabolism like lactic acid, carbon dioxide, etc.
3. Formation and circulation of aqueous maintains the intraocular pressure.
4. Forms an optically clear medium for normal vision.
5. High concentration of ascorbate may help to scavenge free radicals and protects eye from effect of ultraviolet and other radiations.
6. In adverse conditions of infections and inflammations it permits accumulation of immune mediators, by decreasing the production of aqueous humor and changing its composition.

INTRAOCULAR PRESSURE

Eye maintains an intraocular pressure due to the combined activity of the following factors.
- The formation and circulation of aqueous
- Ocular coats and their integrity
- Ocular contents

- Tone of extraocular muscle
- Activity of hypothalamus

Normal Intraocular Pressure

Measurement of intraocular pressure by various methods (tonometry) shows that *IOP normally ranges around 10 to 20 mm Hg*. This is only statistical range of IOP in normal population and is not always applicable to individual patients.

Since, the eyes and especially optic nerve head of different individuals have varied susceptibility to (even damage) to a given intraocular pressure a specific numerical value cannot be fixed as normal. So the *normal intraocular pressure may be defined as that pressure tolerated by the eye and does not lead to optic nerve damage*. Intraocular pressure normally rises to about *2 mm* during early morning and before noon in 40–60% of individuals *(normal diurnal variation)*. Transient raise of IOP also can occur during straining, blinking (extraocular muscle contraction), etc.

There is a slight elevation of IOP at night during sleep in supine position. *An exaggeration of the normal diurnal variation over 5 to 8 mm Hg in an early sign of glaucoma.*

It is abnormal if repeated IOP measurements show a difference more than 5 mm Hg between two eyes.

GLAUCOMA

Glaucoma is an acute or a chronic progressive optic nerve disease caused by a variety of ocular and extraocular conditions—most common of the risk factors known is a raised intraocular pressure.

The diagnosis of glaucoma is made if there are at least, two or three characteristic clinical signs.
- Glaucomatous changes in the optic nerve head
- Characteristic changes in the visual field
- A raised, normal or rarely below normal intraocular pressure
- Risk factors like family history of glaucoma genetic predisposition, systemic disorders, etc.

The type of glaucoma is determined mainly from the clinical features and the status of the anterior chamber angle as seen through a gonioscope.

In open angle glaucoma, the aqueous flow is obstructed due to a resistance in the outflow of aqueous from anterior chamber angle across trabecular meshwork and Schlemm's canal leading to rise of IOP but angle is open and even wide.

In closed angle glaucoma, the AC is shallow and angle is narrow due to various causes which makes the root of iris to move forwards, close the angle and block the trabecular meshwork leading to raise of IOP.

Most treatment options available now (medicines, laser, surgery, etc.) are directed to reduction and maintenance of a tolerable IOP; that is to achieve a target pressure and to protect the optic nerve head its vascular supply.

Baseline Intraocular Pressure

Before taking decision to treat glaucoma in the early stages and also in glaucoma suspect, a baseline IOP has to be found out by assessing diurnal variation and peaking of IOP by checking IOP several times in a day. An IOP more than 21 mm Hg and a diurnal variation of 8 mm Hg with associated symptoms and other signs of glaucoma may be considered sign of glaucoma.

Target Pressure

In the evaluation, diagnosis, management and follow-up of glaucoma patient the parameters like the intraocular pressure, extent of optic nerve damage glaucomatous visual field changes, associated risk factors (diabetes mellitus, cardiovascular diseases, etc.) help the ophthalmologist to consider *a range of intraocular pressure between which glaucomatous damage is not likely to progress. This is the target pressure.*

This target pressure is a range of acceptable IOP level within which the progression of glaucomatous optic nerve damage is expected to be halted or retarded. Studies indicate show that maintenance of IOP between 16 to 18 mm Hg and a fluctuation of about 3 mm Hg is likely to stabilize glaucoma. But this is mainly clinical and not numerical.

This target pressure is again variable according to severity of glaucomatous damage.

- **Mild glaucoma disease:** This mild disease patients are those who have glaucomatous damage of optic nerve, but normal visual field and those with ocular hypertension who are at risk of developing POAG, requires a target IOP reduction of 20% from base values and better kept below 18 mm Hg.
- **Moderate glaucoma disease:** Patients with visual field abnormalities in one hemifield but not within 5 degrees of fixation require a 30% target IOP reduction and IOP maintained below 15 mm Hg.
- **Severe glaucoma disease:** There are patients with visual field abnormalities in both hemifield or field loss within 5° of fixation are severe glaucoma disease patients require a 50% target IOP reduction and better stabilized below 13 mm Hg.

TONOMETRY

Tonometry is a clinical, fairly accurate method of measurement of intraocular pressure. The working pattern of tonometers ia based on the following physical principles.

Applanation (Tonometers)

These tonometers applanate or *flatten a small, 3.06 mm diameter area of cornea,* using a *force of 0.1 g* exerted by a lever system. The instrument has to apply more pressure to applanate the cornea in eyes with high IOP. *Thus intraocular pressure measured in mm Hg is directly proportional to the force* applied and inversely proportional to the area flattened and is equal to the force applied by tonometer multiplied by 10. *The amount of aqueous displaced or squeezed out of eye by this procedure is only minimal—about 0.05 mL and so the IOP is not basically raised by the procedure itself.* Since only a small area of cornea is applanated and the capillary force induced acts in opposite direction, this procedure will not produce a distension of ocular coats during the procedure especially sclera. *So in applanation tonometry measurement of IOP is unaffected by variations of scleral rigidity.*

Corneal Thickness and Intraocular Pressure

Corneal thickness differences can affect the IOP measurements using applanation tonometry. *There can be an overestimation of IOP in eyes with thicker corneas and underestimation of eyes with thinner corneas.* Most of applanation tonometers are designed for an average corneal thickness of 545–600 μm.

The applanation tonometers in common clinical use
- *Goldmann tonometer* is the most clinically accepted and accurate tonometer and is used universally.
- *Perkin's tonometer* is portable and can also be used in bed side, operating room, children, etc.
- *Dreager tonometer* uses a different prism and has same uses as Perkin's tonometer.
- *Makay-Marg* tonometer has a movable plunger and its movements are translated by a transducer and records on a paper. These tonometers are useful in measuring IOP in scarred, irregular and edematous corneas.
- *Tonopen* is small portable battery operated electronic tonometer. It is a modified Makay-Marg tonometer. It is simple and can even be handled by technicians.
- *Pneumatic tonometer* also utilizes the function of a transducer which converts the gas pressure in a sensing gas chamber device covered by a polymeric silicone diaphragm. When the diaphragm touches the cornea, the gas vent through which the gas escapes reduces in size and the pressure in the chamber rises. This gas pressure in the chamber is converted by transducer into an electrical signal and is recorded on paper. Pneumatic tonometer is useful in measuring IOP of eyes with edematous, irregular and scarred corneas and over contact lens. It can also be used for tonography.
- *Noncontact tonometer* utilizes a jet of air for corneal applanation avoiding direct contact of instrument to cornea. Hence procedure does not require local anesthesia and is more useful in glaucoma screening campaigns.

Indentation (Tonometers)

Indentation tonometers not only indent the cornea due to the application of a weight on it, but also the weight can slightly distend the ocular coats especially the sclera in those patients whose sclera has been weakened by diseases like myopia, scleritis, etc. So they are not as accurate as applanation tonometers in tonometry, especially in patients with distensible eyes (low scleral rigidity or low scleral resistance against distention). Indentation tonometers measure IOP as follows:

- *Schiotz tonometer* has a concave foot plate applied to cornea for indentation. The foot plate has a canal in the center through which a metal plunger moves and indents the cornea according the weight. The plunger supports a lever which moves one needle over the scale. The total weight of plunger lever and needle is 5.5 g. The weight can be enhanced to 7.5, 10 or even 15 g by addition. The depth of indentation depends on the resistance against indentation by intraocular pressure and the ocular coats. Each scale unit represents 0.05 mm protrusion of the plunger. The measurements can be observed and recorded from the scale over which needle moves. This measurement is arranged in such a way that when the plunger indents the cornea more, needle moves to a higher reading but represents or indicates a lower the IOP. This relationship between weight used for indentation, scale reading and IOP measurement in mm Hg can be obtained from the table of calibration, provided the scleral rigidity is normal.

The intraocular pressure as recorded by Schiotz tonometer in normal eyes is between 10–20 mm Hg and has to be mentioned especially as mm Hg Schiotz in record. The measurement of IOP with this method can give falsely high IOP measurement results in patients with increased scleral rigidity as in high hypermetropes, nanophthalmos, ARMD and those have irregular, steep and thick corneas and those on miotics and vasoconstrictors. There can be an underestimation of IOP in patient with low scleral rigidity (sclera less rigid) as in myopia, those on miotics and vasodilators, and those who underwent intraocular surgery especially, RD surgery and vitrectomy, when indentation method is used.

TABLE 1: Calibration for Schiotz tonometer.

Scale reading	Tonometer plunger load			
	5.5 g	7.5 g	10.0 g	15.0 g
	IOP mm Hg	IOP mm Hg	IOP mm Hg	IOP mm Hg
0.0	41.5	59.1	81.7	127.5
0.5	37.8	54.2	75.1	117.9
1.0	34.5	49.8	69.3	109.3
1.5	31.6	45.8	64.0	101.4
2.0	29.0	42.1	59.1	94.3
2.5	26.6	38.8	54.7	88.0
3.0	24.4	35.8	50.6	81.8
3.5	22.4	33.0	46.9	76.2
4.0	20.6	30.4	43.4	71.0
4.5	18.9	28.0	40.2	66.2

Contd...

Contd...

Scale reading	Tonometer plunger load			
	5.5 g	7.5 g	10.0 g	15.0 g
	IOP mm Hg	IOP mm Hg	IOP mm Hg	IOP mm Hg
5.0	17.3	25.8	37.2	61.8
5.5	15.9	23.8	34.4	57.6
6.0	14.6	21.9	31.8	53.6
6.5	13.4	20.1	29.4	49.9
7.0	12.2	18.5	27.2	46.5
7.5	11.2	17.0	25.1	43.2
8.0	10.2	15.6	23.1	40.2
8.5	9.4	14.3	21.3	38.1
9.0	8.5	13.1	19.6	34.6
9.5	7.8	12.0	18.0	32.0
10.0	7.1	10.9	16.5	29.6
10.5	6.5	10.0	15.1	27.4
11.0	5.9	9.0	13.8	25.3
11.5	5.3	8.3	12.6	23.3
12.0	4.9	7.5	11.5	21.4
12.5	4.4	6.8	10.5	19.7
13.0	4.0	6.2	9.5	18.1
13.5		5.6	8.6	16.5
14.0		5.0	7.8	15.1
14.5		4.5	7.1	13.7
15.0		4.0	6.4	12.6
15.5			5.8	11.4
16.0			5.2	10.4
16.5			4.7	9.4
17.0			4.2	8.5
17.5				7.7
18.0				6.9
18.5				6.2
19.0				5.6
19.5				4.9
20.0				4.5

- **Electronic intentation tonometry** can produce a continuous, magnified permanent record of IOP as in tonography.

Facility of Outflow of Aqueous

The ease with which aqueous drains out of eye through angle of AC is the facility of outflow. It is the volume of aqueous flows out of eye per unit of time and depends on the pressure gradient in angle of AC. This facility is decreased in most types of glaucoma especially primary open-angle glaucoma.

TONOGRAPHY

Tonography is the clinical method of assessing facility of outflow. The basic pathogenesis of many types of glaucoma, particularly primary open angle glaucoma is considered as an increase resistance to the outflow (facility) of aqueous through trabecular meshwork. Tonography is a technique by which ophthalmologist can detect this embarrassment to aqueous outflow in the diagnosis of glaucoma in its early stages which have border line or fluctuating IOP. But, since there are other sophisticated techniques for early diagnosis of glaucoma, now tonography is not routinely used by many clinicians.

Present Status of Tonography among Modern Methods of Early Diagnosis of Glaucomas

Once developed, glaucoma is a continuous process which can produce progressive damage of retinal ganglion cells. At present the only risk factor of glaucomatous damage which can be treated effectively is IOP. We have to lower the IOP to a level which will retard or halt the further ganglion cell damage and loss. It is unfortunate that, before field changes appear in the standard white to white automated perimetry 40% and even more ganglion cells would have been damaged or lost due to glaucoma. For early diagnosis and follow-up of these latent or preperimetric glaucomas a number of **sophisticated tests** *like short wavelength automated perimetry (SWAP), evaluation and demonstration of damage of retinal nerve fiber layer (RNFL) by scanning laser ophthalmoscopy, scanning laser polarimetry and optical coherence tomography* are available. But these tests are expensive and carried out mainly in tertiary ophthalmic centers. Thus, tonography can be considered.

- In situations where a patient cannot afford or reach such facilities. Then tests like tonography can be considered and utilized as a preliminary method for the early diagnosis of latent glaucomas.
  Single tonometric measurement of IOP may not be contributory in the early stages especially of primary open-angle glaucoma. In such situations establishment of an abnormal facility of outflow by tonography can be a warning signal before constant rise of IOP leading optic nerve damage occur.
- Tonography combined with gonioscopy is helpful to differentiate open and angle closure glaucoma.

- Some glaucoma patients have normal (normal tension glaucoma) or below normal (low tension glaucoma) but increased resistance to aqueous outflow. By tonometry alone these glaucomas cannot be diagnosed but tonography can reveal such latent glaucomas.

Tonography can be performed using an ordinary or electronic Schiotz tonometer with a recording device or a pneumotonometer (pueumatonography).

Technique of tonography: When a weighted tonometer (Schiotz) is placed on cornea for about 4 minutes, after an initial small sudden rise of IOP, there will be a lowering of IOP over that period (due to squeezing out of aqueous by the weight) and then becomes steady. The rate at which IOP reduces during this time interval gives the facility of outflow. In normal eyes the resistance to the outflow of aqueous is less, more aqueous flows out and IOP falls considerably. *In eyes with increased resistance (glaucoma) IOP fall is less than normal eyes. From the initial scale reading (and corresponding IOP) and the final reading at the end of 4 minutes (and the corresponding IOP), coefficient of facility of outflow can be found out from a chart. Charts for 5.5 g. 7.5 g and 10 g weight are available. The coefficient of outflow facility represented by the* **symbol 'C'** *and the value is expressed in microliters per minute per mm Hg IOP. Normal C value ranges between 0.22–0.3 microliter per minute per mm Hg.*

$$\text{Coefficient of outflow} = P_o/C$$

P_o is the intraocular pressure at the beginning of test and C is the coefficient of facility outflow.

The ratio of P_o/C is more useful than 'C' alone in the early diagnosis of glaucoma. P_o/C value less than 100 is normal. Value between 100 and 150 is suspicious. Value above 150 is abnormal.

For example: if P_o of eye is 20 mm Hg and 'C' value is 0.1

Then $P_o/C = 20/0.1 = 200/1 = 200$ indicates glaucoma

Q. How to find out 'C' value from initial and final scale reading of tonography using 'C' value chart?

After tonography, from initial and final scale reading of Schiotz tonometer (at the end of 4 minutes), C value can be directly read from a chart prepared by Moses, Becker and modified by Leydhecker).

Initial scale reading at the onset of tonography is given in the left hand column of chart. The change in scale reading (difference of initial and final reading) is shown on the top column of table. Corresponding 'C' value is noted on the columns given on next page.

Location of 'C' value from chart with initial and final scale reading of tonography with 5.5 g weight.

Measurements of Anterior Chamber

Initial Scale reading	Change in the scale reading (IOP) during tonography (4 minutes)																		
	0.50	0.75	1.00	1.25	1.50	1.75	2.00	2.25	2.50	2.75	3.00	3.25	3.50	3.75	4.00	4.25	4.50	4.75	5.00
C values																			
0.50	0.06	0.10	0.14	0.19	0.24	0.32	0.39	0.50	0.61	0.78	0.94								
0.75	0.06	0.09	0.13	0.17	0.22	0.29	0.35	0.44	0.53	0.66	0.78								
1.00	0.05	0.08	0.12	0.16	0.21	0.26	0.32	0.40	0.47	0.57	0.66	0.80	0.94						
1.25	0.05	0.80	0.12	0.15	0.19	0.24	0.29	0.36	0.42	0.51	0.59	0.70	0.81						
1.50	0.05	0.08	0.11	0.14	0.18	0.23	0.27	0.32	0.38	0.46	0.53	0.62	0.71	0.83	0.94				
1.75	0.05	0.08	0.11	0.14	0.17	0.21	0.25	0.30	0.35	0.42	0.48	0.56	0.64	0.74	0.83				
2.00	0.05	0.07	0.10	0.13	0.16	0.20	0.24	0.29	0.33	0.38	0.44	0.51	0.58	0.66	0.74	0.84	0.93		
2.25	0.05	0.07	0.10	0.13	0.16	0.19	0.23	0.27	0.31	0.36	0.41	0.47	0.53	0.61	0.68	0.76	0.84		
2.50	0.04	0.06	0.09	0.12	0.15	0.18	0.22	0.26	0.30	0.34	0.39	0.44	0.49	0.56	0.62	0.69	0.76	0.84	0.92
2.75	0.04	0.06	0.09	0.12	0.15	0.18	0.21	0.25	0.28	0.32	0.37	0.42	0.46	0.52	0.58	0.64	0.70	0.77	0.84
3.00	0.04	0.06	0.09	0.11	0.14	0.17	0.20	0.23	0.27	0.31	0.35	0.40	0.44	0.49	0.54	0.60	0.65	0.72	0.78
3.25	0.04	0.06	0.09	0.11	0.14	0.17	0.20	0.23	0.26	0.30	0.33	0.38	0.42	0.47	0.51	0.57	0.62	0.68	0.74
3.50	0.04	0.06	0.08	0.11	0.13	0.16	0.19	0.22	0.25	0.29	0.32	0.36	0.40	0.44	0.49	0.54	0.59	0.65	0.70
3.75	0.04	0.06	0.08	0.11	0.13	0.16	0.19	0.22	0.25	0.28	0.31	0.35	0.38	0.43	0.47	0.52	0.56	0.61	0.66
4.00	0.04	0.06	0.08	0.11	0.13	0.15	0.18	0.21	0.24	0.27	0.30	0.34	0.37	0.41	0.45	0.50	0.54	0.59	0.63
4.25	0.04	0.06	0.08	0.11	0.13	0.15	0.18	0.21	0.24	0.27	0.30	0.33	0.36	0.39	0.43	0.48	0.52	0.56	0.60
4.50	0.04	0.06	0.08	0.10	0.12	0.15	0.17	0.20	0.23	0.26	0.29	0.32	0.35	0.38	0.42	0.46	0.50	0.54	0.58
4.75	0.04	0.06	0.08	0.10	0.12	0.15	0.17	0.20	0.23	0.25	0.28	0.31	0.34	0.37	0.41	0.44	0.48	0.52	0.56

Contd...

Contd...

Initial	Change in the scale reading (IOP) during tonography (4 minutes)																			
Scale reading	0.50	0.75	1.00	1.25	1.50	1.75	2.00	2.25	2.50	2.75	3.00	3.25	3.50	3.75	4.00	4.25	4.50	4.75	5.00
C values																			
5.00	0.04	0.06	0.08	0.10	0.12	0.15	0.17	0.19	0.22	0.24	0.27	0.30	0.33	0.37	0.40	0.43	0.47	0.51	0.54
5.25	0.04	0.06	0.08	0.10	0.12	0.15	0.17	0.19	0.22	0.24	0.27	0.30	0.33	0.36	0.39	0.43	0.46	0.50	0.53
5.50	0.04	0.06	0.08	0.10	0.12	0.14	0.16	0.18	0.21	0.23	0.26	0.29	0.32	0.35	0.38	0.42	0.45	0.49	0.52
5.75	0.04	0.06	0.08	0.10	0.12	0.14	0.16	0.18	0.21	0.23	0.26	0.29	0.32	0.35	0.38	0.41	0.44	0.47	0.50
6.00	0.03	0.05	0.07	0.09	0.11	0.13	0.15	0.18	0.20	0.22	0.25	0.28	0.31	0.34	0.37	0.40	0.43	0.46	0.49
6.25	0.03	0.05	0.07	0.09	0.11	0.13	0.15	0.18	0.20	0.22	0.25	0.28	0.31	0.34	0.37	0.40	0.43	0.46	0.49
6.50	0.03	0.05	0.07	0.09	0.11	0.13	0.15	0.18	0.20	0.22	0.25	0.27	0.30	0.33	0.36	0.39	0.42	0.45	0.48
6.75	0.03	0.05	0.07	0.09	0.11	0.13	0.15	0.18	0.20	0.22	0.24	0.27	0.30	0.33	0.36	0.39	0.41	0.44	0.47
7.00	0.03	0.05	0.07	0.09	0.11	0.13	0.15	0.18	0.20	0.22	0.24	0.26	0.29	0.32	0.35	0.38	0.40	0.43	0.46
7.50	0.03	0.05	0.07	0.09	0.11	0.13	0.15	0.17	0.19	0.22	0.24	0.26	0.29	0.32	0.34	0.37	0.39	0.42	0.45
7.50	0.03	0.05	0.07	0.09	0.11	0.13	0.15	0.17	0.19	0.22	0.24	0.26	0.29	0.32	0.34	0.37	0.39	0.42	0.45
8.00	0.03	0.05	0.07	0.09	0.11	0.13	0.15	0.17	0.19	0.22	0.24	0.26	0.29	0.31	0.34	0.37	0.39	0.42	
8.50	0.03	0.05	0.07	0.09	0.11	0.13	0.15	0.17	0.19	0.21	0.23	0.26	0.28	0.31	0.33	0.36	0.39		
9.00	0.03	0.05	0.07	0.09	0.11	0.13	0.15	0.17	0.19	0.21	0.23	0.26	0.28	0.31	0.33				
9.50	0.03	0.05	0.07	0.09	0.11	0.13	0.15	0.17	0.19	0.21	0.23	0.26	0.28						
10.00	0.03	0.05	0.07	0.09	0.11	0.13	0.15	0.17	0.19	0.21	0.23								
11.00	0.03	0.05	0.07	0.09	0.11	0.13	0.15												

Source: Moses, Becker and Leydhecker

Example:
The initial scale reading of tonography with 5.5 g weight of one eye is 4 (IOP 20.5 mm Hg Schiotz) and after 4 minutes of tonography the scale reading has changed to 6 divisions (IOP reduced to 14.5 mm Hg Schiotz). From this the change in scale reading 2 of divisions on scale, the C value can be located from the chart and is 0.15.
- Initial reading   : 4
- Final reading   : 6
- Change in scale reading   : 2
- C value   : 0.15

This table is useful only if the ocular rigidity is normal. When rigidity is abnormal the table of Dreger may be used to get the correct C value.

Incision Planes for Anterior Chamber Entry in Various Surgeries

Surgical entry into AC is an essential part of many intraocular surgeries like paracentesis, peripheral iridectomy, cataract surgery, antiglaucoma surgery, etc. The incision for the AC entry can be done at various levels (Fig. 6).

- **Vertical incision at the corneolimbal junction:** It passes vertically through peripheral cornea at its junction with semitraslucent limbal stroma (corneolimbal junction) and is ideal for paracentesis, peripheral iridectomy, etc. It enters directly into the narrowest portion of anterior chamber opposite last roll of iris, from which a small portion of iris can be excised and removed (peripheral iridectomy). Just behind this region vitreous has its strongest attachment its base so that vitreous will not move forwards and block the iridectomy hole. Thus, a peripheral iridectomy is immune to block by vitreous (than other types iridectomies) and provide a good alternative communication between posterior and anterior chamber due to pupillary block from various causes leading to glaucomas.

  This incision plane has other *advantages* also.
  1. Limbal stroma is avascular.
  2. Deep various plexus and the functioning part of trabecular meshwork in filtration angle is avoided.

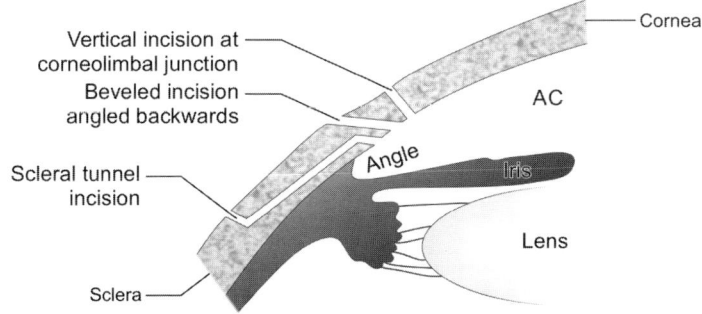

Fig. 6: Anterior chamber entry incision planes for various surgeries.

- **Beveled incision angled backwards:** Section angled backwards has an additional benefit of being a self-sealing incision.
- **Scleral tunnel incision:** 2 or 3 mm behind the limbus through sclera through a scleral tunnel into the anterior chamber is the ideal incision for small incision cataract surgery, trabeculectomy, etc.

Intraocular Pressure—Normal and Abnormal Variations (Summary)

- Normal : 10–20 mm Hg
- Normal diurnal variation : 2 mm Hg above normal
- Glaucoma : 21 mm and above with signs of optic nerve damage
- Normal tension glaucoma : Normal range of IOP (below 21 mm Hg) with signs of optic nerve damage
- Low tension glaucoma : Lower than normal range of IOP (below 20 mm Hg) with signs of optic nerve damage
- Baseline IOP : 21 mm Hg and a diurnal variation over 5–8 mm Hg
- Target pressure : 16–18 mm Hg
  - Mild glaucoma disease : Need a 20% reduction from baseline IOP and better kept below 18 mm
  - Moderate glaucoma disease : Need 30% reduction from baseline IOP and maintain below 15 mm Hg
  - Severe glaucoma disease : Require a 50% reduction from baseline IOP and stabilized below 13 mm Hg
- Ocular hypertension : Above 21 mm Hg without signs of optic nerve damage
- Ocular hypotony : Below 8 mm Hg

CHAPTER 7

Measurements of Posterior Chamber

Posterior chamber (PC) is the space in the anterior segment of eye between iris and lens, filled with aqueous. It is bordered by posterior surface of iris, posteromedial surface of ciliary body, portions of anterior surface of vitreous, zonules and lens (Fig. 1).

PARTS OF POSTERIOR CHAMBER

Posterior chamber is divided into three portions by zonules. But they freely communicate each other as the partitions are not complete. They are prezonular portion, zonular portion and retrozonular portion (Fig. 2).

Prezonular Portion

Prezonular portion is between iris and lens. It is almost triangular in shape. The base is formed by the ciliary processes and the spaces between them

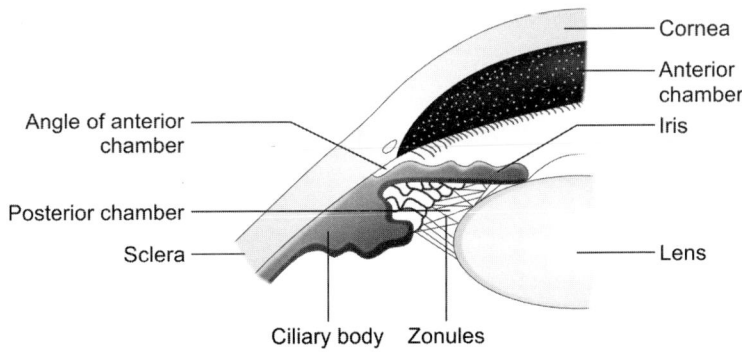

Fig. 1: Boundaries of posterior chamber.

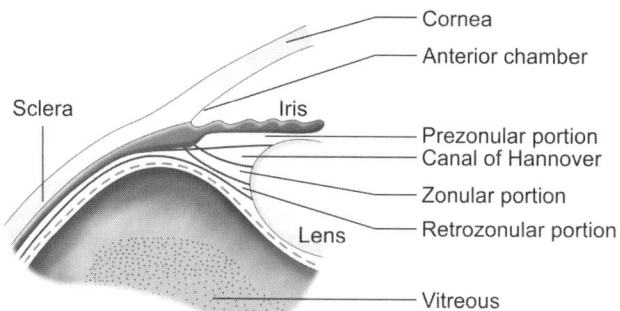

Fig. 2: Parts of posterior chamber.

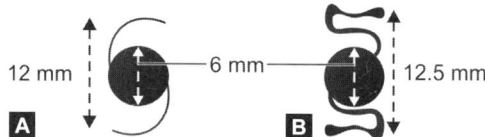

Figs. 3A and B: Overall size of a rigid (A) posterior chamber IOL and (B) anterior chamber IOL.

(recesses of Khunt). Apex is at the point where the pupillary margin and lens meet. Anterior boundary is pigment epithelium of iris and posterior boundary is zonules and lens. Aqueous is formed from ciliary body into the prezonular portion of posterior chamber and flows through pupil into anterior chamber under a pressure gradient. The contact of iris lens is maximum in middilatation and explain the mechanism of primary angle closure angle glaucoma. The volume of prezonular compartment becomes small and the access to AC large in maximum dilatation of pupil.

Ciliary sulcus is the grove between the root of iris and adjacent portion of ciliary body. *The average diameter of ciliary sulcus is 11.25 mm.* This sulcus often forms a support for fixation of haptic of intraocular lens (sulcus fixation of IOL).

Average overall diameter of a rigid posterior chamber IOL is 12 mm. The size of the optic is 6 mm and haptic is 6 mm. The average overall diameter of AC IOL is about 12.5 mm (Figs. 3A and B).

Zonular Portion

Zonular portion is the part of posterior chamber between anterior and posterior groups of zonules.

Retrozonular Portion

It is the part of posterior chamber between zonules and anterior vitreous face. It is slit-like and is called retrozonular space of petit. Peripherally, the space extends up to the attachment of vitreous base to ora serrata. Centrally, it is limited by a ligament like attachment of posterior capsule of lens (condensation of vitreous) to anterior face of vitreous called hyaloideocapsular ligament (ligament of Weiger).

BOUNDARIES OF POSTERIOR (SUMMARY)

Anteriorly : Posterior chamber is bounded by posterior surface of iris.
Peripherally : Posterior chamber is bordered by posterior medial surface of ciliary body.
Posteriorly : Posterior chamber is lined by anterior face of vitreous, zonules and lens.

FUNCTIONS OF POSTERIOR CHAMBER

- Aqueous is formed by ciliary body into posterior chamber.
- Posterior chamber provides the space for the changes in the size and shape of lens in its growth and the function of accommodation.
- In situations of pupillary block PC space is utilized for collection of aqueous and a timely peripheral iridectomy or iridotomy to produce an alternative communication between PC and AC, resulting in relief of glaucoma (Figs. 4 and 5).
- Gives a provision for sulcus fixation of IOL (Fig. 6).

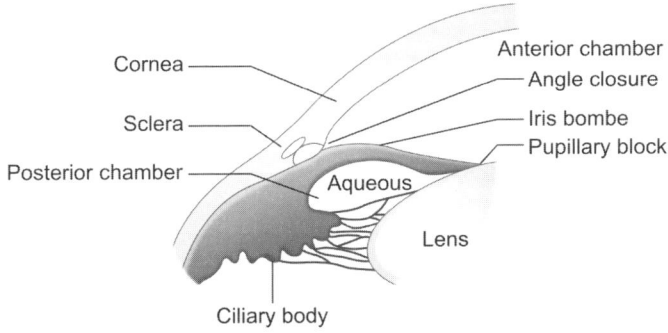

Fig. 4: Pupillary block glaucoma.

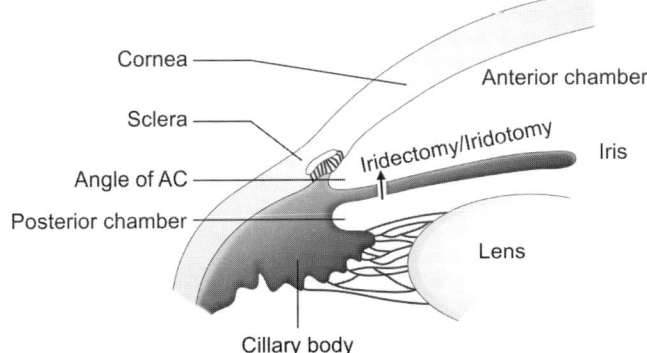

Fig. 5: Pupillary block relieved by peripheral iridectomy/laser iridotomy.

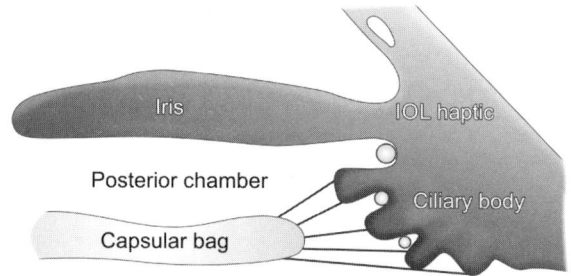

Fig. 6: Possible positions of sulcus fixated IOL in posterior chamber.

DIMENSIONS OF POSTERIOR CHAMBER

- Volume of posterior chamber is about : 0.06 mL
- Ciliary sulcus—diameter : 11.25 mm.

CHAPTER 8

Measurements of Uveal Tract

Uveal tract is the middle layer of the ocular wall. It is the most vascular portion of eye and provides nutrition to many parts of eyeball. This middle coat has three anatomically continuous, but functionally different portions—iris, ciliary body and choroid anteroposteriorly (Fig. 1).

IRIS

Iris, the most anterior portion, is a circular diaphragm separating anterior and posterior chamber and attached slightly below the anteromedial surface of ciliary body, where it is most thin and can be torn easily.

Structure (layers) of Iris (Fig. 2)

- *Single layer of endothelial cells:* The front surface of iris is covered by a single layer of endothelial cells which is absent at the crypts and get atrophied in

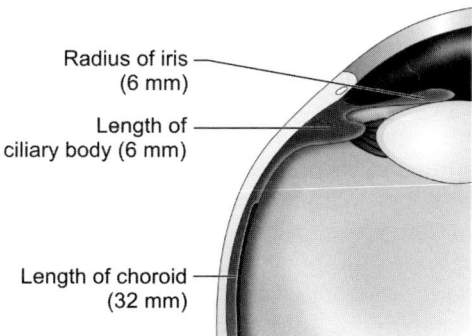

Fig. 1: Parts and general dimensions of uveal tract.

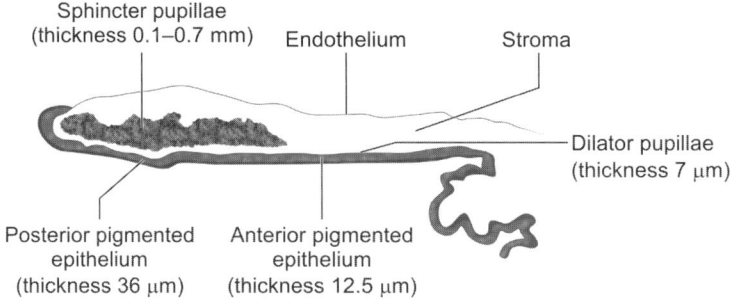

Fig. 2: Structure (layers) of iris.

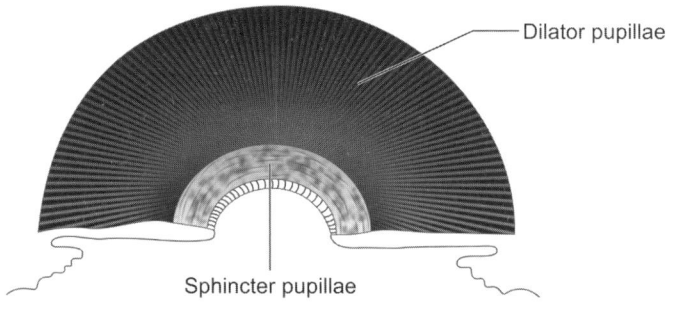

Fig. 3: Muscles of iris.

adults. This is bordered posteriorly a condensation of connective tissues which contain fibroblasts and pigment cells (melanocytes) arranged parallel to surface and deep to fibroblasts.

- *Stroma:* Stroma consists of loose collagen bundles arranged in curved clockwise and anticlockwise arcades. This arrangement permits free diffusion of aqueous, facilitate movement of pupil but get easily waterlogged in inflammatory conditions producing sluggish pupillary reactions. Stroma contains blood vessels, nerves and muscles.

The size of the pupils and the pupillary reactions are governed by two smooth muscles of ectodermal origin, within the iris (intrinsic) and controlled by nerves from autonomous nervous system.

- *Sphincter pupillae* (Fig. 3): *It is a flat strip of smooth muscle having a width of 0.75 mm and a thickness of 0.1–0.17 mm.* It lies close to pupillary margin deep in stroma but separated from underlying dilator pupillae and anterior epithelium by a thin sheet of stromal collagen to which it is bound firmly. Because of this, even if a portion of iris and sphincter are removed (sector iridectomy) the remaining portion of pupillary margin can react to stimuli. When stimulated produces, contraction of pupil and is supplied by parasympathetic fibers orginating from Edinger-Westphal nucleus situated in midbrain and fibers reaching the muscle via the oculomotor nerve.
- *Dilator pupillae*: It is a thin sheet of radially arranged smooth muscle fibers of *about 60μm long and 7μm wide situated in depth of iris* in close relation with the anterior pigment epithelial lining of iris and extends from the margin of pupil and peripherally get attached to ciliary body. It is supplied

by sympathetic nerve fibers through long ciliary nerves and dilates pupil on stimulation.
- *Anterior epithelium:* Posterior surface of iris is bordered by two layers of pigmented epithelium which become continuous at pupillary margin and are embryologically an extension of anterior lip of optic cup with a potential space in between them. *Anterior epithelium is narrow, lightly pigmented,* represent the outer layer of optic cup, is made of a single layer of flattened cells and lies just under dilator pupillae muscle. *It is about 12.5 µm thick.*
- *Posterior epithelium:* Thicker, heavily pigmented and is the source pigment dispersion in normal and various clinical conditions like pigmentary glaucoma. It consists of a layer cuboid cells of about 36–55 µm height and 16–25 µm width. It corresponds to inner layer of optic cup. There is a gradual decrease of pigmentation of posterior epithelium towards periphery of iris and become continuous with the nonpigmented posterior epithelial lining of ciliary body. Desmosomes produce adhesion between anterior and posterior pigment epithelium. When posterior synchiae are broken using mydriatics, portion of epithelium left on lens contain both layers and pigmented (Figs. 4A and B). But when epithelial cysts of iris are formed in the potential space between two layers, they separate as in retinal detachment.

Circumference and Diameter of Iris

Circumference of iris is 38 mm and diameter is about 12 mm (Fig. 5). Iris is perforated in the center by a circular opening called pupil, which controls the amount of light entering the eye.

During pupillary constriction and mid-dilation, pupillary margin reaches more close to the lens. It is away from lens when pupil is fully dilated. This fact is important in understanding pathogenesis and treatment of uveities and glaucomas.

*The anterior surface of iris is divided into an outer ciliary zone and inner pupillary zone by an interrupted circular ridge called collarette which lies 1.6 mm from pupillary **margin** and overlies circulus vasculosus iridis minor* (Fig. 6).

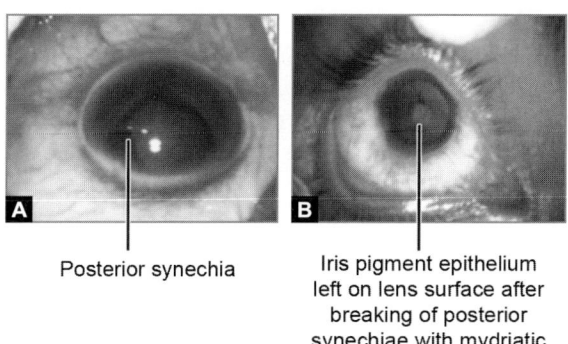

A: Posterior synechia
B: Iris pigment epithelium left on lens surface after breaking of posterior synechiae with mydriatic

Figs. 4A and B: Posterior synechia and iris epithelium in acute iridocylitis.

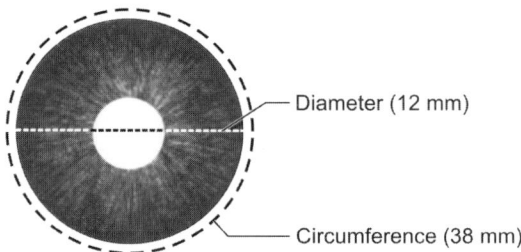

Fig. 5: Circumference and diameter of iris.

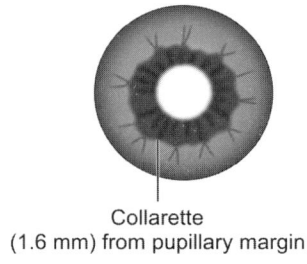

Collarette
(1.6 mm) from pupillary margin

Fig. 6: Position of collarette.

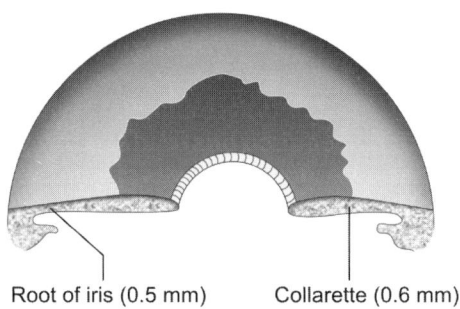

Root of iris (0.5 mm)   Collarette (0.6 mm)

Fig. 7: Thickness of iris.

Thickness of Iris

The thickness of iris is about 0.6 mm (thickest) at collarette and 0.5 mm at iris root (Fig. 7). Smaller folds extend from pupillary margin to about 1mm peripherally and this gives a slightly uneven border to the pupillary margin.

Functions of Iris

- Avoids glare, aberrations and sharpen the image.
- Act as a diaphragm separating anterior chamber and posterior chambers.
- Participates in aqueous humor circulation.
- Provides nutrition to lens and cornea.
- Heat is absorbed by pigments of iris and ciliary body.

Dimensions of Iris (Summary)

- Circumference : 38 mm
- Diameter : 12 mm
- Area : 110 mm^2
- Distance of collarette from
- pupillary margin : 1.6 mm
- Thickness of collarette : 0.6 mm
- Pupillary zone width : 1.6 mm
- Ciliary zone width : 2.4 mm
- Thickness of root of iris : 0.5 mm
- Sphincter pupillae : Width : 0.75 µm
  - : Thickness : 0.1–0.7 µm
- Dilator pupillae : Height : 60 µm
  - : Width : 7 µm

PUPIL

Pupil is a nearly round hole almost in the center of iris. It has following *functions:*
- Control the amount of light entering the eye.
- Sharpening of image formed in retina.
- Constriction of pupil during accommodation helps to improve depth of focus and reduce spherical aberration.
- Circulation of aqueous: Pupil form a communication between posterior chamber (PC) and anterior chamber (AC) and so become the main path of aqueous circulation.
- Abnormal pupillary reactions help in the diagnosis of ocular and neurological disorders.

Size of Pupil (Figs. 8A and B)

The pupil is only approximately circular in shape and placed slightly nasal to the center of iris. In ordinary intensities of light (room light) the *normal diameter of pupil varies between 2.5–4.5 mm.* Though the usual pupillary diameter is around *3.5 mm*, the image of pupil appear 1/8th enlarged due to the refraction of normal corneal surface, and appears clinically as *4 mm.* The size of pupil changes constantly depending on the amount of light entering the eye and dependent on changing balance between tone of sphincter and dilator muscle. When the pupillary reactions are elicited, the two pupils have to be illuminated with same amount of light and the angle of incidence of light on each eye must be same.
- *An enlargement of pupil size (normal and abnormal) more than 4 mm is mydriasis and an abnormal constriction to less than 2 mm is miosis.*
- In the newborn, pupil is small due to the lack of development of sympathetic system and this size is retained till the first year. Pupil acquires the maximum size in childhood or adolescence. It again becomes miotic in the old age.

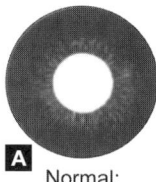 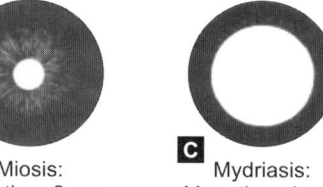 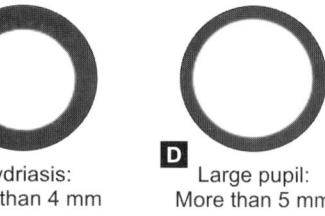

A	B	C	D
Normal: 2.5–3.5 mm	Miosis: Less than 2 mm	Mydriasis: More than 4 mm	Large pupil: More than 5 mm

Figs. 8A to D: Size of pupil.

- Pupil is large in blue eyes and small in dark eyes. *Myopes have larger pupil (probably due to the decreased or absence of stimulus for accommodation which make sphincter muscle atrophied) than hypermetropes. Pupils of two eyes of a person are normally equal in size but a slight difference of 0.25 mm between two pupils (anisocoria) is considered as physiological in the static condition.*
- *Physiological anisocoria*—can occur in lateral illumination of one eye; pupil of more illuminated eye is smaller than its fellow.
- *Tournay's reaction—when the eyes are suddenly turned to one side, the pupil of abducting eye dilates and there is a miosis in the adducting eye. The difference is around 0.5 mm and remains so, as far as the lateral gaze is maintained.* This reaction has been reported to be lost in syphilis.

Pupil is contracted during sleep due to decreased sympathetic tone to dilator and diminished tone of inhibitory impulses from constrictor center. The small pupil in sleep is a constant phenomenon and it helps to differentiate true from simulated or false sleep which has normal size.

Pupillary Diameter and Pupillary Reactions (Normal and Abnormal)

- Normally reacting dilated pupil occur in:
  - Impaired muscle tone
  - Nervous excitement
  - Darkness or dimlight
  - Myopia
- Normally reacting small pupil is seen in:
  - Babies
  - Old age
  - Bright light
- Mid-dilated large nonreacting pupil is a sign of:
  - Diseases of retina, optic nerve
  - Oculomotor nerve paralysis
  - Irritation of cervical sympathetic
- Very large nonreacting pupil can result from:
  - Pharmacological, excessive use of mydriatics

- Small nonreacting pupil is due to:
  - Miotics
  - Morphine
  - Iritis
  - Irritation of oculomotor nerve
  - Palsy of sympathetic system
- *Loss of direct reaction to light with retained consensual reaction/Afferent pupillary defect (Marcus Gunn pupil)* indicate severe retinal and optic nerve disease.
- *Hemianopic reaction:* When one-half of retina is stimulated using light (ideally a slit lamp light beam reduced to a spot) pupil reacts briskly than when other half of retina is similarly stimulated. This pupillary abnormality occur due to a lesion in the optic tract.
- *Loss of both light and convergence reaction (absolute pupillary paralysis):* Is due to a lesion in oculomotor nerve.
- *Argyll Robertson pupil:* Small pupils which do not react to light but react on convergence (light near dissociation due to damage in pupillary pathways in tectum between afferent and efferent tracts) result from syphilitic disease.
- *Tonic pupil of Adie:* This is a unilateral mid-dilated pupil with a sluggish reaction to light and ill-sustained (with a long latent period) reaction to convergence usually occurring in young women. Adie's pupil may resemble Argyll Robertson pupil, but the former is of unknown etiology. The involved eye often has mild accommodative paralysis and asthenopia and two eyes do not work together in near activities.

Normal and Abnormal Size of Pupils

- Normal diameter : 2.5–3.5 mm
- Physiological anisocoria : 0.25 mm difference between two eyes
- Mydriasis : Abnormal dilation to more than 4 mm
- Miosis : Abnormal constriction to less than 2 mm

Pupil can be dilated to 8 mm or even more pharmacologically. Ideal pupillary diameter required for cataract surgery is about 6 mm.

CILIARY BODY

Ciliary body is the broadest, middle portion of uveal tract and has complex functions. It lies on the inner aspect of sclera following its curvature and extends from the level of scleral spur to the level of ora serrata, the teeth shaped anterior end of retina (Fig. 9).

The ciliary body is *triangular in shape* with its base forward. The plicated, broad anterior portion is *pars plicata* and smooth posterior portion is the *pars plana*.

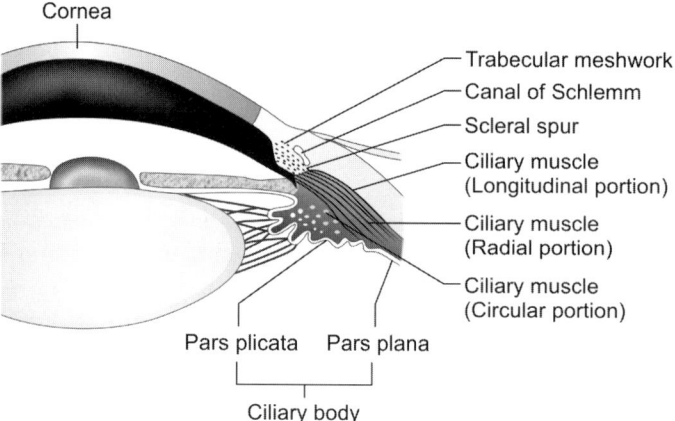

Fig. 9: Parts of ciliary body.

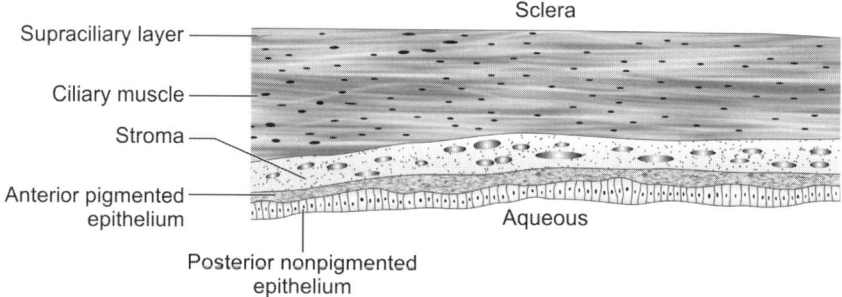

Fig. 10: Structure of ciliary body.

Structure of Ciliary Body (Fig. 10)

Structurally, ciliary body has following layers from surface to depth.
- *Supraciliary layer:* Supraciliary layer is a layer of collagen strands getting attached to the overlying scleral collagen framework. This forms a route for the exit of aqueous (uveoscleral outflow). It can enlarge and form a potential space for collection of exudate or transudate in ciliary body, in inflammatory conditions and choroidal detachment.
- *Ciliary muscle:* The triangular shape of ciliary body may be due to the architectural arrangement of ciliary muscle bundles. It consists of three groups of smooth muscle fibers probably originating from scleral spur.
  - Longitudinal or meridional portion—is the outer most, is close to sclera and pass from scleral spur posteriorly into the stroma of choroid. The muscle participates in the function of accommodation.

- *Intermediate radial or oblique portion*—radiate from the scleral spur and get inserted probably on the posterior part of uveoscleral portion of trabecular meshwork and involved in the facility of outflow of aqueous through trabecular meshwork. Its contraction in response to miotics increases the pore size of trabecular meshwork.
- *Circular or sphincter portion*—is the deepest and inner most portion of ciliary muscle. Its muscle bundles run parallel to limbus like a sphincter and lie close to the lens. This portion is very much involved in accommodation.

Accommodation

Accommodation is the phenomenon in which eyes increase their power from that for distance to see near object (clearly). In the act of accommodation there occur contraction of ciliary muscle occurs, especially longitudinal and circular portion of ciliary muscle pulling the ciliary body forwards resulting in the relaxation of zonules thereby making the lens become more convex and increasing its refractive power, when one looks at nearer objects.

Summary of changes occurring in the function of accommodation:
- Contraction of ciliary muscles (longitudinal and circular)
- Loosening of zonules
- Increase in the anterior curvature (from 10 mm to 6 mm) and posterior curvature of lens.
- Increase in the sagittal thickness of lens
- Decrease in the equatorial diameter of lens
- Slight forward movement of lens axially
- The dentations on the equator of lens adjacent to the zonular attachments almost disappear during accommodation when the zonular tension is relaxed.
- Some pupillary constriction sharpens the image
- *Stroma:* Stroma is made of collagenous connection tissue. It contains muscles, blood vessels and nerves. Stroma separates the muscle bundles. The arterial suply to ciliary body comes from long posterior ciliary arteries and anterior ciliary arteries and form the circulus arteriosus iridis major. This vascular circle is situated in the stroma behind the root of iris and in fornt of circular portion of ciliary muscle.
- *External limiting membrane:* It is a thin membrane (anterior basement membrane) and is supposed to be produced by the underlying pigmented ciliary epithelium. It extends anteriorly to basement membrane of dilator pupillae and posteriorly to basement membrane of retinal pigment epithelium.
- *Ciliary epithelium* (Fig. 11): Posterior surface of ciliary body is lined by two layers of epithelium which are continuation of epithelial lining of iris. In ciliary body only the outer layer is pigmented and inner layer is nonpigmented (but both layers are pigmented in iris). Ciliary epithelium play an important role in secretion of aqueous and is an essential part

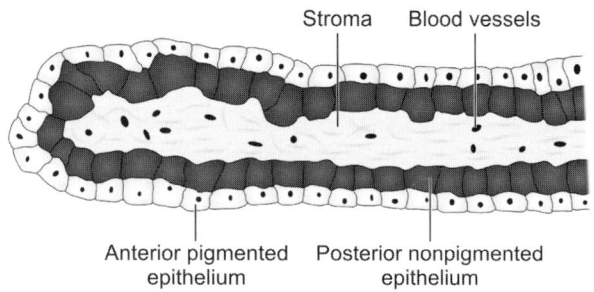

Fig. 11: Structure of ciliary process.

of blood ocular barrier. About 90% of total aqueous formed is probably due to secretory activity (powered by the metabolic function) of ciliary epithelial cells.
- Anterior pigmented epithelium *is made of cells of 8-10 μm wide and height of about 8-12 μm in pars plicata and 10-15 μm in pars plana.* It is pigmented and continues anteriorly with corresponding layer of iris and posteriorly with retinal pigment epithelium.
- Posterior nonpigmented epithelium consists of a layer of non-pigmented cuboid cells of 12-15 μm width and 10-15 μm height in pars plicata and columnar cells of 6-9 μm width and 30 μm height in pars plana.

Dimensions of Ciliary Body

The anteroposterior length of ciliary body (CB) is 6.0-6.5 mm and extends more inferotemporally than superonasally.
- Temporal quadrant of CB extends about 6.5 mm posteriorly from sclerolimbal junction
- Nasal quadrant is about 5.7 mm
- Superior quadrant is about 6.1 mm
- Inferior quadrant is about 6.2 mm.

Of this pars plicata shares the anterior 2 mm and pars plana the next posterior 4-4.5 mm. The CB is shorter and pars plana is more anterior in infants.

Pars Plicata

The anterior broad portion of ciliary body is pars plicata. This portion is about *2 mm long, 0.5 wide and has a height of 0.8-1 mm. Pars plicata has about 70-80 macroscopic plications around it's circumference* (hence the name pars plicata). Microscopic examination shows many smaller folds—ciliary processes, each of which is made of stroma, tufts of blood vessels, the whole being covered by two layer of epithelium—outer pigmented and inner nonpigmented. Ciliary process contains no muscle, but very vascular (veins and capillaries of 15-30 μm diameter) and are very much involved in the formation of aqueous by ultrafiltration (blood vessels) and secretion (ciliary epithelium).

Pars Plana

Pars plana is the posterior narrow, smooth *4–4.5 mm portion of ciliary body* and is lined by two layers of epithelium on inner surface which are the continuation of that of pars plicata.

The posterior group of zonular fibers originates from an 1.5 mm wide area of pars plana lying 1.5 mm in front of ora serrata. Part of vitreous base is attached to the epithelium of pars plana over an area, 1.5–2 mm forward from ora serrata.

Surface Marking of Ciliary Body

The measurements of CB on the surface of eyeball (surface marking) are made *from the level of corneolimbal junction posteriorly* and its localization from outside is important in:
- Pars plana surgical approaches
- Cyclodestructive procedures
- Intravitreal injections.

Ciliary body is slightly posterior in relation to apparent limbus in superior quadrant and inferior quadrant.

Pars plicata surgical procedures (cyclocryotherapy and transcleral laser cyclophotocoagulation), etc. are better done *about 1.5–2 mm* behind corneolimbal junction to get the desired effect.

Pars plana surgical procedures are done *about 4 mm behind corneolimbal junction in phakic eyes and 3 mm behind in pseudophakic eyes.*

Pars plana is preferred for posterior segment surgical entry, because:
- This region is relatively avascular and so the chance of intraocular bleeding is minimal during surgical procedures.
- Least possibility of retinal injury during surgical entry.

Functions of Ciliary Body

- Supports lens: Lens is attached to and held in position by ciliary body.
- Ciliary muscles play an important role in accommodation.
- About 90% of the aqueous is formed due to activity ciliary epithelium.
- Blood ocular barrier: Ciliary epithelium is an essential part of blood ocular barrier.
- Pars plicata can form a support for IOL fixation (sulcus fixated IOL) on certain occasions.

Summary of Dimensions of Ciliary Body

- Total length of ciliary body   : 6–6.5 mm
  (widest inferotemporally and
  narrowest superonasally)
- Average posterior limit of CB from
  corneolimbal junction.
  – Temporal quadrant   : 6.5 mm
  – Nasal quadrant   : 5.7 mm

- Superior quadrant : 6.1 mm
- Inferior quadrant : 6.2 mm
- Pars plicata
  - Length : 2 mm
  - Width : 0.5 mm
  - Height : 0.8–1 mm
  - Number of plications : 70–80

  Equator of lens is about 0.5 mm from plications.
- Pars plana

  Length : 4–4.5 mm

Posterior group of zonular fibers take origin from pars plana, about 1.5 mm anterior to ora serrata.

Ciliary portion of vitreous base (broad band of vitreous strongly attached to epithelium of pars plana) extends 1.5–2 mm forward from ora serrata.

CHOROID

Choroid is the thinnest and most posterior portion of the uveal tract, composed mainly of blood vessels. It provides nutrition to the posterior layers of retina especially rods and cones. Choroid is sandwiched between sclera and retina and extends from the level of ora serrata anteriorly and to the level of optic nerve posteriorly. It is anchored firmly to sclera around optic nerve and less firmly in the regions of passage of vortex veins, posterior ciliary artery and ciliary nerves. The anchoring to sclera is strongest behind equator and so the choroidal detachment usually limits anterior to this and rarely extends behind equator.

Dimensions of Choroid

- *Length of choroid*—is about 32 mm
- *Thickness of choroid:* The thickness of choroid decreases gradually from its *posterior portion 0.1–0.22 mm in the anterior portion. It is thickest in the region against macula (0.5–1 mm)*: Choroid gets thinner in disease conditions like chronic glaucomas, buphthalmos and myopia.

Structure of Choroid (Fig. 12)

Structurally, choroid has the following layers from surface to depth which has been described below.

- *Suprachoroidal lamina (Lamina Fusca):* It is a thin sheet of delicate collagen network running from sclera to choroid. It is more firmly attached to sclera posteriorly and so choroidal detachments usually never spread behind equator. The long and short ciliary arteries and nerve which supply uveal tract run in this lamina. As a whole, the attachment of this lamina to sclera is not so firm, so that a potential space can form between them called epichoroidal or suprachoroidal space.

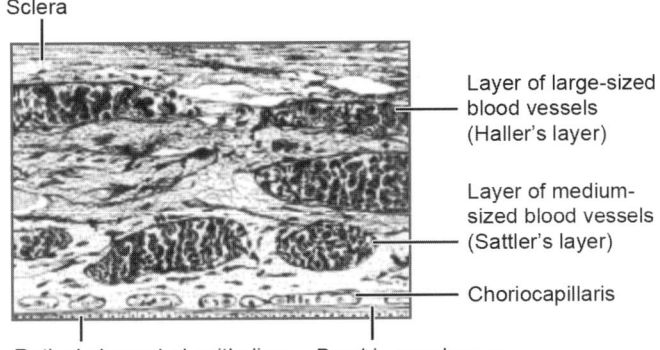

Fig. 12: Structure of choroid.

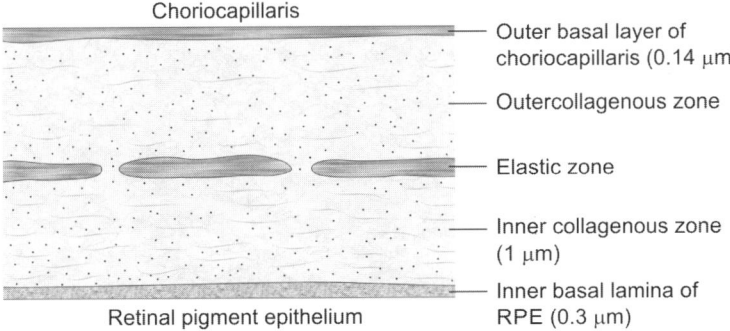

Fig. 13: Structure of Bruch's membrane.

- *Stroma:* It is made of connective tissue containing melanocytes, fibrocytes and contain blood vessels and nerves.

  The main mass of choroid is constituted by blood vessels arranged in three layers, the size of blood vessels decreases in size from out to inwards.
  1. *Haller's layer:* It is the outer layer of large vessels.
  2. *Sattler's layer:* It is middle layer of medium-sized vessels.
  3. *Choriocapillaris:* Inner most layer of small vessels (capillaries) the arterioles of which come from short posterior ciliary arteries. It is a dense fenestrated capillary plexus. The vessels of choriocapillaris overlying macula is denser than other areas. *Arterioles have a lumen of 20–40 µm. Capillaries have wide bore of 20–25 µm.*
- *Bruch's membrane* is a very thin, noncellular connective tissue lamina closely bound to choriocapillaris over it and retinal pigment epithelium (RPE) under it, so that in retinal detachment, RPE remains attached to choroid (Fig. 13).

  It extends from level of ora serrata to that of optic disk margin. *The thickness of Bruch's membrane in adult is about 2 µm, and thickness increases with age. It is thickest near optic disk margin (2–4 µm) and becomes thin near the ora serrate (1–2 µm).*

Its ultrastructure is complex and has five layers.
1. *Outer basal lamina (of choriocapillaris):* It is an interrupted sheet in contact with the choriocapillaris and is 0.14 mm thickness.
2. *Outer collagenous zone:* It has almost same structure as inner basal lamina.
3. *Elastic zone:* It is made of interrupted rod-like fibers which have a dense cortex and collagenous core.
4. *Inner collagenous zone:* It is 1 μm thick (thicker anteriorly towards ora) and is made of collagen fibers.
5. *Inner basal lamina (of RPE):* 03 μm thick is just over the retinal pigment epithelium (formed from it) but separated from it by a zone of 100 μm width.

Functions of Choroid

- Choroid gives nutrition to outer layers of retina especially rods and cones.
- It helps to conduct blood vessels to anterior segment of eye.
- Choroid blood flow participates to a certain extent in the regulation of intraocular pressure.
- Bruch's membrane of choroid is an important part of blood ocular barrier.
- Pigments of choroid absorb any excess light reaching the retina and avoid light reflection.

Summary of Dimensions of Choroid

- Length : 32 mm
- Surface area : 1180 mm^2
- Thickness : 0.1 mm anteriorly
  : 0.22 mm posteriorly
- Macular region : 216 μm
- Subfoveal : 300 μm (thickest)
- Volume : 10 μL
- Thickness of Bruch's membrane : 2 μm (average)
  - Near optic disk : 2–4 μm (thickest)
  - Near ora serrata : 1–2 μm (thickest)
  - Inner basal lamina : 0.3 μm
  - Inner collagenous zone : 1 μm
  - Outer basal lamina : 0.14 μm

CHAPTER 9

Measurements of Lens

Eye has a biological, biconvex, transparent lens situated behind iris and in front of vitreous, attached to ciliary body by zonules performing important functions of accommodation and focussing light on retina (Fig. 1).

For practical purposes, eyeball may be divided arbitrarily into a small anterior and a large posterior portion along the level of *lens zonule diaphragm*. The portion of eyeball including lens, zonules and the structures in front of them are often called as the *anterior segment of eyeball* and the structures behind that level as posterior segment of eyeball.

DIMENSIONS OF LENS

Diameter of Lens

- *Normal diameter*—of lens is about 6.5 mm at birth and increases to *9 or 10 mm at the age of 20* and remains so until old age (Fig. 2).

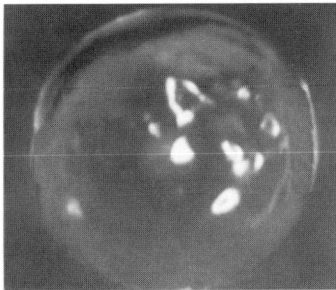

Fig. 1: Normal lens. (*For color version, see Plate 2*)

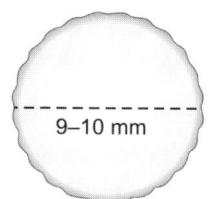

Fig. 2: Normal diameter.

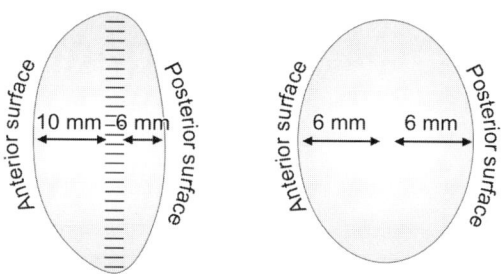

Figs. 3A and B: Change in curvature, thickness and diameter of lens in accommodation. (A) Unaccommodated; (B) Accommodated.

Anterior and posterior surfaces of lens meet at the *equator, which is about 0.5 mm away from ciliary processes.*
Diameter can vary in normal and diseased conditions.
- The equatorial diameter lens *decreases during accommodation.*
- The diameter lens is smaller in *microphakia, a congenital anomaly of lens.*
- *Colobomatous lens* has a notch, usually in its inferior part and the diameter is smaller in that portion of lens.

Radius of Curvature of Lens (Figs. 3 A and B).

Radius of curvature of anterior surface of lens is about 10 mm and that of posterior surface is 6 mm. In accommodation, the anterior surface becomes more curved and reaches even 6 mm in strong accommodation. Lens surfaces are more curved in microspherophakia, lenticonus and displacements of lens.

Thickness of Lens (Figs. 4 A to D)

- *Normal thickness or width of lens in adult is about 4.5 mm. Thickness increases with age. It is about 3.5–4 mm broad at birth. Breadth increases to 4.5 mm by the age of 40 and becomes 4.75–5 mm in old age.*
  Thickness of lens can vary in physiological and pathological situations.
- There is an *increase* in sagittal thickness during *accommodation.*
- In *Morgagnian cataract and intumescent cataract,* due to cortical hydration, the lens swells and becomes extremely thick reaching to *even to 7 mm,* consuming the space of anterior chamber, making it shallow and even leading to secondary angle closure glaucoma.

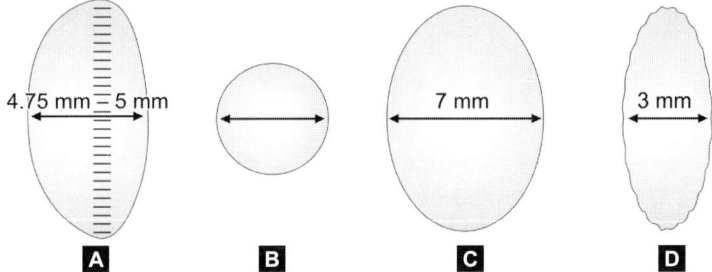

Figs. 4A to D: Thickness—normal and abnormal. (A) Normal; (B) Microspherophakia; (C) Intumescent lens; (D) Hypermature shrunken lens

- *Hypermaturity* of cataract sometimes can make lens shrink (shrunken cataract) thereby decreasing its thickness to *2.5-3 mm*. Then the AC becomes deep and iris tremulous.
- *Microspherophakia* is a congenital anomaly in which lens as a whole is small in size and more spherical (surfaces more curved).
- In **lenticonus,** only curvature of lens is abnormal, surfaces are more curved.
- Displacement of lens can produce change in shape, size and curvature of lens.
- Long-standing dislocated lens becomes more spherical.

Power of Lens

- *Dioptric power of lens is about +20D (between +16D to +20D)*
- *At birth, accommodative power is about +15 to +16 diopters and decreases to about +8D around the age of 25 and reduce again to +2D or less by the age of 50.*

Weight of Lens

At birth the weight of lens is about 65 mg. The weight increases to 180 mg by the age of 25 and 258 mg.

Refractive Index of Lens

Normal refractive index of lens is 1.39, slightly more than aqueous and vitreous (1.33) and is due to the high protein content of lens fibers.

Transparency of lens is maintained by:
- Regular arrangement of lens fibers.
- Homogenous structure of its fibers.
- Epithelial cells are not rich in organelle and lens fibers are devoid of organelle.
- Small size of extracellular space (under 1% of lens volume)
- Regulation of ionic and water content by a pump system of lens.

Functions of Lens

- Lens transmits light (80% of light between 400 nm and 1400 nm is transmitted into the eye).
- 35% of refractive power of eye is contributed by lens and shares in converging light rays on retina.
- Takes part in accommodation.
- Indirectly lens forms a support for iris.

STRUCTURE AND SURGICAL ANATOMY OF LENS (FIG. 5)

Lens has following parts from its surface to center.
- Pericapsular membrane (zonular lamella)
- Capsule
- Epithelium
- Cortex
- Nucleus.

Pericapsular Membrane (Zonular Lamella)

This is an incomplete membrane covering only a narrow area around the equator of lens, where zonules are attached. It is often considered as the superficial layer of the underlying capsule of lens. *Zonular lamella is about 0.6–0.9 μm thick*. Structurally, it is fibrogranular, the *component fibrils are about 1–3 nm wide but the fibrils of zonules are thicker, about 10 nm*. Zonular lamella has zonular adhesive mechanism. The fibronectin content of zonular lamella provides adhesive property to zonules.

True exfoliation is the exfoliation of zonular lamella. Due to prolonged exposure to infrared radiation, zonular lamella breaks and gets exfoliated as large sheets, of thin transparent membrane which float in aqueous, and curl out. It is seen only in the pupillary area of anterior surface of lens. Similar appearance can occur in intraocular inflammation, ageing and without any cause.

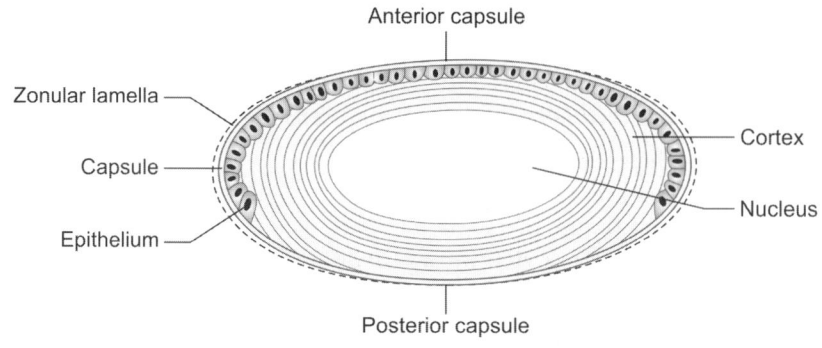

Fig. 5: Structure of lens.

Pseudoexfoliation: The zonular lamella and lens capsule are almost normal in pseudoexfoliation. In *pseudoexfoliation syndrome,* an exfoliative material of unknown origin gets deposited on the lens surface and this occur as a result of the part of widespread degenerative changes in the uvea particularly ciliary region, angle, iris and lens. Clinically these flakes are evident on the midperipheral region of anterior surface of lens (where anterior capsule is rubbed by iris). Pseudoexfoliation is often associated with glaucoma.

Lens Capsule (Fig. 6)

Capsule covers entire surface of lens. The lens capsule has a lamellar structure (about 40 lamellae), each lamella has a thickness of 40 nm. It is considered as a basement membrane of underlying epithelium. Lens is anchored to ciliary body by zonules which are attached to the lens capsule, at the equator and periphery of lens in a crisscross pattern.

The thickness of capsule is not uniform in its all portions. The capsule is thickest just in front of the equator. It is thin at the poles and equator. It is thinner at the anterior pole and thinnest at the posterior pole.
- Anterior capsule is:
  - 15–25 μm thick, 3 mm in front of equator (thickest)
  - 10–15 μm thick in the center of anterior capsule
- Equator capsule is about 14–18 μm thick
- Posterior capsule is:
  - 17–20 μm near the insertion of posterior zonular fibers
  - 3–4 μm at the center of posterior pole (thinnest).

The diameter of capsular bag is 10–11 mm. The overall diameter of the posterior chamber IOL is 12 mm (optic size 5 to 7 mm and haptic 6 mm). The overall diameter of AC IOL is 12.5 mm.

Lens Capsule and Cataract Surgery

The anatomical and functional integrity of lens capsule is critical in many stages of cataract surgery like capsulotomy, hydrodissection, nucleus management, cortical aspiration, intraocular lens (IOL) implantation, etc.

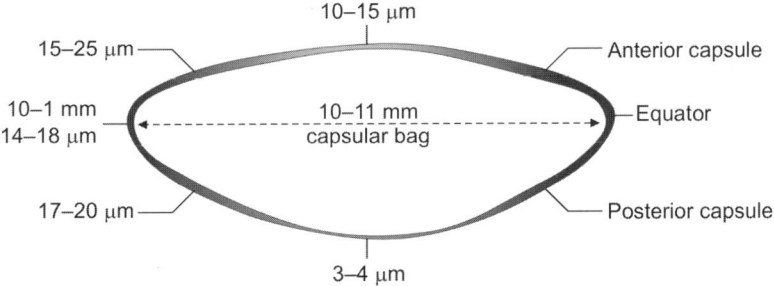

Fig. 6: Thickness of various portions of lens capsule.

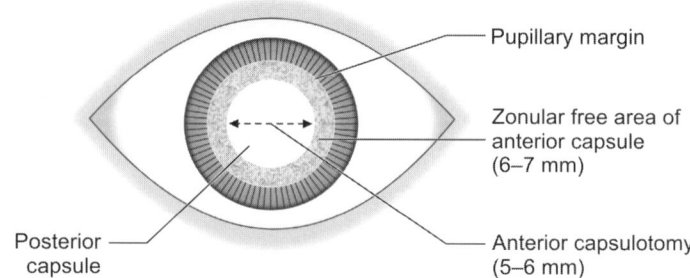

Fig. 7: Anterior capsulotomy.

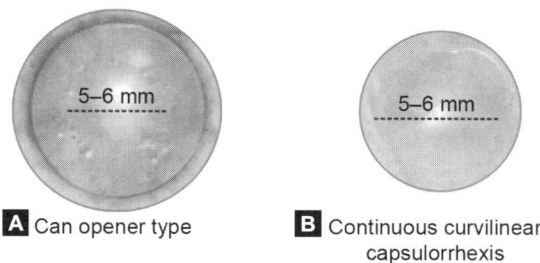

Figs. 8A and B: Anterior capsulotomy (diameter).

Anterior capsulotomy (Figs. 7, 8A and B): It is the surgical removal of 5–6 mm of anterior capsule during cataract surgery. Lens capsule is more elastic in the young than in adults, and so during capsulotomy in children it stretches more before tearing. It becomes firmer as age advances, so that a controlled capsulotomy is more effective between 40 to 60 years of age. In elderly persons, hypermature cataract, and hard nuclear cataract capsule become atrophic, fibrotic and calcified. The zonules are attached to the lens, mainly in the equator and adjacent areas of anterior and posterior surfaces of lens.

Normally, the zonular insertion on anterior and posterior capsule extend 1.5 mm and more anterior to equator and the zonular free areas are the central 6–7 mm of the capsule. So, ideally capsular opening (anterior capsulotomy) may be done safely in the *central zonular free area of 5–6 mm of anterior surface of lens. The size of ideal anterior capsulotomy is around 6 mm*, but 0.5–1 mm larger than the optical portion of iris. Very large or more peripheral capsulotomies can cut or strip zonular attachment leading to zonulodialysis. Generally, a larger capsulotomy is preferred in manual small incision cataract surgery (SICS) for easy nucleus manipulation.

Posterior capsulotomy (Figs. 9A and B): During cataract surgery in children below 8 years a primary posterior capsulotomy (with or without anterior vitrectomy) is usually done to avoid visual axis opacification (VAO). In children, the anterior capsule is highly elastic and it may not be easy to attain a capsulotomy of desired size. With the help of highly viscous ophthalmic viscoelastic devices, it is possible to perform a smaller-size capsulotomy. Once

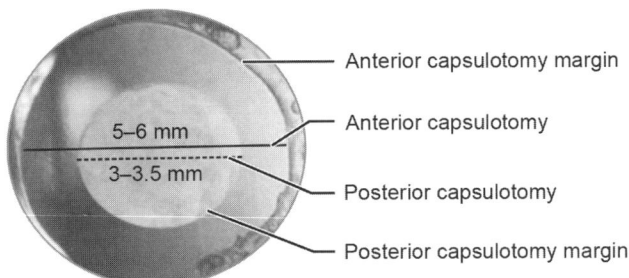

Figs. 9A and B: Anterior and posterior capsulotomy.

capsular flap is removed, it will attain a little larger size than the original due to its elasticity. The size of posterior capsulotomy should be sufficiently large to maintain a clear visual axis and also small enough to get a peripheral capsular support for IOL. So we have to aim a *central, circular, posterior capsulotomy of 1–1.5 mm smaller than the optic size of IOL. The preferred size of posterior capsulorrhexis is 3–3.5 mm.*

Lens Epithelium

Under the capsule, the lens has a monolayer of about 5,00,000 cuboid epithelial cells in an immature lens. *The lens epithelium is present only under the anterior capsule and extends up to the equator.* But epithelium is absent beyond that level over the posterior capsule, as this portion of epithelium occupies the center of lens due to its invagination during the development of lens. New lens fibers are formed from this epithelium from the pre-equatorial region of lens. These cells (germinative zone) produce new cells by mitosis and then differentiate loosing organelles and become transparent lens fibers. Epithelium secretes lens capsule and control the passage of electrolytes and nutrients to lens fibers. It plays an important role in the metabolism of lens and is very vulnerable to injuries.

Lens Cortex

This is a broad zone of lens fibers under the epithelium anteriorly (anterior cortex) and over lens capsule posteriorly (posterior cortex). *Anterior cortex is thicker than posterior cortex.*

Cortex has mainly two regions in adults, which can be dissected separately during surgery by hydroprocedures called hydrodissection and hydrodelineation, respectively.
- *Peripheral cortex* (Fig. 10): It is under the anterior capsule and over the posterior capsule. New lens fibers are added from epithelium to peripheral cortex during life. This subcapsular cortex in the young slowly gets converted into supranuclear cortex. During cataract surgery, by *hydrodissection*—we

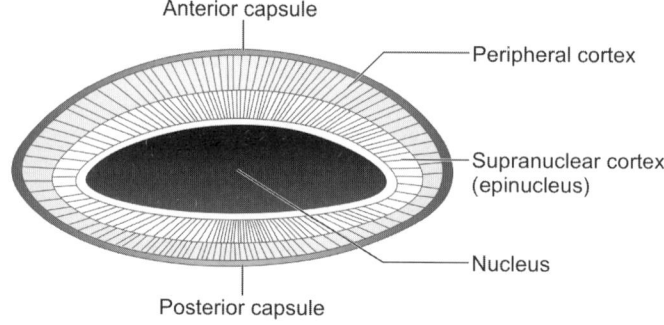

Fig. 10: Surgical anatomy of lens.

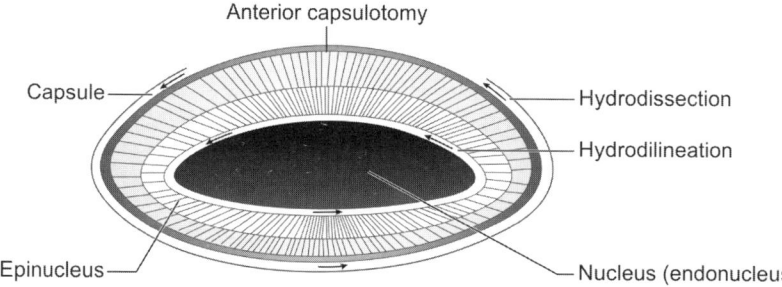

Fig. 11: Hydroprocedures.

can separate peripheral cortex from lens capsule. In this procedure we inject fluid (BSS) under lens capsule to separate the peripheral cortex from capsule. This steps helps in easy cortical aspiration and cortical clearance especially in surgical management of immature cataract.
- *Supranuclear cortex (epinucleus):* It is that portion of cortex inner to peripheral cortex adjoining nucleus and covering it. By the procedure of *hydrodilineation/delamination*—we can separate the supranuclear cortex (epinucleus) from nucleus. In this procedure we inject fluid (BSS) between epinucleus and (endo) nucleus. This can reduce the size of nucleus, which can be easily delivered through a small incision.

Hydroprocedures (Fig. 11) reduce the stress exerted on capsule, zonular apparatus, cortex and nucleus during cataract surgery. They can separate the cataractous lens into the capsule, cortex, epinucleus and nucleus and this separation facilitates nucleus rotation and its easy delivery. Again epinuclear plate protects posterior capsule as a cushion during nucleus manipulation in phacoemulsification.

Nucleus (Endonucleus)

Nucleus has mainly *three concentric layers* which present as different areas of light scattering during slit-lamp examination in the clear adult lens.

1. Embryonic nucleus—is the innermost (core) portion
2. Fetal nucleus—is the next portion
3. Adult nucleus—is the outermost portion and is under the epinucleus.

Surgically three portions are met in nucleus.
1. Softer peripheral shell
2. Densely sclerotic middle portion
3. Less sclerotic central core.

The size of nucleus and the size of lens itself are larger in nuclear cataract than cortical cataract. As the age advances the density of nucleus increases and the densest part is displaced to the deepest part of nucleus. So during phakoemulsification it is better to continue trenching up to its 90% thickness especially in nuclear cataract before cracking is attempted.

SUMMARY OF DIMENSIONS OF LENS

- *Diameter*
  - Normal diameter of lens : 9–10 mm

  Diameter is less in accommodation, microphakia and displaced lens.
- *Area*
  - Anterior surface : 83 mm^2
  - Posterior surface : 87 mm^2
- *Circumference* : 31.4 mm
- *Radius of curvature*
  - Anterior surface : 10 mm
  - Posterior surface : 6 mm

  In accommodation, mainly the anterior surface becomes more curved and approach 6 mm.

  Anterior and posterior surfaces are more curved in microspherophakia, lens displacements and lenticonus.
- *Volume*
  - Average : 140 µL
  - Between 20–40 year age : 163 µL
  - Between 80–90 years age : 240 µL
- *Weight*
  - At 25 years : 180 mg
  - At 90 years : 250 mg
- *Thickness*
  - Normal : 4.75–5 mm

  Thickness increases in accommodation
  - Intumescent lens : 7 mm
  - Hypermature cataract (Shrunken) : 3 mm
- *Refractive index*
  - Cortex : 1.38
  - Nucleus : 1.41
  - Overall : 1.42

- *Power*
  - Dioptric power : +16D to +20D
  - Accommodative power :
    - At birth : +15 to 16D
    - Age of 25 : +8D
    - Age of 50 : less than +2D

CHAPTER 10

Measurements of Zonules (of Zinn)

Lens is suspended from ciliary body and held in position by strands of fibers called zonules (suspensory ligament of lens). Through these structures ciliary muscles exert their functions on lens (Fig. 1).

Zonules are bundles of fibers. They pass start from ciliary body very near ora serrata and run in various directions crossing each other passing over pars plana, then through the grooves of pars pilcata and finally get attached to the lens capsule where they join zonular lamella.

DIMENSIONS AND EXTENT OF ZONULES

- Zonules *orginate from ciliary body from about 1.5 mm anterior to ora serrata.*
- **Insertion** *of zonules form a 2.25 mm band over equator of lens and extend further 1.5 mm band over anterior surface of lens and 1 mm on the posterior surface of lens.*

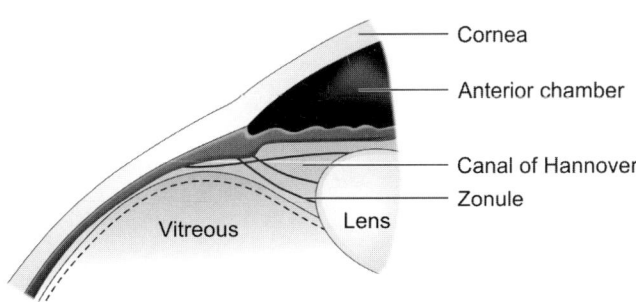

Fig. 1: Zonules.

- **Length** *of zonular fibrils vary from 2 to 7 mm.*
- Each zonular fiber is compose of fibrils. *Thickness of zonular fibril is around 10 nm.*
- **The resistance** of zonules to rupture is 100 gram in children and 60 gram in elderly. The point of least resistance is at the insertion of zonules to lens capsule.

PARTS OF ZONULES

Zonules have four portions from pars plana to lens capsule.
1. **Pars orbicularis** orginating from and lying under pars plana.
2. **Zonular plexus** portion passing between ciliary process.
3. **Zonular fork** where zonules bend over to ciliary valleys
4. **Anterior, equatorial and posterior limbs of zonules**—which gets attached to lens capsule.

ZONULAR BUNDLES (FIG. 2)

According to origin and the site of insertion on lens, they are grouped into:
- *Anterior zonular bundles:* Originate from pars plana as far back as ora serrata, run in close contact with ciliary body, then curve towards the equator of lens and get *attached to it, about 1.5 mm in front of equator.* They are stronger than posterior bundles.
- *Posterior zonular bundles:* Originate far forwards from the summits of ciliary body and sides of ciliary processes and pass backwards behind equator of lens, then *get attached on posterior surface lens, 1 mm behind equator.* Posterior bundles are more numerous and finer than anterior bundles. This zonular bundle runs between ciliary processes and no fibers originate from ciliary processes themselves.
  The space between anterior and posterior group of zonules is **the canal of Hannover.**
- *Equatorial zonular bundles* pass from pars plicata to the equator of lens.

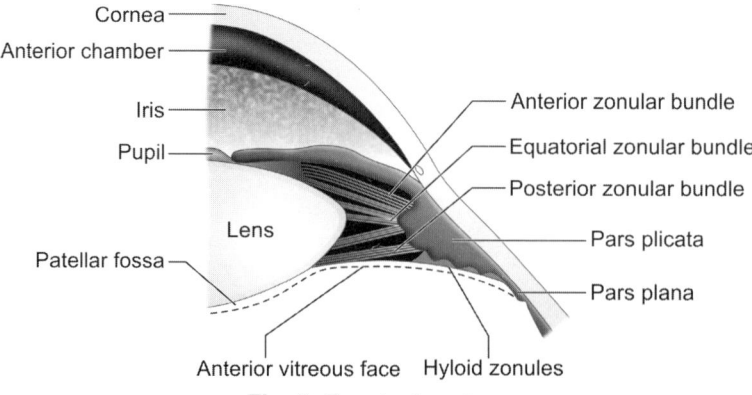

Fig. 2: Zonular bundles.

- *Hyaloid zonules* are very fine fibers extending from pars plana and get attached to the lens at the edge of patellar fossa and Weigers ligament.

As a whole the zonules form a ring around lens and in meridional section, it is triangular in shape. The base of triangle faces the equator of lens and apex is long curved and extends along the portions of ciliary body to ora serrata.

FUNCTIONS OF ZONULES

- Zonules take part in accommodation by transferring the action of ciliary muscle to lens.
- Hold lens in position.
- Lens zonules diaphragm divide eyeball into anterior and posterior segment which carry out different functions.
- Zonules divide the posterior chamber into prezonular, zonular and retrozonular portions.

SUMMARY OF DIMENSIONS AND EXTENT OF ZONULES

Length of zonular fibrils: *2–7 mm*
Thickness of zonular fibrils: *About 10 nm*
Resistance of zonular rupture is *100 g in children and 60 g in elderly.*
Attachment:
- **Anterior zonulr bundles** originate from the pars plana and get attached to anterior capsule of lens *about 1.5 mm and more in front of equator.*
- **Posterior zonular bundles** arise from pars plicata and get attached to posterior lens capsule *about 1 mm and more behind equator.*

CHAPTER 11

Measurements of Vitreous Humor

Most of the space of posterior segment of eyeball is occupied by a semisolid, transparent gel called vitreous which transmits and permits light rays to focus on retina and protects it. It is bordered anteriorly by lens, zonules and ciliary body and posteriorly by retina and optic nerve head. *Vitreous constitutes about posterior 4/5th of the volume (80%) of the eyeball. It is shaped almost like an anteroposteriorly compressed sphere.*

STRUCTURE OF VITREOUS (FIG. 1)

Vitreous is a gel consisting of *99% water and 1% solid. Solids are collagen*, hyaluronic acid and inorganic salts. Collagen forms a delicate meshwork which intertwines hyaluronic acid providing rigidity and viscosity to vitreous. *These fibrils have 60–25A° diameter and periodicity between 120A° and 300A°.*

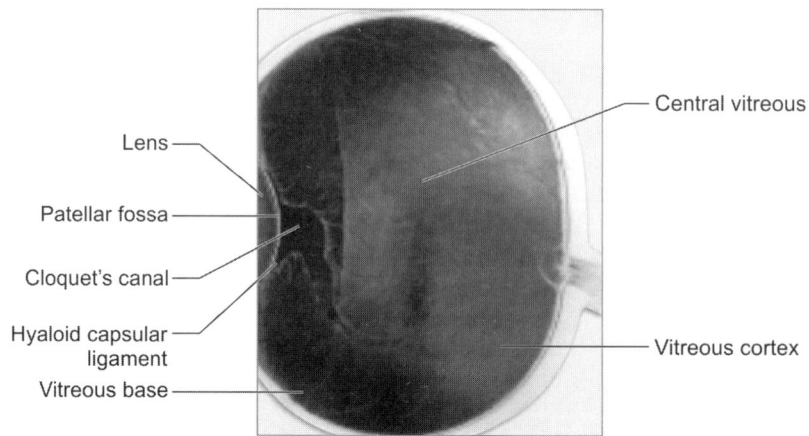

Fig. 1: Structure of vitreous.

Maximum concentration of hyaluronic acid is seen in the periphery of vitreous, particularly in its posterior cortical layers.

Basically vitreous has two portions which are slightly different structurally.
- Vitreous cortex
- Central or core vitreous.

Vitreous Cortex

Vitreous cortex is the *peripheral 0.2-0.3 mm broad dense* vitreous zone adjoining retina and covering entire vitreous body. The vitreous base divides vitreous cortex into anterior and posterior parts. The constituent collagen fibers in the cortical vitreous are more densely packed in a felt-like network. They are oriented almost parallel to the inner surface of retina. Microscopically the *fibers of vitreous cortex are 12 nm wide and insert* into the internal limiting membrane of retina. Mucopolysaccharides occupy the spaces between the fibers. Vitreous cortex also has cells—wandering leukocytes and hyalocytes embed in it. Hyalocytes are seen more in vitreous base. They produce hyaluronic acid and have phagocytic activity.

Anterior and posterior hyaloid membranes are fibrous condensations covering outer surface of vitreous cortex. *Anterior cortex* or *anterior hyaloid membrane* extend from vitreous base to posterior surface of lens. *Posterior hyaloid membrane* is 2-3 µ thick, glassy, made of thick collagen fibers and is nearer the retina firmly joining to margins of optic disk, fovea and retinal blood vessels. Contraction of these fibers can result in detachment of vitreous from internal limiting membrane of retina.

Central or Core Vitreous

In central vitreous, cells are few, fibers are thin, loosely bound to hyaluronic acid and do not attach to peripheral structures. Wide separation of collagen fibers provide more transparency to central vitreous (less dense optically).

PRIMARY, SECONDARY AND TERTIARY VITREOUS

Vitreous is formed during three periods of its development—as primary, secondary and tertiary vitreous:
- *Primary vitreous*: It is formed from neural ectoderm and the formation becomes complete when embryo is about 13 mm long. Later when secondary vitreous is formed, primary vitreous gets shifted and crowded to the center of vitreous cavity into a canal space—*Cloquet's canal* bordered by superior and inferior plicated membranes.
- *Secondary vitreous:* Develops from neural ectoderm when the embryo grows to 70 mm length in the 3rd month and fills two-thirds of optic cup. It contributes the major portion of adult vitreous growing around primary vitreous.
- *Tertiary vitreous:* It is formed during *3rd-6th month (70-190 mm stage)* from neuroectodermal layer of developing ciliary body. It elongates, groups into bundles and grows towards lens and get attached to it *as zonules*.

VITREOUS TOPOGRAPHY (FIG. 2)

Topographically vitreous has various features and relationships with adjacent structures.

Anterior Vitreous Face

On biomicroscopic examination, anterior vitreous face is seen as a definite layer of condensed vitreous extending from ora serrata to posterior capsule of lens up to Wieger's ligament. It is also called anterior hyaloid membrane and follows the contour of ciliary body, zonules and lens.

Behind the zonules, peripheral to Wieger's ligament there are *two potential spaces* in front of anterior surface of vitreous which may get opened in pathological conditions.

- *Petit's canal:* It is a potential space between zonules and posterior lens capsule in front and anterior vitreous face behind. In some diseased conditions this space will be occupied by blood, pigments or inflammatory cells.
- *Berger's space:* It is also called *Erggellet's space* is an expansion of anterior end of cloquet's canal. This space may be formed in anterior vitreous detachment associated with trauma (organized blood) and Marfan's syndrome.

Cloquet's Canal and Plicated Membranes

Cloquet's canal is a tubular structure in adult vitreous body representing fetal hyaloid artery and contains the vestiges of primary vitreous which get localized within the canal due to growth of secondary vitreous around it. It passes almost through the center of vitreous body from patellar fossa to optic disk. The contents of canal are more liquid than other parts of vitreous. Peripheral vitreous is more gelatinous. Anterior and posterior ends of this canal are wider and funnel-shaped.

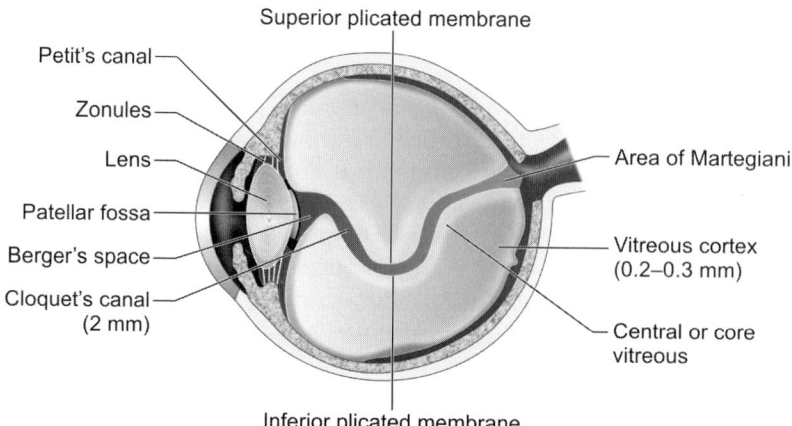

Fig. 2: Vitreous and its attachments.

Cloquet's canal is divided into three portions—an anterior postlenticular portion, middle portion and a posterior peripapillary portion. Anteriorly, it starts from the postlenticular space of Berger and ends in front of optic disk as a funnel-shaped space called *area of Martegiani*. *Cloquet's canal is about 2 mm wide,* larger in elderly due to vitreous liquefaction and posterior vitreous detachment. The size can vary according to eye movements, refraction and volume of primary and secondary vitreous. Infants cloquet's canal is almost straight. The canal of adult has a sinous course. The anterior expanded portion slightly sags below, runs posteriorly and nasally, rises a few mms above visual axis in the center of vitreous, becomes narrow, there again deviates temporally to macula and then bends nasally to join the margins of optic disk.

Superior and inferior plicated membranes are condensations of vitreous around, cloquet's canal and form boundaries of the canal. These membranes move according to the mobility of eye. The movements are rapid in conditions of vitreous liquefaction like old age, myopia and healed uveitis.

Though cloquet's canal appears optically empty under biomicroscopic examination, the retrolental portion can contain the remnants of hyaloid vessels and may appear as cork screw like structures attached to posterior pole of lens and dense opacities like Mittendorf's dots.

Posterior Vitreous Surface

As different from anterior vitreous face, posterior vitreous surface is larger. Adjacent posterior vitreous cortex is thickest peripherally and thinnest towards optic disk. There is no definite space between retina and posterior cortex. Sometimes a fibrous condensation can be seen under high magnification in this region due to vitreous shrinkage.

Boundaries and Attachments (Fig. 3)

- **Anteriorly** vitreous is closely related to the following structures.
  - *Lens:* It is the most important structure to which it is related and attached anteriorly and centrally. Vitreous has a concavity on its anterior surface (*patellar fossa*) in which lens is placed. There is a capillary space between them (*Bergers space*). Thus, lens is attached firmly to the anterior face of vitreous only along the margins of patellar fossa by the *hyaloideocapsular ligament of Wieger*. The attachment of this ligament gives a circular or semicircular white outline visible mainly on the temporal half to the posterior (capsule) surface of lens called *Egger's line* (Fig. 4). It is about *8 mm in diameter*. This ligament is strong in the young, becomes weak as the age advances and is weakest in elderly around age of 60. The hyaloid group of zonules gets attached to this ligament.
  - **Ciliary processes and zonules**—form the immediate anterior boundary of vitreous on either side of lens.

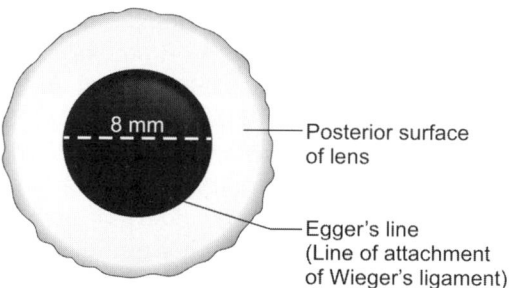

Fig. 3: Posterior surface of lens.

- **Anteroperipherally:**
  - **Vitreous base:** Vitreous base is the junction between vitreous and the surrounding structures. Here it has its strongest attachment at the posterior part of pars plana and immediate portion of ora serrata. *The vitreous base is a ring of 2–4 mm wide condensed vitreous straddling about a 2 mm of posterior part of pars plana and adjacent 2–4 mm of ora serrata.* Vitreous fibers from base, run in a fan like fashion towards posterior and central vitreous and may condense to form a fibrous layer. In infants, vitreous base lie just posterior to ora. As age advances it broadens anteriorly and posteriorly. Vitreous base forms a dividing line between anterior and posterior vitreous cortex. It is very difficult to disinsert the fibers during surgery from the structures to which it is attached. The attachment is so firm that attempt to separate vitreous base can only result in tearing of corresponding attached portion of ciliary body and peripheral retina. Anterior border of vitreous base is smooth but posterior border has tongue-like extensions into peripheral retina in some areas. Vitreous collapse can produce a horse-shoe tear in these areas.
- **Blood vessels of retina:** Posterior to vitreous base, vitreous is in close relationship with retina proper but separated from it by internal limiting membrane by a potential space called subhyaloid space. Vitreous has a stronger attachment along the blood vessels of retina.
- **Posteriorly** the vitreous has attachment to:
  - **Macula:** Vitreous has a definite attachment of *about 2–3 mm diameter around fovea*. This attachment is strong in young and tenuous in older persons.
  - **Optic disk:** Vitreous is attached to the margins of optic disk (not the surface) posteriorly. This attachment is sometimes called *posterior vitreous base*. In posterior vitreous detachment, this appears as a glial tissue ring around optic disk on the posterior surface of detached vitreous.

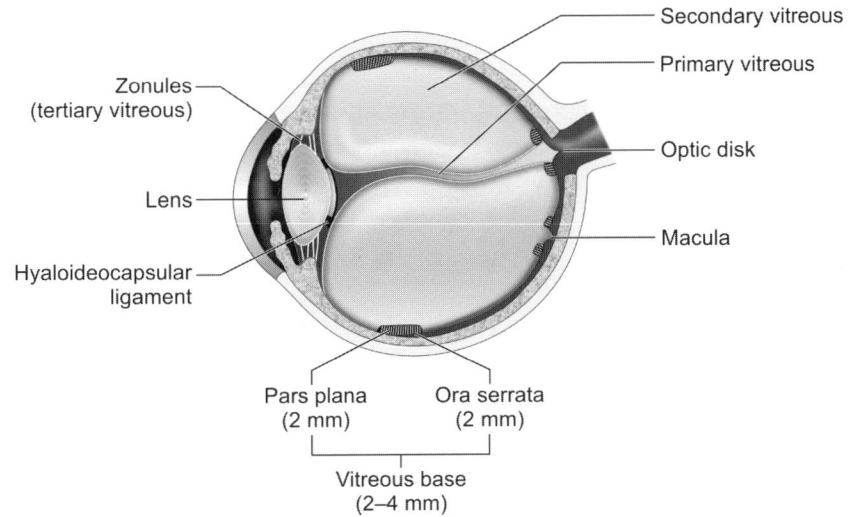

Fig. 4: Vitreous and its attachments.

Transparency of Vitreous Humor

Vitreous is transparent due to:
- High water content (99%), allowing maximum transmission of light. It transmits 90% of light rays between 300 nm and 1400 nm.
- Solid component is very low (1%). They are randomly distributed and are smaller than the wavelength of visible light and so minimal scattering of light.
- Light absorption is negligible since the gel is colorless.
- The formed elements of blood are not allowed to enter into the vitreous cavity by the blood ocular barrier.

Functions of Vitreous

- Vitreous forms part of the transparent media of eye and permit the light to focus ultimately on retina.
- Vitreous protects the retina, optic nerve and lens system from shake (shock absorber) due to its elasticity.
- Vitreous contributes to the structural integrity of the globe.
- During development it helps in the growth of the eye.
- Vitreous forms a medium through which nutrients diffuse between ciliary body, lens and retina.
- In many situations vitreous act as a barrier between anterior and posterior segments of eyeball with different functions.

Summary of Vitreous Parameters

- *Volume:* The normal volume of vitreous humor in adult is slightly less than 3.9 mL.

- *Weight:* Weight of vitreous humor is about 3.9 g. It accounts for 2/3rd to 3/5th of the weight and volume of eyeball.
- *Specific gravity:* 1.0053
- *Oncotic pressure:* Zero (25 mm of Hg in plasma)
- *Refractive index:* 1.3349 (almost same as aqueous)
- *Viscosity:* Two or four times of water
- *pH:* pH of vitreous is between 7 and 7.5.

Dimensions of Vitreous

- Hyaloideocapsular ligament (Wieger) : *8 mm in diameter*
- Vitreous cortex : *0.2–0.3 mm broad and dense area*
- Vitreous base : *2–4 mm wide (pars plana 2 mm and ora sarrata 2–4 mm)*
- Cloquet's canal : *2 mm wide*
- Collagen fibers : *3–5 nm thick*
- Posterior hyaloid membrane : *2–3 nm thick*

VITRECTOMY MEASUREMENTS

Vitrectomy is the surgical removal of vitreous (as a therapeutic and diagnostic technique) for restoration of vision in a variety of vitreoretinal disorders like:
- Nonresolving vitreous hemorrhage and vitreous opacities (vitreous membranes, debris, floaters, asteroid hyalosis).
- Traction retinal detachments associated with proliferative diabetic retinopathy, vasculitis, retinal vein occlusion, relinopathy of prematurity (ROP), sickle cell retinopathy, etc.
- Primary retinal detachment with giant retinal tear, posterior breaks, recurrent detachments, etc.
- Posteriorly dislocated lens, IOL, nucleus, cortex, capsular tension ring.
- Vitreous prolapse or loss during cataract surgery, penetrating injuries, etc.
- Corneal decompensation due to vitreous incarceration in wound
- Macular pucker
- Macular hole surgery
- Epiretinal membrane surgery
- Endophthalmitis
- Removal of intraocular foreign body
- Intraocular cysticercosis
- Diagnostic vitrectomy in endophthalmitis, intraocular tumors (lymphoma, reticulum cell sarcoma).

Important Anatomical Measurements for Vitrectomy

A surgeon performing vitrectomy should be well aware of the location and measurements of internal structures like ciliary body, ora serrata, retina proper, vitreous base, etc. in relation to the external landmarks like limbus, extraocular muscles, vortex veins, etc. (Fig. 5).

- *Pars plicata of ciliary body extends to a level of 2.5 mm behind limbus.*
- *Pars plana of ciliary body extends about 3.5 mm behind from the level of pars plicata on nasal side and 5 mm on temporal side (even more in myopia).*
- *Approximate distance of limbus to ora serrata is 5 mm on nasal side and 7 mm on temporal side.*
- *Retci muscle insertions are about 6–8 mm away from the limbus. Insertion distance of medial rectus is 5.5 mm behind limbus (nearer to limbus) and that of superior rectus is about 7.7 mm (farthest from the limbus).*
- *Thus, approximately the anterior insertion points of recti muscles almost coincide the junction of pars plana and ora serrata (Fig. 6).*
- *There are about 7 vortex veins in each eye and most of them exit sclera about 10–14 mm behind ora serrata and 14–18 mm posterior to limbus.*
- *Distance of limbus to equator is about 9–12 mm.*
- *Posterior pole of the eye is about 29–32 mm away from the limbus.*

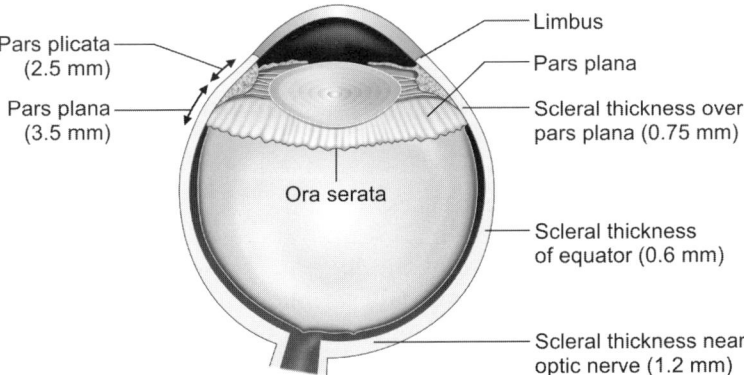

Fig. 5: Distance of pars plicata and pars plana from limbus and measurements reverent to vitrectomy.

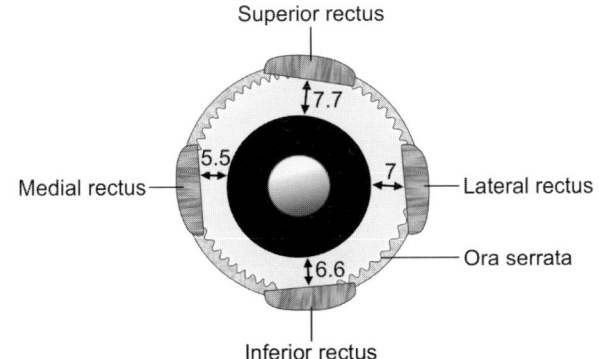

Fig. 6: Relationship between extraocular muscle insertion and their distance from ora serrata.

- *Short ciliary arteries and nerves enter sclera at a distance of 1-2 mm close to optic nerve.*
- *Average thickness of sclera is 1 mm near the limbus. The thickness is 0.75 mm over pars plana, 0.3 mm under extraocular muscle insertion, 0.6 mm at the equator and 1.2 mm near the optic disk.*

Types of Vitrectomies

Basically, there are three types of victrectomies according to the site of surgical approach to vitreous and the techniques:
1. Limbal (anterior) or open sky vitrectomy
2. Pars plana (closed) vitrectomy
3. Pars plicata vitrectomy

Limbal (Anterior) or Open Sky Vitrectomy (Fig. 7)

In 1962, Kasner performed the first (open sky) vitrectomy using cellulose sponge and scissors (by courageously entering the area which was considered forbidden at that time), as a therapeutic measure without damaging the integrity of globe.

This procedure is easy, but not safe, and is associated with many complications.
- Damage to iris and cornea
- Do not allow retropupillary access
- Limited visibility of vitreous
- Limited accessibility to vitreous cavity
- Risk of damaging vitreous base and peripheral retina.

So, open sky vitrectomy is attempted only on rare occasions by anterior segment surgeons through a limbal route of entry or already existing corneal or limbal wound, as a part of emergency management of:
- Vitreous loss during intraocular surgeries like cataract surgery to remove vitreous from incision wound, anterior chamber (AC), etc.
- Penetrating injuries with vitreous prolapse or incarceration to the wound.

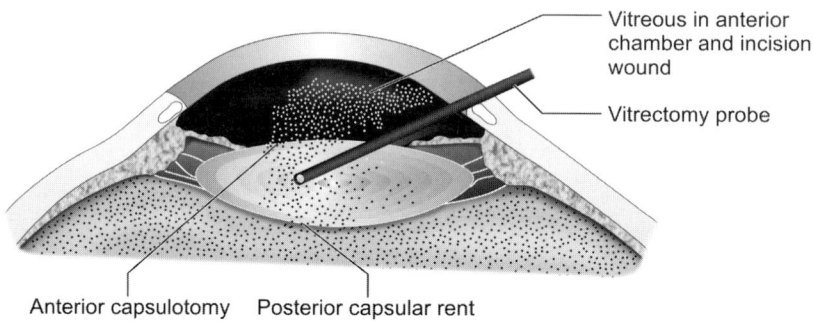

Fig. 7: Limbal (anterior) or open sky vitrectomy.

Pars Plana (Closed) Vitrectomy (Fig. 8)

This is the most ideal and perfect vitrectomy technique and was first attempted and popularized by Robert Machemer and his colleagues in 1970. The technique is commonly carried out by posterior segment surgeons, and allow retropupillary access to vitreous. In this method vitreous cavity is approached through a pars plana sclerotomy or self-sealing scleral tunnel incision placed at:
- *Average distance of 3.5 mm behind limbus in any eye as measured by a caliper.*

  Incision made anterior than 2.5 mm from limbus is likely to injure pars plicata resulting in intraocular bleeding. Incision done farther than 5 mm from limbus is likely to injure retina.
- About 4 mm behind limbus in phakic to avoid trauma to lens and retina.
- Almost 3 mm behind limbus in pseudophakic or aphakic eyes.
- About 2–3 mm behind limbus in children below 7 years as pars plana is narrow and not well developed in children.

  Pars plana approach has many advantages over open sky technique.
- Pars plana approach provides a closed and controlled system for vitreous removal avoiding collapse of eye and least trauma to neigbhoring structures.
- This technique facilitates the introduction of many more vitrectomy related functions into the vitreous cavity thereby improving the surgical quality and visual result.
    - *Continuous infusion (using cannulas of 23 or 25 or 27 gauge), cutting (ocutome with 23 or 25 or 27 gauge) and aspiration.*
    - Excellent visibility as the procedure is carried out under magnification provided by operating microscope with coaxial illumination and X (nasal to temporal) movement and Y (superior inferior) movement in relation to patient's eye.
    - Visibility further enhanced by wide angle visualizing systems or contact (Volk Rolls) and non-contact (BIOM, PWOR) which produces excellent panoramic view of retinal periphery even through hazy media and small pupil.
    - Illumination augmented by fiber optic lighting system which provides endoillumination.
    - Miniature vitreoretinal scissors to cut vitreous bands.

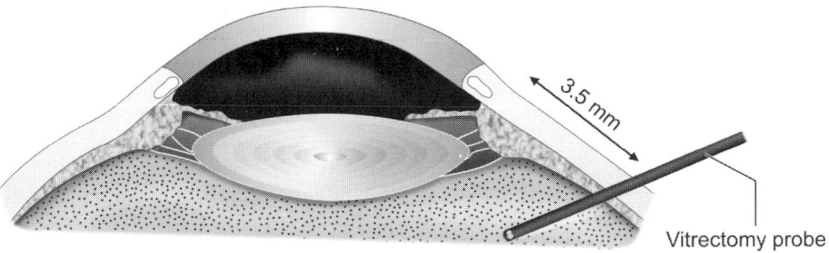

Fig. 8: Pars plana vitrectomy.

- Vitreous pick and forceps to remove epiretinal membrane by gentle peeling
- Ultrasonic fragmenter to remove dislocated lens and nuclear fragments.
- Endodiathermy to coagulate bleeding intraocular vessels
- Cryotherapy
- Endophotocoagulation with fibroptic probe delivering diode laser
- Facility for internal tamponade of retinal breaks using silicon oil, sulfahexaflouride/air mixture
- Intravitreal foreign body forceps and intravitreal magnet for removal of intraocular foreign bodies.

Measurements and Architecture of Pars plana Vitrectomy Incisions

In general three self-sealing sclerotomies or scleral tunnel incisions are made for vitrectomy, about 3.5 mm behind limbus which enter vitreous cavity through pars plana. They are (Figs. 9, 10A and B):
- For introduction of cannula for infusion.
- For introduction of instrument for suction and cutting of vitreous (ocutome)
- For introduction of fibroptic light source for endoillumination.

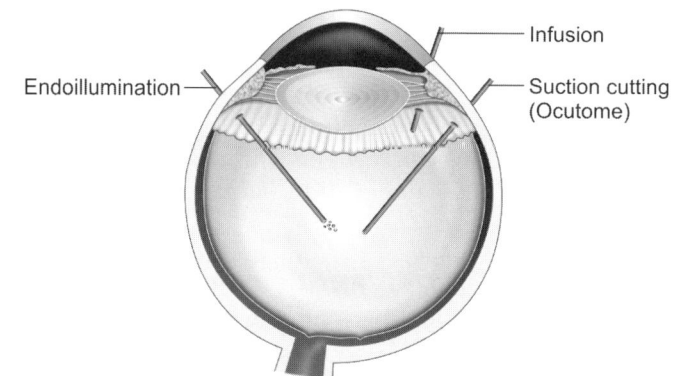

Fig. 9: Parts for pars plana vitrectomy.

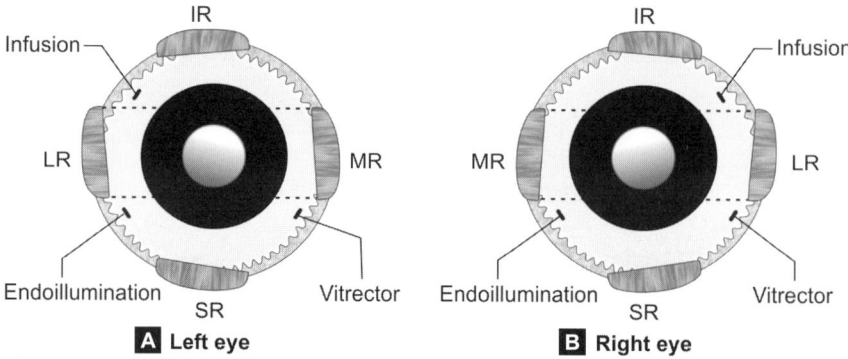

Figs. 10A and B: Relative positions of vitrectomy probes in right and left eye. (LR: lateral rectus; IR: inferior rectus; MR: medial rectus; SR: superior rectus)

Size of the incision: It depends on the gauge of the probes 20, 23, 25 or 27 and is made using MVR blade or Torchar. *Usual size if incision for introduction of 20-23 gauge probe is between 2.5-1 mm.*

Recent microincisional vitrectomy surgeries or minimally invasive vitreous surgeries (MIVS) are performed through 0.5 mm incisions which avoids the need of scleral or conjunctival sutures.

Incisions can be stab incisions or tunnel incisions.

- *Stab incisions*—are weak and associated with postoperative hypotony and endophthalmitis. Their intrascleral length is only 0.5 mm (Fig. 11).
- *Tunnel incisions*—have an entry incision and intrascleral path (Figs. 12A and B).

They have advantages of appositional collapse and water-tight closure and are preferred in MIVS.

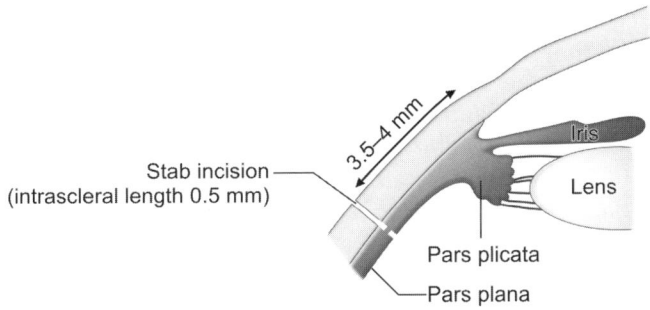

Fig. 11: Stab incision.

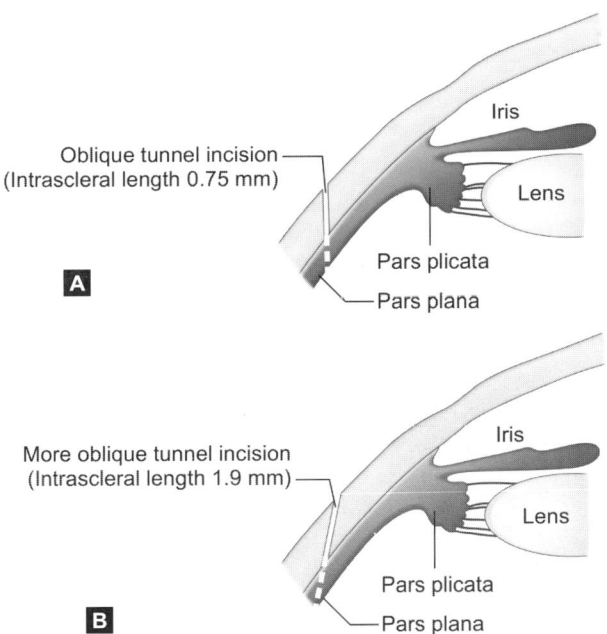

Figs. 12A and B: (A) Oblique tunnel incision; (B) More oblique tunnel incision.

An oblique tunnel incision makes an angle between external and internal surface of sclera. When the tunnel becomes more oblique, tunnel length increases. The intrascleral length of tunnel incision is 0.75–1.93 mm. Such tunnels are more water/air proof.

Radial tunnel incision has an entry incision parallel to limbus and intrascleral tunnel running anterioposterior.

In circumferential tunnels, entry incision is perpendicular to limbus and intrascleral tunnel parallel to it (Fig. 13).

Radial tunnels can injure ora serrata and lens. So generally circumferential tunnels are preferred.

Pars Plicata Vitrectomy (PPAV) (Fig. 14)

This rare vitrectomy technique is carried out by approaching vitreous through pars plicata. The procedure is not a safe one as it can injure the major vascular arcade leading to intraocular bleeding and also can cause injury to lens. A forcible entry can sometimes produce iridodialysis. Even then this technique is very rarely selected by anterior segment surgeons in following situations:
- During phacoemulsification complicated by inadvertent posterior capsular rupture (PCR) resulting in retained cortical lens matter and vitreous in torn capsular bag. The procedure is performed to remove vitreous from anterior chamber, posterior chamber and capsular bag and prevent further vitreous prolapse and its ineration in the wound and to facilitate IOL implantation.

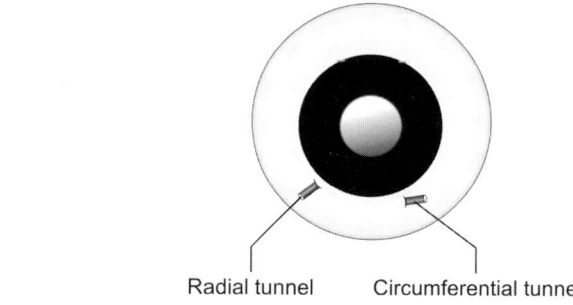

Fig. 13: Radial and circumferential tunnels for minimally invasive vitreous surgery.

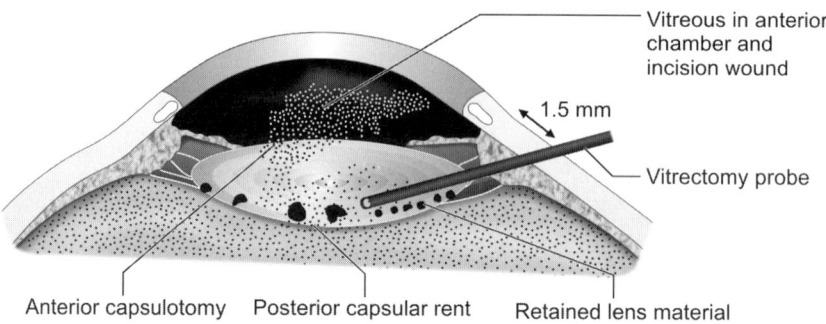

Fig. 14: Pars plicata vitrectomy.

- Anterior vitrectomy through this route is also tried during intrascleral fixation of IOL.
- A pars plicata approach is also selected in children with ROP as pars plana is not be well developed at this age.

Use of the pre-existing corneal wound for pars plicata vitrectomy is not safe as it may not be large enough for introduction of vitrectomy probe. So another sclerotomy is done after closure of primary incision for cataract surgery and filling AC with viscosurgical device.

The incision for pars plicata vitrectomy is usually done 1.5 mm behind limbus using 20 guage MVR blade, tip being directed obliquely down towards the mid vitreous cavity. But site of sclerotomy can be slightly varied according to the site of primary incision for cataract surgery and extend of posterior capsular rent.

CHAPTER 12

Measurements of Retina

Retina is the only tissue in the body which can perceive light and forms the innermost layer of ocular wall. As the word meaning of retina says (Rete = net) it is almost a network like arrangement of cells in 10 layers mainly consisting of retinal pigment epithelium, photoreceptors, two order of neurons, their connections and limiting membranes arranged in order, from out, in wards between choroid and vitreous. They are (Fig. 1):
- Retinal pigment epithelium.
- Photoreceptors layer carrying the cell bodies of receptors of light—rods and cones.

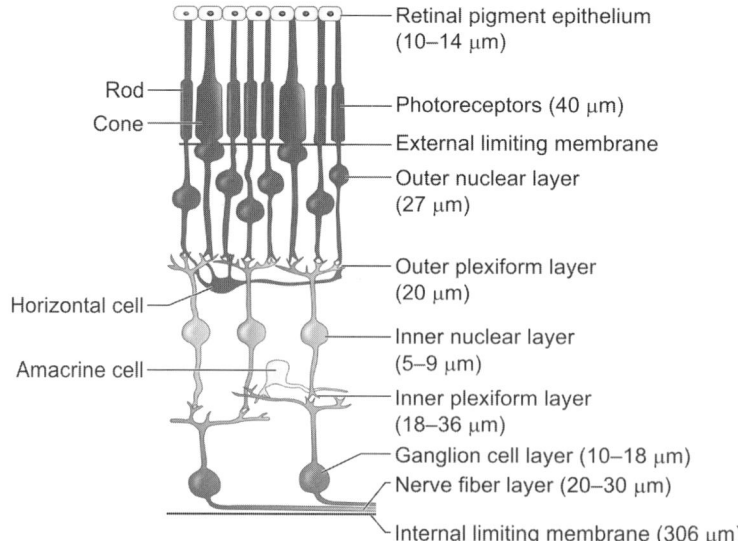

Fig. 1: Layer-by-layer structure and thickness of retina.

- External limiting membrane
- Outer nuclear layer—made of nuclei of rods and cones
- Outer plexiform layer constituted by the synaptic connections between rods and cones and the first order of neurons, bipolar cells
- Inner nuclear layer—the cell bodies of bipolar cells
- Inner plexiform layer formed by the synaptic connections of bipolar cells and the second order of neurons, the ganglion cells
- Layer of ganglion cells, comprising the cell bodies of ganglion cells
- Nerve fiber layer, made of the axons of ganglion cells
- Internal limiting membrane, the membrane lining the inner surface of nerve fiber layer, separating it from vitreous.

GENERAL STRUCTURE (ARCHITECTURE) OF RETINA

Most regions of retina have the above basic ten-layered structure (Fig. 2).

Retinal Pigment Epithelium

Retinal pigment epithelium (RPE) is the outermost layer of retina. It is a continuous sheet of approximately **5 million hexagonal cells** extending from optic disk to ora serrata. Each cell has four sides and is about 12–18 µ wide and 10–14µ thick. RPE is firmly attached to Bruch's membrane on one side (outside) and cell bodies of photoreceptors on the other side (inner side). The inner apical surface of RPE cells have microvilli that surround the outer segment of rods and cones. Their apex have *melanin pigment granules of size 2–3 nm*. Nucleus is situated in the base of the cell.

Functions of Retinal Pigment Epithelium

- RPE forms part of blood retinal barrier and selectively transport nutrients from blood of choriocapillaris to photoreceptors.
- It helps in the storage of vitamin A and its conversion to a form that can be utilized for synthesis of photopigment (recycling of vitamin A).
- Cells of RPE are involved in phagocytosis and degradation of lamellar disks of photoreceptors.
- It absorbs scattered light.

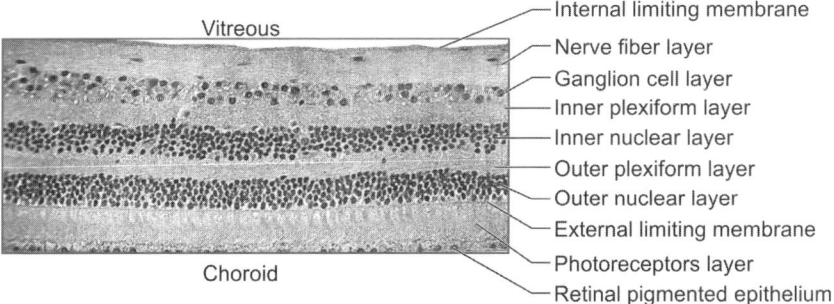

Fig. 2: Histological structure of retina.

- RPE help in the adhesion between it and neurosensory retina. They remain attached because of the biological adhesive—acid mucopolysaccharide between them. RPE cell sheath hold retina mechanically.

Photoreceptor Layer

This layer consists of outer segments of rods and cones and villi of RPE surrounded by mucoprotein extracellular substance. *The photoreceptor layer has a mean thickness of 40 μm. There are about 125 million photoreceptors in the eye. Number of rods are approximately 92 million and cones are about 6 million. The outer and inner segments of rods are 40-60 μm long. Cones in the retinal periphery are 40 μm long and those in the fovea are 80 μm long.* But rods and cones vary in their density in different individuals and in different zones of retina of the same eye.

Cone population varies between *1,00,000 to 3,24,000/mm² in different zones of retina. Fovea has the maximum cone density of about 1,99,000/mm².* Cone population is 40-45% more on nasal retina than temporal retina. Again density of cones is more in inferior than superior retina.

Rod population is more dense in a broad horizontally oval area of retina which has the same eccentricity as the center of optic disk and extending towards nasal and superior retina. *Nasal retina has more (20-25%) rods than temporal retina. Inferior retina has 2% less rods than superior retina. In an area 0.5 mm nasal and temporal, and 0.4 mm superior and inferior to the center of fovea there is an one rod one cone arrangement. The rods are completely absent in an average horizontal diameter of 0.35 mm area at fovea (rod-free zone).*

The visual pigment is a combination of a supportive protein portion, opsin and a reactive chromatophore, nonprotein portion cis retinal derived from vitamin A which preferentially absorbs light. *Rhodopsin is the visual pigment of rods and is maximum sensitive to light of wavelength of 493 nm.* Rods are concerned with scotopic vision. Pigments of cones are not fully understood and supposed to contain one of the three different iodopsin pigments which preferentially absorb light peak of wavelength at *440 nm (blue), 540 nm (green) and 577 nm (red).* Cones are concerned with photopic vision, form sense, stereopsis and color vision.

Photoreceptors convert light energy of wavelength of between 397 and 723 nm into chemical energy and then to electrical impulses which are propagated through neurons of retina and visual pathway to occipital cortex.

External Limiting Membrane

External limiting membrane is formed by the junctional complexes that unite photorreceptor inner segments and Muller's cells. This membrane appears to separate photoreceptor layer from outer nuclear layer. It is not a complete or true membrane.

External limiting membrane not only acts as a selective barrier for nutrients but also stabilizes the outer segments of photoreceptors.

Outer Nuclear Layer

Outer nuclear layer is about 22-50 μm thick and made of nuclei or cell bodies of photoreceptors. Rod nuclei are oval and is *5.5 nm wide*. Nuclei of cones are *5-7 μm wide*, oval and situated *3-4 μm inner* to external limiting membrane. The width of this layer varies in different areas of retina according to the number of rods and cones nuclei. Near the nasal edge of optic disk there are 8-9 rows of nuclei and is *about 45 μm thick*. Temporal to optic disk outer nuclear layer has only four layers of nuclei and so the thickness is only 22 μm. *The thickness increases to 50 μm in foveal region as there are 10 rows of cone nuclei in this region.*

Outer Plexiform Layer

This layer is constituted by the axons of photoreceptors and their synaptic junction between bipolar cells and Muller's cells. Its outer 2/3rd is made of inner fibers of photoreceptors and processes of Muller's cells and the inner 1/3rd is formed by the dendrites of bipolar cells, horizontal cells and Muller's cell processes. *The average thickness of this layer is about 20 μm and becomes thickest at macular region (51 μm).* In this region the constituent fibers are oblique as they are formed by the deviated fibers of fovea (Henle's fiber layer). The fibers of outer plexiform layer are arranged loosely to form a delicate network. In diseased conditions large amount of edema fluid, exudates and blood can collect easily in this potential space.

Inner Nuclear Layer

The nuclei of bipolar cells, horizontal cells, amacrine cells and Muller's cells contribute this layer. It is thinner than outer nuclear layer. The retina has about 35,67600 bipolar cells. *Their cell bodies are about 9 μm diameter at fovea and 5 μm at retinal periphery.*

- *Bipolar cells* function as the first order of neurons of visual pathway. They relay the information from photoreceptors to ganglion cells radially in retina.
- *Horizontal cells*—form a network of fibers, which modulate and integrate the information received from photoreceptors horizontally.
- *Muller's cells*—are the largest cells of retina and extend between external and internal limiting membranes. Muller's cells are seen in highest concentration in foveal region and decrease in number towards periphery. The mean cell density is around *8000-13000 cells/ mm^2*. Muller's cell play an important role in the metabolism of retinal tissue. They have a role as K^+ electrode and contribute to the b-wave of electroretinogram.
- *Amacrine cells*—are flask-shaped cells situated in the inner nuclear layer and have the size of *12 μm*. They are absent in fovea. They produce neurotransmitter.

Inner Plexiform Layer

Inner plexiform layer is constituted by the synaptic connections between bipolar cells and ganglion cells. This layer also contains the process of Muller's cells and amacrine cells. The inner plexiform layer is about 18–36 μm thick and has an average 2 million synapses per mm^2 area. This layer is absent in the fovea.

Ganglion Cell Layer

There are about 1.2 million ganglion cells in eye, separated from each other by process of Muller's cells and neuroglia. Each ganglion cell is a large round or *oval cell of 10–30 μm size* and has a single long axon. The axons from all the ganglion cells converge at the optic disk and go out of eyeball through scleral canal and as optic nerve and reach up to lateral geniculate body. Most of the regions of retina have only one layer of ganglion cells. But from the temporal edge of optic disk it becomes two layered. *The number of layers of ganglion cell layer then increases towards the macular region and becomes maximum at the edge of fovea (6–8 layers). But at fovea and optic disk ganglion cells are absent.*

There is 1 to 1 relationship between photoreceptors and ganglion cells in the fovea leading to quick transmission of impulses. In retinal periphery many receptors have correspondence to one ganglion cell leading to progressive loss of resolution.

The thickness of ganglion cell layer varies from 10–20 μm at nasal retina to even 60–80 μm in the macular region. The density of ganglion cells is maximum in the macular region (32–380000 cells/mm^2) especially in a 04 2.00 mm horizontal oval area from edge of foveola. In the peripheral retina density is more in nasal quadrant than temporal and superior quadrant than inferior.

Nerve Fiber Layer

Nerve fiber layer (NFL) is made of the axons of ganglion cells delineated by Muller's cells and other glial cells. *Each fiber is about 0.6–2.00 μm in diameter.*

Most of the nerve fibers run a radial and parallel course to enter the edge of optic disk. The fibers arising from region immediately temporal to optic disk (fovea) enter directly to the temporal edge of optic and are called the papillomacular bundle. It is thinnest portion of nerve fiber layer. In the nasal edge of the optic, the nerve fibers are more crowded and is the first portion of the optic disk to be affected in papilledema and the temporal edge last. The nerve fibers arising from ganglion cells temporal to fovea take an arcuate course, over papillomacular bundle and enter the superior and inferior edge of optic disk. These superior and inferior fibers are separated at their origin by a horizontal raphae. This raphe extends from fovea to extreme periphery of retina. The nerve fibers are nonmyelinated up to lamina cribrosa. Thickness of NFL varies according to the area, age and disease. It is thicker above the superior and inferior poles of optic disk (polar areas), than temporal and nasal sectors. *The average thickness of nerve fiber layer varies between 0.16 mm to*

0.23 mm. Thickness of nerve fiber layer is about 20–30 μm at the nasal edge of optic disk (thickest).

Internal Limiting Membrane

Internal limiting membrane (ILM) is mainly made of the basal lamina of Muller's cells. It is attached and merges to cortical vitreous. Its thickness varies in different zones. It is thin *(51 nm) in the region of vitreous base.* It then progressively *becomes thick, 306 nm at equator and 1887 nm posteriorly.* But it gets attenuated, or is absent at the fovea, optic disk and over major blood vessels.

The long axons of ganglion cells collect in the posterior part of retina to form the optic nerve (axons of second order of neuron) and go out of eyeball as optic nerve which then passes through orbit and enters the cranial cavity through the optic canal to optic chiasma. The fibers from the nasal half of retina cross over to opposite side in the chiasma and pass to the optic tract of opposite side and then to lateral geniculate body of that side. The fibers from the temporal half of the retina entering the optic chiasma do not cross and pass into optic tract of same side and then to the lateral geniculate body of the same side. The the second order of neurons end at the lateral geniculate body. Third order of neurons arises from lateral geniculate bodies and reaches the occipital cortex through optic radiations.

In the retina, an inverted image of the object is formed in each eye. After stimulation of retina by light the visual impulses pass through visual pathways and reach the *occipital cortex by about 124 milliseconds* where the inverted image formed in the retina of each eye which are everted and the two images are fused into one and we enjoy all the qualities of binocular single vision.

SUMMARY OF MEASUREMENT OF RETINAL LAYERS

(Layer-by-layer measurements of retina)
- **Retinal pigment epithelium**
  Thickness : 10–14 μm and has about 5 million cells
- **Photoreceptor layer**
  Thickness is about 40 μm and has about a total of 92 million rods and 5 million cones
  - Length of rods : 40–60 μm
  - Length of cones : 40–80 μm
- **Outer nuclear layer**
  - Average thickness : 27 μm
  - Near nasal edge of optic disk : 45 μm
  - Near temporal edge of optic disk : 27 μm
- **Outer plexiform layer**
  - Average thickness : 20 μm
  - Macular region : 51 μm
- **Inner nuclear layer**
  - Thickness fovea : 9 μm
  - Periphery : 5 μm

- **Inner plexiform layer** : 18–36 μm thick
- **Ganglion cell layer**
  - Nasal retina : 10–20 μm thick
  - Macular region : 80 μm thick
- **Nerve fiber layer**
  - Average thickness : 20–30 μm
- **Internal limiting membrane**
  - Vitreous base region : 51 nm thick
  - Equator : 306 nm thick
  - Posteriorly : 1887 nm thick

GROSS MEASUREMENTS AND GENERAL FEATURES OF RETINA

Shape and Extent of Retina (Fig. 3)

In the living eye, the retina is a transparent neural membrane having a *surface area of* 266 mm². It is not exactly circular in outline as seen with ophthalmoscope but retina extends more anteriorly on the nasal side than temporal side. This may be one of the reasons for the wider field of vision (90) outwards. Also inferior part of retina extends slightly more anterior than superior. Again, *retina is not a flat structure but shaped like a cup or a globe open anteriorly. It has a diameter of 24 mm at equator and 20 mm at the level of ora serrata*. It extends posteriorly from optic disk to ora serrata anteriorly ending in tooth like margins (dentate process) with bays in between (oral bays) which are prominent nasally but progressively straightening temporally. These oral bays are actually extensions of pars plana into the retinal periphery.

Thickness (Fig. 4)

Thickness of retina varies in different zones. Retinal thickness is about *0.56 mm near optic disk*. Retina is thinnest at fovea and is only *0.25 mm thick*. It becomes *thin at the equator (0.8 mm)*. At the *ora serrata it is only 0.1 mm thick*. Thin areas of retina are more prone to degenerations and breaks.

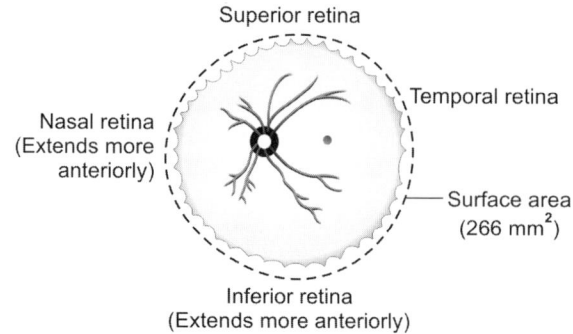

Fig. 3: Surface area and extent of retina.

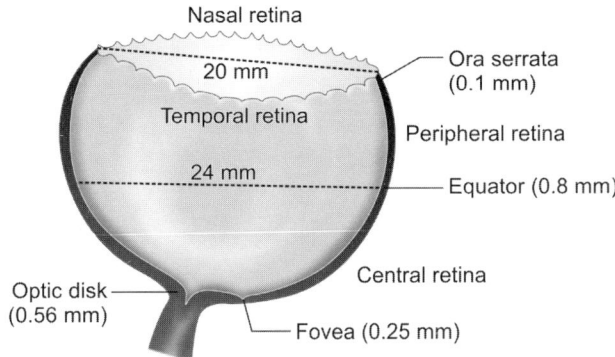

Fig. 4: Dimensions, shape and thickness of retina.

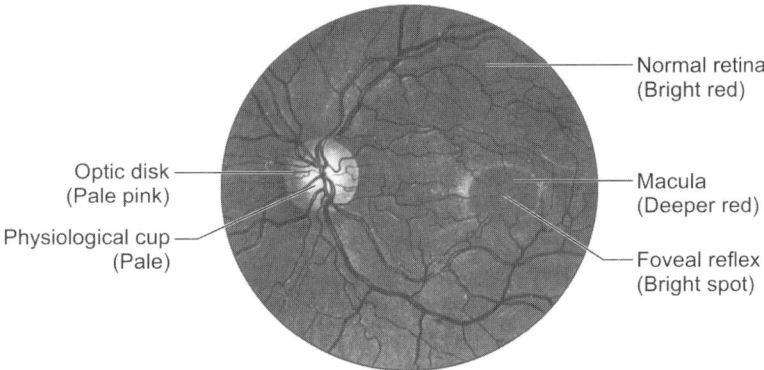

Fig. 5: Color of portions of normal retina.

Color of Normal Retina (as seen with Ophthalmoscope) (Fig. 5)

Living retina is a transparent membrane. But when retina is examined with ophthalmoscope:
- The normal retina appear bright red in color due to red reflex from blood circulating in the choroidal vessels behind. In dark complexioned people retina is darker red, and in fair skinned people, light red
- As a whole optic disk is pale pink in color. Again temporal half of disk is paler than nasal
- Macula is deeper red in color than surrounding retina
- Foveal reflex is the bright spot in the center of macula.

Topography of Retina (Areal Subdivisions of Retina) (Fig. 6)

Retina does not have the ten layered composition in all areas, but some regions show structural differences and so perform different functions.

So clinicians divide retina into two main portions—*a posterior retina (central retina) and an anterior retina (peripheral retina) along an imaginary line passing through the equator of eyeball.* This division helps in documentation

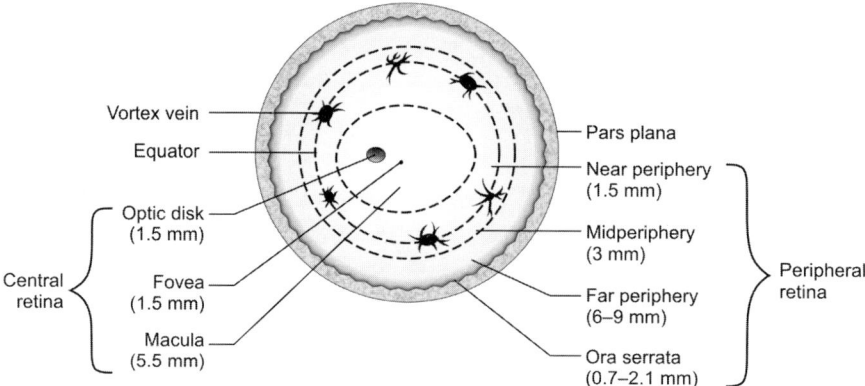

Fig. 6: Areal subdivisions of retina.

and a better diagnosis, localization and treatment of retinal and choroidal disorders. *This line can be imagined as if passing along the anterior borders of ampullae of vortex vein (when we examine retina with the ophthalmoscope).* Such internal measurements can be correlated and mapped on the scleral surface for practical purposes.

Posterior or Central Retina

Posterior or central retina is an approximately *6–10 mm* posterior portion of the retina extending up to equator anteriorly. It has again different areas.
- Optic disk—*is a vertically oval or round 1.5 mm area of posterior retina.*
- Macular area—*is about 5 mm horizontally elliptical area temporal to the optic disk slightly below horizontal meridian.*
  Macular area is again *subdivided* into three smaller areas—central foveola and three concentric portions of retina surrounding it.
    - Foveola : *0.35 mm floor of the foveal pit (central point is the umbo)*
    - Fovea (fovea centralis): *It is an 1.5 mm central area of retina (shallow round pit) around foveola situated 4 mm temporal to optic disk and 0.8 mm below horizontal meridian*
    - Parafovea: *It is a 0.5 mm wide area of retina around fovea*
    - Perifovea: *It is a further 1.5 mm area of retinal belt around parafovea.*

Anterior or Peripheral Retina

Constitute the rest of the retina which has a larger *10–15 mm area,* extending probably from equator to extreme anterior periphery of retina.
  Peripheral retina is again subdivided into four concentric regions around central retina—near periphery, midperiphery, far periphery and ora serrata.
- *Near periphery*—is concentric 1.5 mm belt of retina around perifovea and starts almost from equator. The retina in the region (imaginary) of equator of retina is often called equatorial retina
- *Midperiphery*—*is a 3 mm of retina around near periphery*
- *Far periphery*—is not uniformly concentric, but nasal retina extends, more anteriorly than temporal retina.

- *Ora serrata*—is the anterior extremity of retina. It is the border between the retina and the pars plana in the far periphery.
  Thus, ora serrata is more near the limbus on nasal side and can be located on the surface of eyeball approximately near the insertion medial rectus and farther from limbus on the temporal side and can be located near the insertion of lateral rectus. Also, ora serrata and adjacent retina on temporal side are more easily visible with indirect ophthalmoscope than nasal side. This asymmetry may probably due to position of optic nerve which leaves the eyeball 3 mm medial to posterior pole.

CLINICAL AND FUNCTIONAL DIFFERENTIATIONS AND MEASUREMENTS OF OPTIC DISK, MACULA AND PERIPHERAL RETINA

All regions of retina do not have the same clinical appearance, but three regions, optic disk, macula (fovea) and peripheral retina (ora serrata) have different clinical features and functions.

Optic Disk

Optic disk is the 1.5 mm circular or oval portion of posterior retina and is the only ophthalmoscopically visible part of the optic nerve. It is situated in the nasal part of the retina 3-4 mm from the fovea. It is color appears pale pink on ophthalmoscopic examination. Structurally of the ten layers of retina, optic disk has only one layer—nerve fiber layer; all other layers stop at its edge. Since receptors are absent, this area does not perceive light stimulus, and appears, as a blind spot in visual field *about 15° from fixation point. The optic disk is usually oval in shape; vertical diameter 9% longer than horizontal. Mean vertical diameter of disk is 1.9 mm and horizontal diameter is 1.7 mm. Area of optic disk is about 2.6 mm^2. Larger disks (macrodisks) having an area more than 4.09 mm^2 can occur in morning glory syndrome, high myopia and buphthalmos (20 mm^2). Small disks (microdisks) of less than 1.29 mm^2 area can occur in highly hypermetropic eyes and optic nerve drusen. There is slight crease in size from –5 D to +5 D in refractive errors. Abnormal shape of optic disk is suggestive of astigmatism or amblyopia.*

Physiological Cup

Optic disk has a central depression called physiological cup. It is funnel-shaped and slightly eccentrically placed towards the temporal side of disk. The size of disk is determined by the amount of atrophy of the Bermingsters papilla during development of vitreous. *The diameter of the cup is about 0.92 mm horizontally and 0.84 mm vertically. Cup volume is about 0.34 mm^3. Depth is around 0.23 mm. Optic cup is deep in 25%, medium in 31% and shallow in 23% of individuals.* Some individuals do not have physiological cup. Retinal vessels reach the retinal surface from the medial side of cup slightly displaced superonasally. Temporal arteries take an arcuate course than nasal.

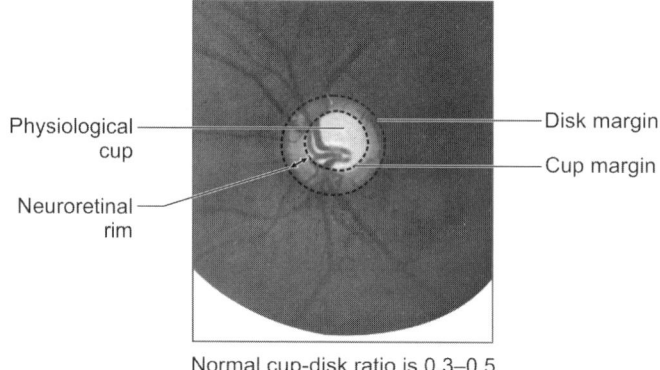

Normal cup-disk ratio is 0.3–0.5

Fig. 7: Cup-disk ratio.

Cup-Disk Ratio (Fig. 7)

If optic disk is divided into ten parts, about three parts of the disk are occupied by physiological cup (0.3:1). Cup disk ratio, is the ratio of cup diameter to disk diameter, usually measured in vertical meridian. Normally cup disk ratio is between 0.3 to 0.5 and do not alter more than 0.1 between two eyes. Enlargement of cup indicate loss of optic nerve fibers leading of narrowing of neuroretinal rim. Cup-disk ratio can be assessed and measured roughly using ophthalmoscope with a graticule. The thickness or height of disk is measured using white scleral ring as a reference landmark. An enlarged cup-disk ratio more than 0.5 especially in vertical axis (as early neuroretinal rim loss occur in glaucoma in upper and lower part of disk) or an asymmetry of cup-disk ratio more than 0.2 between two eyes is suggestive of glaucoma. If persons with microdisks like hypermetropia who do not usually have physiological cup develop a cup disk ratio 0.2–0.3 later is suggestive of glaucoma. Conversely in persons with macrodisk, cup-disk ratio of 0.8 can be considered normal if there are no other signs of glaucoma.

Neuroretinal Rim (Fig. 8)

Neuroretinal rim (NRR) is the part of optic disk between cup and edge of disk. Axons of ganglion cells occupy this area of the optic disk. The contour of neuroretinal rim is determined by the shape of scleral canal through which the axons pass out of eyes. *Scleral canal is 0.5 mm long.* Its directions may be straight or slightly deviated nasally, temporally or downwards.

The breadth or thickness of NRR normally varies in its different sectors of optic disk.
- Inferior disk region   : Thickest (I)
- Superior disk region   : Thick (S)
- Nasal disk area   : Thin (N)
- Temporal disk region   : Thinnest (T)

This is the ISNT rule.

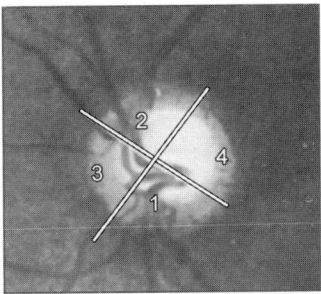

Fig. 8: Variations in thickness (breadth) of different regions of optic disk. (*For color version, see Plate 2*)

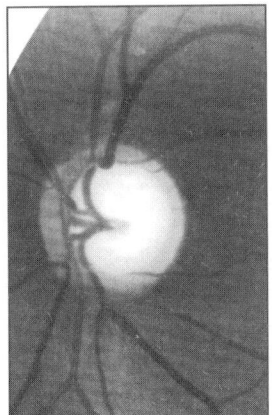

Enlarge vertically oval cup
cup-disk ratio >0.7

Fig. 9: Glaucomatous cupping. (*For color version, see Plate 3*)

In glaucoma there is progressive thinning of NRR (due to neuronal loss) leading to enlargement of cup in all directions. It predominantly occurs in vertical direction leading to loss of NRR at superior and inferior poles. Inferior pole never remains thickest in glaucoma. For early diagnosis of glaucoma, one should give more attention to the inferior temporal than superior temporal disk sectors. If the thickness of the superior and inferior sectors are equal or thinner than nasal portion, it is highly suspicious. A focal NRR notching is also suggestive of glaucoma (Figs. 9 and 10).

Disk Diameter (DD) and Diopter (D) Elevation (Fig. 11)

Using ophthalmoscope a quick and approximate measurement of dimensions —size, depth, elevations, etc. of retinal and choroidal lesions can be made in terms of disk diameter (size) and diopter (elevation).

 1 DD = 1.5 mm width or diameter
 1 D = 0.33 mm elevation (+) or depression (−)

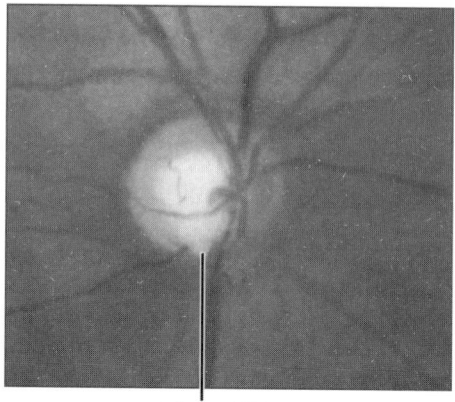

Inferior NRR

Fig. 10: Thinning of inferior neuroretinal rim (NRR) in glaucoma.
(*For color version, see Plate 3*)

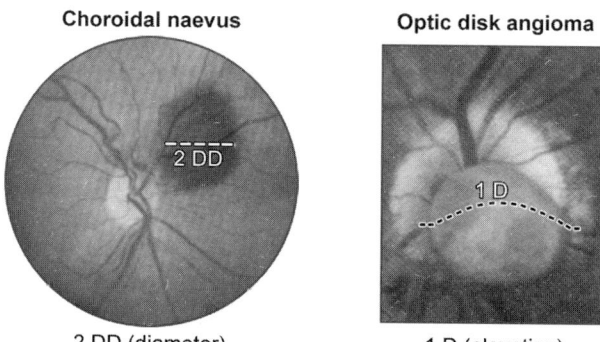

2 DD (diameter)   1 D (elevation)

Fig. 11: Disk diameter (DD) and diopter (D) elevation.
(*For color version, see Plate 3*)

More accurate measurements can be done using ultrasonography, optical coherence tomography (OCT) and Heidelberg retina topography (HRT).

Color Variations of Optic Disk (Normal and Abnormal)

Normally, the optic disk appears pale pink in color, on ophthalmoscopic examination. NRR is broad pink and vascularized. Center of the disk is pale (physiological cup). Temporal part of the disk is paler than nasal.

The color of optic disk can become red, yellow, grey, pale or even white and brown or black in various clinical conditions.

- Optic disk can become *hyperemic or red and swollen*—in *optic neuritis*, early *papilledema* and pseudo-neuritis (Fig. 12).
- *Yellowish, waxy pale* in *consecutive optic atrophy*. Disk edge is clear and surrounding retina abnormal (Fig. 13).
- *Papery white in primary optic atrophy*, disk margin is sharply defined. There is stippling of laminar cribrosa, shallow saucer shaped cup and normal surrounding retina (Fig. 14).

- *Dirty gray color in postneuritic optic atrophy.* Disk margins are blurred, cup filled with fibrous tissue, vessels constricted with perivascular sheathing and surrounding retina show permanent changes of damage.
- *Pale or white disk with large wide cupping* and very narrow neuroretinal rim—in *glaucomatous optic atrophy.* The vessels show considerable bending and apparent discontinuity of blood vessels at disk margins (bayoneting). If the pallor exceeds cupping the visual loss is probably not due to glaucoma but paleness is due to neurological or other causes (Fig. 16).
- *Pallid disk edema* occurs in *anterior ischemic optic neuropathy (Fig. 17).*
- *Yellow swollen disk* is indicative of *optic nerve head drusen* (Fig. 18).
- *Dark brown or black swollen disk* occur in *melanocytoma of optic disk* (Fig. 19).

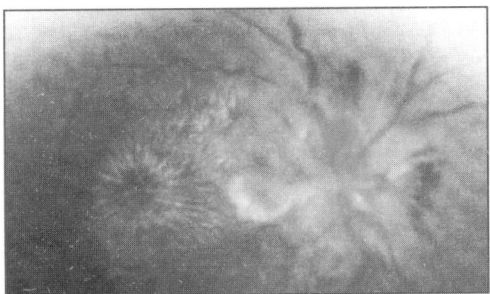

Fig. 12: Red swollen disk (papilledema). (*For color version, see Plate 3*)

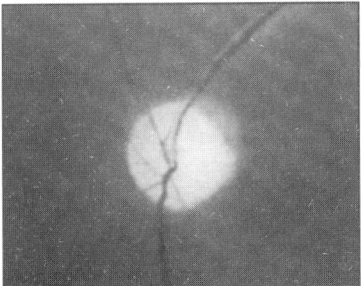

Fig. 13: Consecutive optic atrophy (yellowish waxy pale disk).
(*For color version, see Plate 4*)

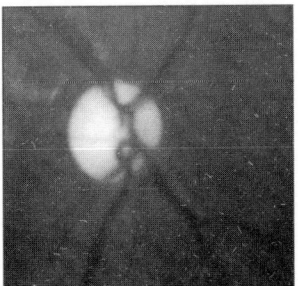

Fig. 14: Primary optic atrophy (papery white disk).
(*For color version, see Plate 4*)

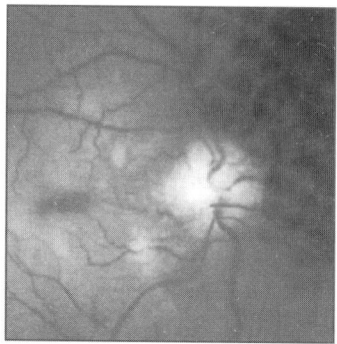

Fig. 15: Postneuritic (secondary) optic atrophy dirty gray color.
(*For color version, see Plate 4*)

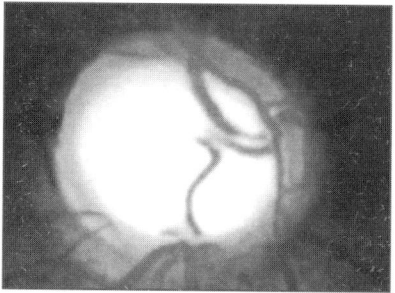

Fig. 16: Pale disk with deep wide (glaucomatous) cupping.
(*For color version, see Plate 4*)

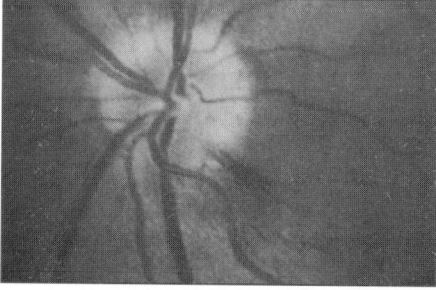

Fig. 17: Anterior ischemic optic neuropathy (pallid disk edema).
(*For color version, see Plate 4*)

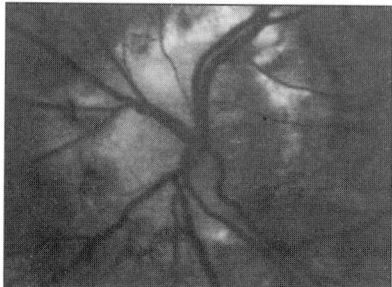

Fig. 18: Optic disk drusen (yellow swollen disk).
(*For color version, see Plate 4*)

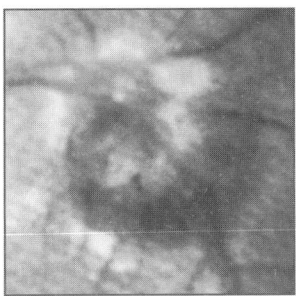

Fig. 19: Melanocytoma of optic disk (dark brown/black swollen disk).

Macula

Macula is *a 5.5 mm ill-defined horizontally oval area of posterior retina starting from temporal edge and 0.8 mm inferior to the center of optic disk bordered by superior and inferior temporal vascular arcades.* Clinically, (ophthalmoscopically) this area appears darker red than other parts of retina (bright red). This area has the special functions of visual acuity, color vision and stereopsis. Histologically, macula has following features which are different from other parts of retina (Fig. 20).
- High density of cones—incidence of cones increasing towards center and decrease of rods
- Ganglion cells are more than one layer in thickness
- Contain xanthophyll (yellow pigment) mainly in outer plexiform layer of this region.

Macula has following structurally and functionally different regions.
- **Foveola:** It is the central *0.35 mm floor of the foveal pit within the fovea and forms the center of macula.* When examined with ophthalmoscope the light reflected from its floor produce a bright spot of foveal reflex. Here the cones are most densely packed. The elongated cones of foveola produce a slight bowing internally, the Umbo (naval). In the foveola there are only three layers for the retina—RPE, layer of cones and nerve fiber layer, all other layers are shifted to sides. There are no rods in this region.
- **Fovea:** *It is the central 1.5 mm area of the macula* where inner surface of retina suddenly slopes into a concave region. It has the special functions of form sense and color vision due to the high density of cones.

  The central 0.5 mm (0.4–0.6 mm) area of the fovea is devoid of blood vessels and is called foveal avascular zone (Fig. 21). This is the center of macula, point of fixation and is an important landmark in fluorescein angiography.
- **Parafovea:** *It is a 0.5 mm area of macula around fovea* where inner nuclear layer, outer plexiform layer and ganglion cell layer are thickest. Each cone is separated from the other by one rod.
- **Perifovea:** *It includes a ring of 1.5 mm area around parafovea* and form the transitional zone of central and peripheral retina.

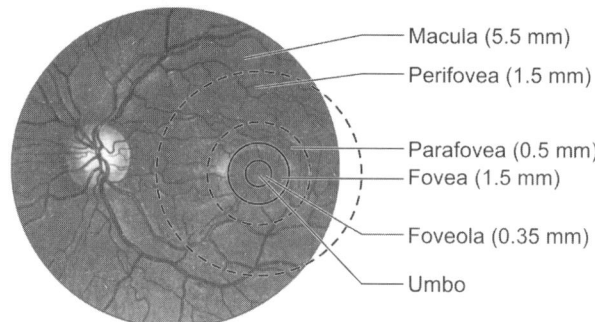

Fig. 20: Portions of macula. (*For color version, see Plate 4*)

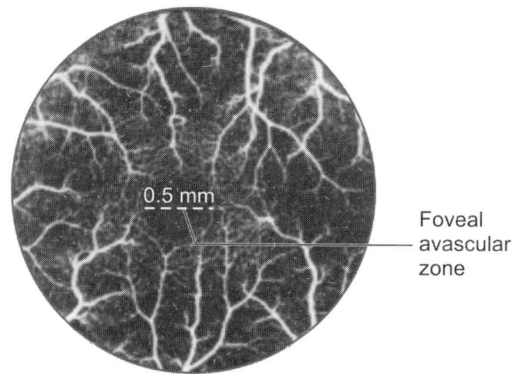

Fig. 21: Foveal avascular zone.

Layer-by-Layer Structural and Functional Differentiation of Central Retina (Macular Region) (Fig. 22)

Retinal pigment epithelium: The component cells of RPE in the macular region are taller, *(11–14 μm) narrow*er and more regularly arranged than other parts of retina. The pigmentation is more dense and pigment granules are distributed throughout their cytoplasm. This gives a dark appearance to macula in fluorescein angiography due to the masking of the choroidal flush.

Photoreceptor layer: The photoreceptor cells of macula are taller and narrower than other parts of retina thus, the margin of fovea form the thickest part of retina. The density of cones is more in the macular region and concentration of cones increases as from parafovea to fovea. In the foveola there are only cones and they are more numerous and density packed; providing maximum form sense (visual acuity) color sense and stereopsis. The foveal cones are separated by 2 μm which provides a visual angle of 25 seconds of arc and is the basis of visual acuity testing.

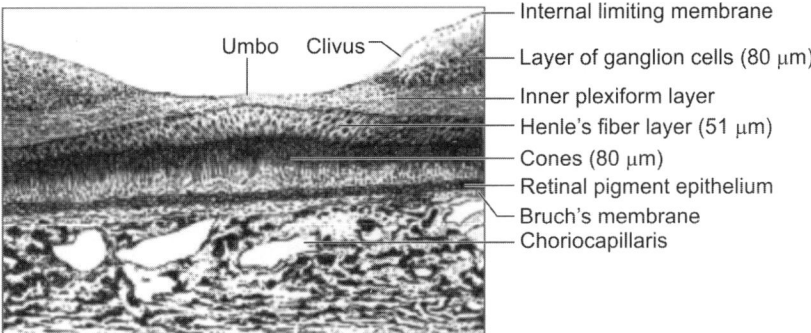

Fig. 22: Structure of fovea.

In the foveola there is dense packing of 2,500 specialized cones (the bouquet of central cones of Rochon-Duvigneaud). The length of each cone is about 70 μm, twice of those at the edge of fovea. The thickness varies from 1 to 15 μm.

Under the photoreceptor layer, the other inner layers of fovea are diverted from its center, curving like 's' and the nerve fibers run almost parallel to surface forming a horizontal layer of fibers—Layer of Henle. This layer becomes steeper towards the periphery of fovea at the margin and then the fibers become vertical. Since the fibers are curved outwards, the inner layers of retina are almost absent at the foveola making it a pit. Around margin of fovea layers reappear receiving elements diverted from center and become unusually thick.

Dimensions of Fovea, Parafovea and Perifovea

- **Diameter of fovea**
    - Foveola : 0.3–0.4 mm
    - Foveal pit : 1.5 mm
    - Floor of pit : 0.4 mm
    - Rod-free area : 0.5–0.6 mm
    - Foveal avascular zone (FAZ) : 0.5 mm (0.4–0.6 mm)
- **Depth of fovea** : 240 μm
- **Thickness of fovea** : 130 μm
- **Parafovea** : 0.5 mm area around fovea
- **Perifovea** : 1.5 mm area around parafovea

External Limiting Membrane (Fovea Externa)

Since the foveal cones are longer (taller) than elsewhere they produce a bulge of external limiting membrane outwards in the foveal region, the fovea externa.

Outer nuclear layer: In the foveal region there are *10 rows of cones nuclei and thickness of this layer increases to 50 μm.*

Outer plexiform layer: The outer plexiform layer of macular region is thickest and is formed mainly by the oblique and parallel fibers diverted from fovea (Henle fiber layer). The constituent fibers in this region are loosely arranged compared to other areas and form a delicate network. Thus, it becomes a

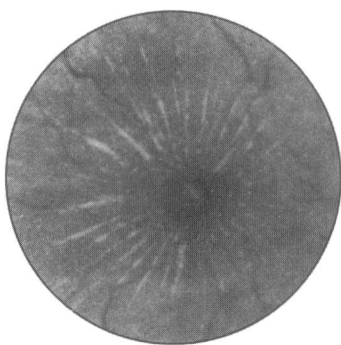

Fig. 23: Macular star. (*For color version, see Plate 5*)

potential space for easy and rapid collection of edema fluid (macular edema). This layer is absent at fovea. The displacement of tissues away from foveola disturbs the normal reticular arrangement of supporting Muller's fibers. Although they are present centrally their processes run horizontally in Henles layer. Thus, the retina in this region loses its compact nature and the resultant laxity enables large quantities of extracellular fluids or exudates to become accumulated in macula region in irritative and inflammatory conditions of retina. The oblique orientation of the outer plexiform layer in the macular region may be the reason for the appearance of *cystoid macular edema*. The *macular star* is probably due to the collection of exudates in Henle's layer where they are molded into a stellate pattern by its radial arrangement of fibers (Fig. 23).

Inner nuclear layer: The cell bodies of bipolar cells of macular region are large and *about 9 μm diameter compared to peripheral retina (5 μm)*. Rod bipolar cells stop almost 1 mm from fovea. Inner nuclear layer is absent at foveola.

Inner plexiform layer: It has the same thickness in all parts of retina except at fovea where it is absent.

Ganglion cell layer: In most of the regions of retina, this layer is one cell thick. But in the macular region the ganglion cells are numerous and become even eight layer thick. The thickness decreases towards fovea where it disappears completely. When edema develops in this thick layer of ganglion cells of macular region as in central retinal artery occlusion or commotion retinae the retina acquire milky white color, but at fovea central is being very thin, through which the red reflex from underlying choroid appears as cherry red spot in contrast to the cloudy white surrounding retinal background.

Nerve fiber layer: It becomes thin in the macular region. At fovea it becomes a very thin network or even disappears entirely.

Internal Limiting Membrane

Over the foveal region it is thin and adherent to vitreous and permeable. Thus, toxins produced due to inflammations of even distant structures like iris, ciliary body and choroid can traverse across vitreous through ILM to foveal region, disturbing its functions and increasing the permeability leading to macular edema.

Structural (Layer by Layer) and Functional Differentiations of Peripheral Retina

In general, the peripheral retina has the following differences from other portions of retina.
- Decreased density of cones and an increased number of rods
- Visual activity function is less and receive only coarse stimuli
- Mainly concerned with vision in dim light
- Increases the field of vision.

The four divisions of peripheral retina have the following differences in structure compared with central retina.

Near periphery: This is a 1.5 mm area of retina around perifovea extending anteriorly from equator area. The cones become more scattered, *density decreases to about 9 to 10 cones per 100 µm.* Cones are thicker than perifovea—outer segment 2.5 µm and inner segment 5-6 µm. The density of rods increases. *There are about 2-3 rods in between two cones in this area.* Outer nuclear layer is thick. Outer plexiform layer fibers becomes vertical in this region and Henle's layer disappears. Ganglion cells are larger and single layered in near periphery.

Midperiphery: Midperiphery is a 3 mm broad area of retina around near periphery. The incidence of cones further decreases to about to 8 per 100 µm. There are 3 rods in between 2 cones. Inner segment of cones is thicker (6-7.5 µm). Rods are thicker than central retina (1.5-2 µm thick). Ganglion cells do not form a continuous layer in this area.

Far periphery: The far periphery portion of retina extends anteriorly from optic disk 9-10 mm on temporal part and 16 mm on nasal part in horizontal meridian. The cones are few and their incidence is only 6-7 per 100 µm. Their outer segments are 3 µm thick and inner segments 8-9 µm thick. There is a wide separation between ganglion cells.

Ora Serrata

Ora serrata, the extreme periphery of retina, is very thin and *is only 0.1 mm thick and resolves into very few layers.* The retinal elements start to disappear in this area. Rods are the first to disappear and become replaced by malformed cones. They are met even up to oral rim. Ganglion cell layer and their fibers stop about 0.5-1 mm from extreme periphery and become replaced by neuroglial cells and Muller's fibers. Structurally, ora is spongy and shows degenerative changes. Ora serrata continues anteriorly as ciliary epithelium.

Distance of Ora Serrata from Limbus (Fig. 24)

A knowledge of distance of limbus to ora serrata and to the different portions of eyeball is important in localization and marking of retinal lesions on ocular

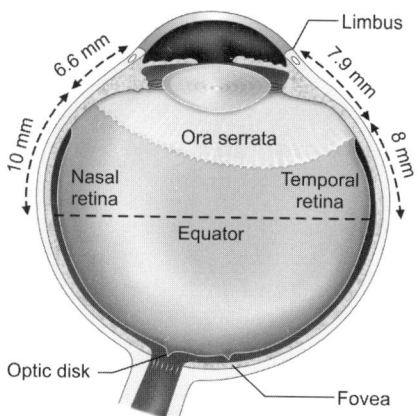

Fig. 24: Extent and surface marking of retina.

surface. The distance can vary in different quadrants of eyeball and also in different refractive conditions. The distance of limbus to ora serrata is:
- On nasal side : 6.6 mm in emmetropes, 6.2 mm in hypermetropes and 7 mm in myopes
- On temporal side : 7.9 mm in emmetropes, 6.7 mm in hypermetropes and 8.4 mm in myopes
- Superiorly : 7.4 mm in emmetropes, 7 mm in hypermetropes and 8.1 mm in myopes
- Inferiorly : 6.99 mm in emmetropes, 6.5 mm in hypermetropes and 8 mm in myopes.

METHODS OF EVALUATION OF DIFFERENT PORTIONS OF RETINA PARTICULARLY THE RETINAL NERVE FIBER LAYER

- *Ophthalmoscopy:* Ophthalmoscopy by direct or indirect method provides a quick and easy method of topographic and specific assessment of different portions of retina.
  Retinal nerve fiber layer (RNFL) is better visualized through a dilated pupil with ophthalmoscopes using red-free green light. The visibility of NFL is more inferotemporally than superotemporally. Superonasal fibers are better visible than infero-nasal. This corresponds with the thickness of NRR. Normal NFL has a *silvery striated appearance* over the retinal background (Fig. 25). When diseased or damaged the silvery striations are lost and the involved area of retina appears darker and deeper red. Slit like defect can occur within the silvery striations in normal retina. *A wedge shaped defect extending to disk margin is abnormal.* It can occur in glaucoma and advanced retinal diseases. Glaucoma can produce *diffuse atrophy of RNFL.*
- *Slit lamp with fundus lenses (Goldmann/Zeiss four mirror contact lens, Hruby lens, 90 D lens, etc.)*

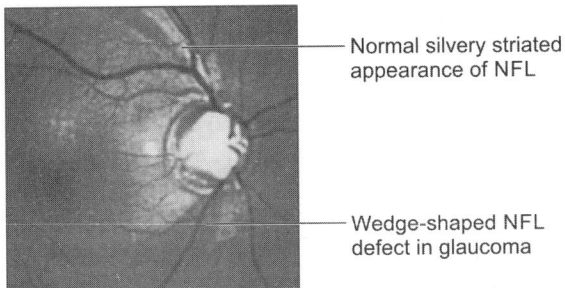

Fig. 25: Ophthalmoscopic appearance of normal and abnormal nerve fiber layer (NFL). (*For color version, see Plate 5*)

These can give a magnified stereoscopic view of optic disk, macula and retinal periphery. But there can be variability in the assessment and opinion about individual cases among different observers. So other objective imaging techniques are preferred.

- *Stereophotography:* This allows quantitative evaluation of optic disk and other portions of retina.

  In glaucoma, detectable changes in the visual field by perimetry occur only after considerable structural RNFL damage (loss of even 40% of ganglion cells) have already occurred. So evaluation of RNFL is often preferred than perimetry or optic nerve head evaluation in early diagnosis (preperimetric) of glaucoma.

- *Imaging technologies:* Three modern imaging technologies are being used for glaucoma evaluation. All the three do not have equal capability of assessment of glaucoma; one better than other. Each have their own advantages and limitations. On a comparative basis:
  - *Optical coherence tomography (OCT)* is more useful in imaging macula, optic nerve head (ONH) and optic nerve fiber layer (ONFL).
  - *Heidelberg retinal tomography (HRT)* is particularly useful in optic nerve head evaluation.
  - *Scanning laser polarimetry (SLP, GDx)* is unique in imaging and evaluating retinal nerve fiber layer.

Optical coherence tomography: It is often considered as a "live biopsy and histopathology" of retina by the use of low-coherence interferometry, so that we can study different layers of retina with near histologic clarity (Fig. 26). It provides a high-resolution cross-sectional image of retina particularly macula, ONH and RNLF layer. When ultrasonography uses sound waves, OCT sends a beam of light into the eye and the reflections returning from the structures of eye are analyzed to produce their images layer by layer. To obtain images of ONH, RNFL and macula (posterior segment OCT) light rays of 830 nm are used. OCT gives posterior segment thickness measurements in an axial resolution of 8–10 microns (Fig. 27).

Heidelberg retinal tomograph (HRT)(Fig. 28): HRT is mainly used in optic nerve head evaluation in glaucoma. HRT utilizes the technology of confocal laser ophthalmoscopy and is designed particularly to obtain a reproducible, rapid

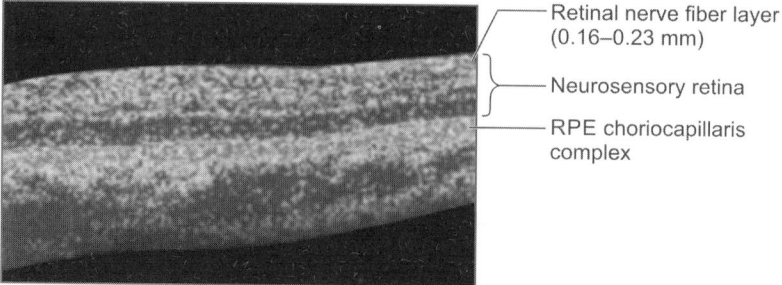

Fig. 26: OCT picture of normal retina

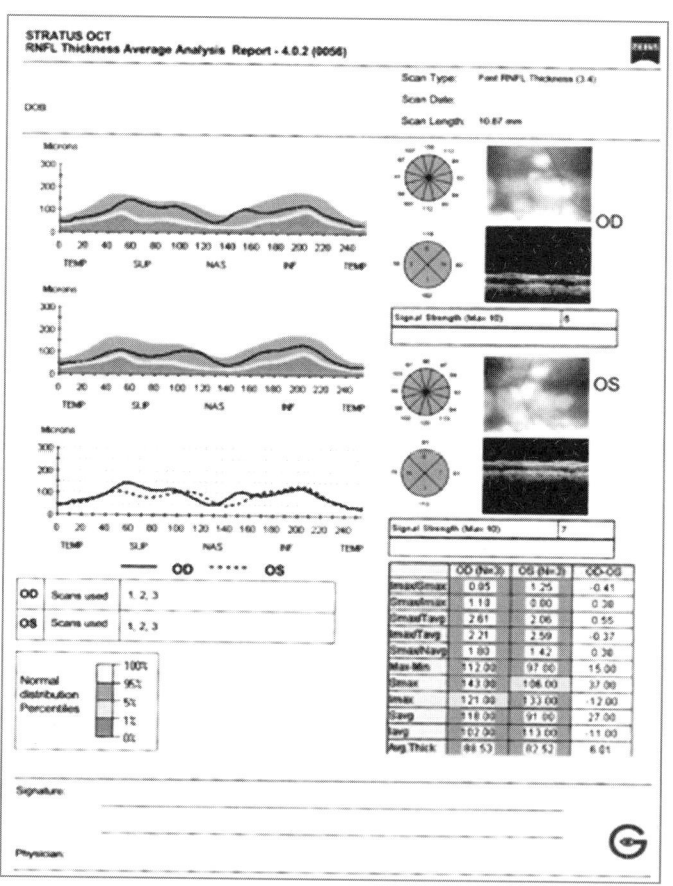

Fig. 27: OCT printout of NFL thickness analysis.

three-dimensional analysis of ONH, RNFL and posterior pole parameters. The technology was introduced commercially by Heidelberg Engineering, Heidelberg, Germany and hence the name. It has three generations, HRT I, HRT II and HRT III. HRT III is superior due to its GPS software. Based on the principle of spot illumination and spot detection, focal plane is adjusted by shifting confocal aperture or pinhole (Fig. 29).

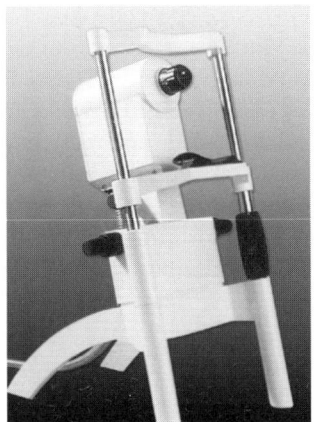

Fig. 28: Heidelberg retina tomograph equipment.

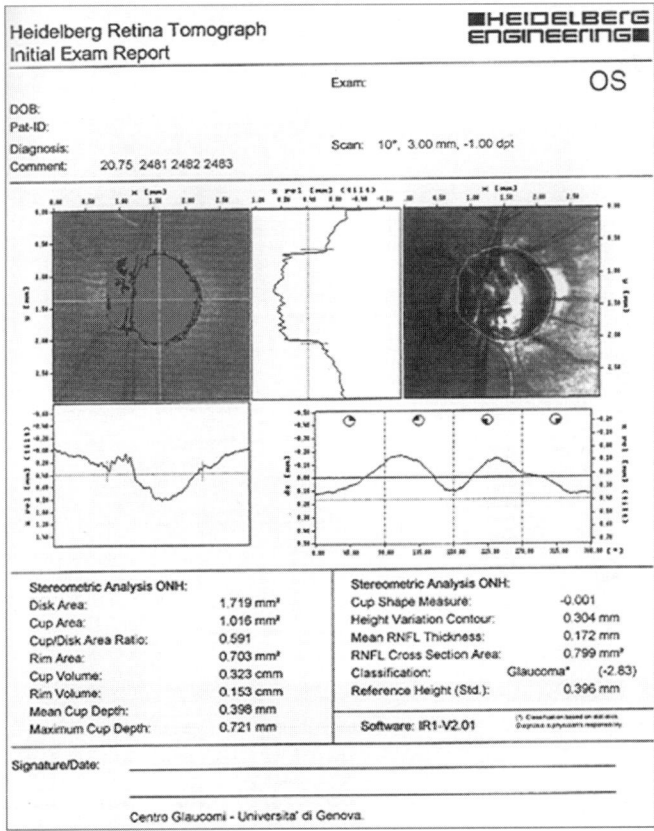

Fig. 29: HRT printout.

Scanning laser polarimetry (SLP), GDx and VCC: Gives a more specific quantitative evaluation of retinal nerve fiber layer thickness using confocal polarimetric scanning ophthalmoscope. GDx is the name of its commercial application.

Retinal nerve fiber layer changes precede visual field changes in glaucoma. Even 40% of ganglion cells would have been damaged before a well-defined scotoma occurs in white-to-white perimetry. Hence RNFL thickness evaluation using SLP or OCT is more superior in early diagnosis and evaluation of glaucoma.

This technique is based on the birefringence of axons of ganglion cells (birefringence is the splitting of one light ray into two in an isometric medium) and measures the rotation of polarized light reflected from retinal nerve fibers, assuming that rotation is proportional to the RNF by birefringence. Total retardation of light is dependent on RNFL by birefringence and to RNFL thickness.

This equipment is particularly useful in assessment of RNFL thickness as an index of glaucoma progression. It is expressed in terms of the parameter— nerve fiber index (NFI) in GDx. Normal eyes have NFI between 0 to 35. NFI between 35 and 44 is boarder line. In advance glaucoma NFI may approach 100 (Fig. 30).

Earlier forms of SLP (GDx NFA, GDx access) with single or double detector had anterior segment birefringence compensation based on fixed values for

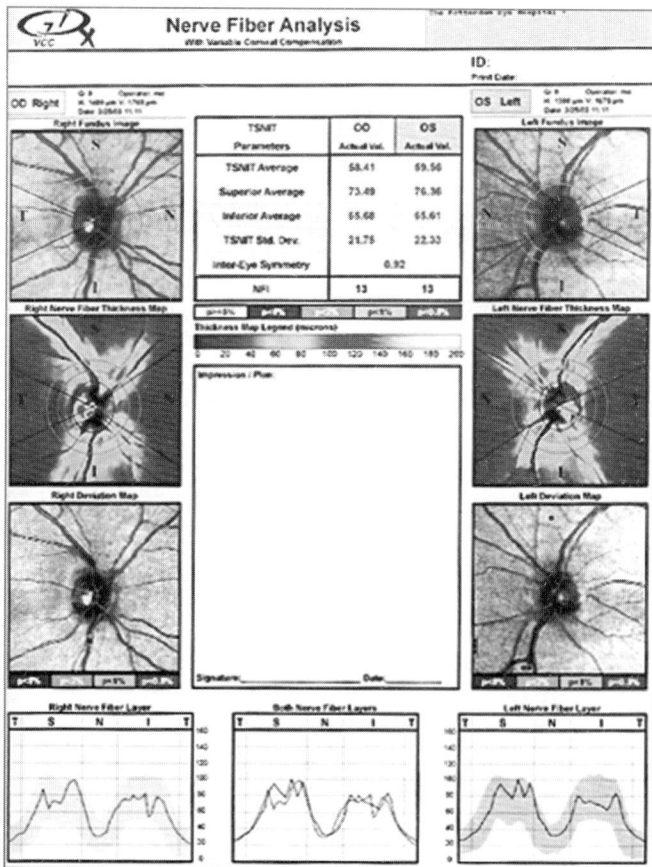

Fig. 30: GDx printout.

its axis and magnitude. But later it was found that the axis and magnitude of birefringence are variable in each individual and is eye specific. The new generation SLP named GDx - VCC (variable corneal compensation), overcomes this variability and compensates individuals variations of anterior segment birefringence using 780–790 nm laser diode.

Evaluation of NFL by the above methods shows that its thickness varies between 0.16 mm and 0.23 mm.

SUMMARY OF MEASUREMENTS OF RETINA

- Surface area of retina : 266 m^2
- Width (diameter) of retina
  - At equator : 24 mm
  - At ora serrata : 20 mm
- Thickness of retina
  - Near optic disk : 0.56 mm
  - Equator : 0.18 mm
  - Fovea : 0.25 mm
  - Ora serrata : 0.1 mm
- Extend of retina in different parts (zones)
  - I. Posterior retina : Average 6 mm in diameter area
    - Optic disk : 1.5 mm
    - Macula : Average 5 mm area
      ◊ Foveola : 0.35 mm
      ◊ Depth of foveola : 130 μm
      ◊ Fovea : 1.5 mm
      ◊ Depth of fovea : 240 μm
      ◊ Parafovea : 0.5 mm
      ◊ Perifovea : 1.5 mm
  - II. Anterior retina (peripheral retina)
    - Near periphery (equator) : 1.5 mm wide area around central retina
    - Midperiphery : 3 mm wide area around near periphery
    - Far periphery : 9.1 mm area extending from temporal edge and 16 mm from the nasal edge of optic disk in horizontal meridian
    - Ora serrata : Extend 2.1 mm on temporal side and up to 0.7–0.8 mm nasally from far peripheral retina.

CHAPTER 13

Measurements of Optic Nerve

Optic nerve, the second cranial nerve transfers the visual neural information from retina to the brain. It is made of *approximately 1.2 million axons arising from ganglion cells of retina which end at lateral geniculate body*. Optic nerve forms a part of the second order of neuron of visual pathway. Anatomically, it extends from optic disk (within eyeball) to optic chiasma situated in the cranial cavity (Fig. 1).

DIFFERENCES OF OPTIC NERVE FROM OTHER CRANIAL NERVES

Though optic nerve is a sensory nerve it has several **differences from other cranial nerves:**
- It is developed as an evagination of forebrain and so forms the part of central nervous system.

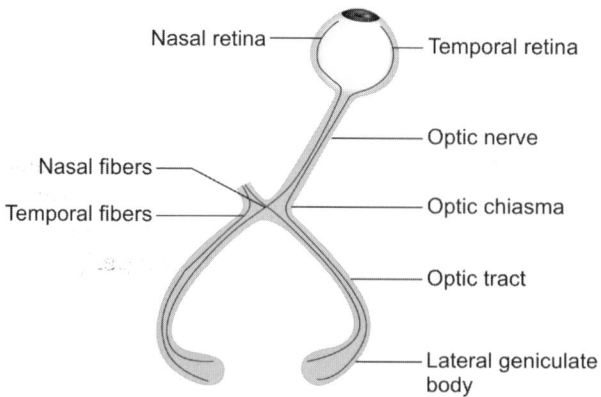

Fig. 1: Extent of optic nerve fibers.

- Its nerve fibers are not covered by Neurilemma sheath and resemble white matter of brain. So once destroyed by injury or disease, the fibers do not regenerate.
- Optic nerve is covered by meninges—dura, arachnoid and pia continuous posteriorly with those of brain.

STRUCTURE AND DIMENSIONS OF VARIOUS PORTIONS OF OPTIC NERVE (FIG. 2)

The total length of optic nerve is about 50 mm. It has four portions.
1. **Intraocular portion:** *It is the smallest portion and extends from optic disk surface to the lamina cribrosa and is about 0.7–1 mm long.*
2. **Intraorbital portion:** *It is the longest portion, about 33 mm long.*
3. **Intracanalicular portion:** *It occupies the optic canal and is approximately 7–10 mm long.*
4. **Intracranial portion:** *It extends to the cranial cavity to about 10 mm.*

Intraocular Portion

Intraocular portion is the part of optic nerve within the eyeball. This portion is about 0.7–1 mm long. This is the only ophthalmoscopically visible portion of the nerve and is called optic disk, clinically. It is not elevated above surrounding retina, and hence the term optic papilla is not very correct. Anatomically, it extends from within the eye from optic disk surface to the posterior limit of lamina cribrosa (posterior scleral surface). Choroid stop at its edge. This portion of optic nerve has four layers which differ in structure, vascular supply and function (Fig. 3).
1. *Nerve fiber layer:* Consisting axons of ganglion cells and astrocytes and perfused by branches of central retinal vessels which anastomose with vessels of prelaminar region.
2. *Prelaminar layer:* It is made of bundles of optic nerve fibers separated by channels made of astrocytes. Unlike retina they are not bound together

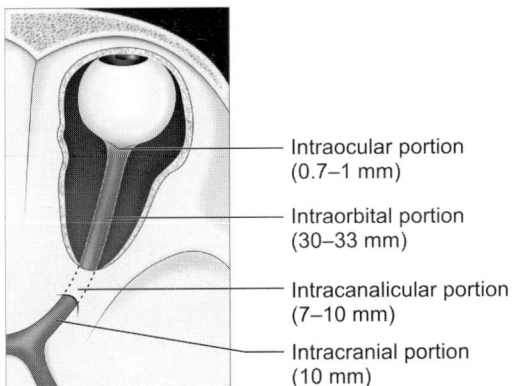

Fig. 2: Portions and dimensions of optic nerve total length = 50 mm.

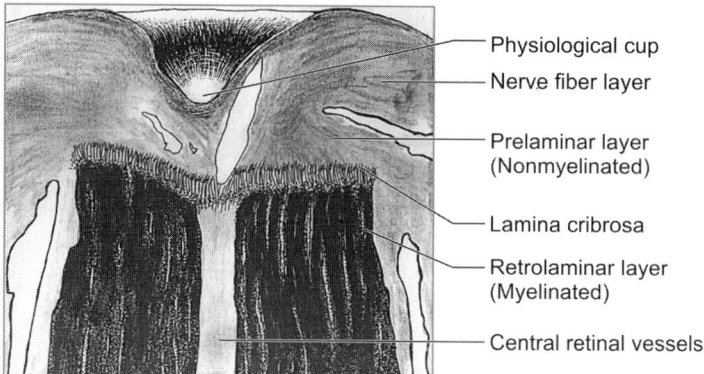

Fig. 3: Structure of intraocular portion of optic nerve (optic disk).

by mullers cells. Thus, optic disk swells easily in papilledema but not so much in the adjacent retina. This layer extends up to the level of choroid. Prelaminar region is supplied by centripetal branches of peripapillary choroidal vessels.

- *Lamina cribrosa:* Consists of *3-10 sheets of perforated scleral (collagen) sheets* through which axon bundles and central retinal vessels pass. The apertures may be round or oval in shape. Pores are larger in the upper and *lower part of lamina cribrosa and so has less structural support for nerve* bundles in this region. Normally, there is a small amount of posterior bowing of lamina cribrosa which should not be mistaken for that of glaucomatous cupping. Lamina cribrosa is supplied by ciliary vessels arising from short posterior ciliary artery and the arterial circle of Zinn and Haller.
- *Retrolaminar layer:* Retrolaminar layer of optic nerve lies just behind lamina cribrosa, gets myelinated and accounts for the *doubling of optic nerve thickness of optic nerve from 1.50 mm within eye to 3 mm more behind the eyeball.* This portion of optic nerve gets covered by meninges. Retrolaminar region is supplied by both retinal and ciliary vessels—centrifugal branches of retinal artery and centripetal branches of pial pluxus.

Intraorbital Portion

Intraorbital portion of optic nerve passes through the orbit from back of eye ball to optic canal. This part is about 33 mm long. *The length of this portion of optic nerve is 8 mm more than the distance between eyeball and optic canal.* This redundancy and the resultant sinuous course of optic nerve facilitates the free movement of eyeball without stretching of the optic nerve. Also this laxity protects optic nerve to a certain extent from stretching which can occur in injuries and proptosis of even 9 mm. *When the eyeball becomes protruded (proptosed) more than 10 mm from its normal position, the optic nerve becomes taut, back of globe becomes tethered and even tended.*

From orbital portion onwards the optic nerve is covered by meningeal sheaths—dura, arachnoid and pia along with the corresponding extension of subarachnoid space around it up to eyeball. The meningeal sheaths blend

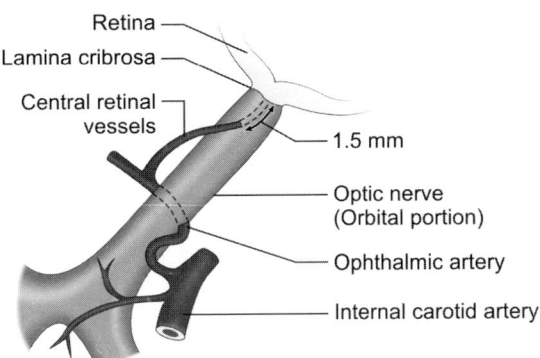

Fig. 4: Optic nerve and central retinal vessels.

anteriorly with sclera. They continue posteriorly with those of brain through optic canal. At the orbital apex it is surrounded by the annulus of Zinn also. Intraorbital portion of optic nerve is supplied by a paraxial system (derived from ophthalmic artery, long posterior ciliary artery, short posterior ciliary artery, lacrimal and central retinal artery before it enters optic nerve) and an axial system of vessels derived from intraneural branches of CRA and the central artery of optic nerve arising from ophthalmic artery.

The dural sheath of optic nerve on its inferomedial surface is *obliquely pierced by central retinal vessels about 12-15 mm behind eyeball.* They cross subarachnoid space and enter optic nerve pass through its axial region to exit at optic disk (Fig. 4).

This crossing of central retinal results across the subarachnoid space around optic nerve is of great surgical importance when we *enucleate the eye with retinoblastoma. During this procedure, it is mandatory to cut the optic nerve at least 10-15 mm behind the eyeball. If the tumor has invaded this part of optic nerve, it is very likely that the tumor had already metastasized to the subarachnoid space.*

But current practice in the treatment of retinoblastoma is salvaging the eyes if possible even in bilateral cases using conservative, eye and vision conserving methods of treatment like brachytherapy, photocoagulation, chemoreduction, thermochemotherapy, thermoradiotherapy, etc.

Intracanalicular Portion (Fig. 5)

Intracanalicular portion of optic nerve occupies the optic canal. It is about *7-10 mm* long. This portion of optic nerve is also covered by meninges and subarachnoid space and containing cerebrospinal fluid (CSF). The dural sheath of optic canal split and the outer layer gets attached to the periosteum. Thus, the optic nerve is free to move in orbit but anchored firmly to optic canal. This bony optic canal occupies sphenoid bone between apex of orbit and cranial cavity. It carries optic nerve from orbit to brain (optic chiasma). Even small

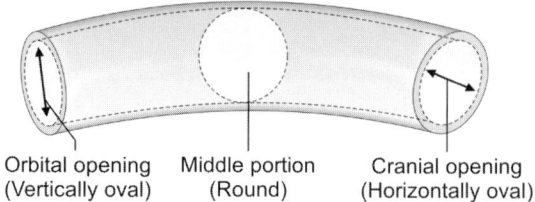

Fig. 5: Optical canal (length and shape)—length = 9 mm, width = 5 mm.

intracanalicular lesions can produce severe compression of optic nerve before they become visible in neuroimaging.

Intracranial Portion

From the posterior opening of the optic canal, the intracranial portion of optic nerve pass into cranial cavity running *posteriorly and medially ascending at an angle of 45° to join the optic chiasma*. In cross-section it is pear shaped, medial side being broader than lateral. It occupies the subarachnoid space of middle cranial fossa in cranial cavity. This portion is about *10 mm long*. It connects the canalicular portion of optic nerve to optic chiasma. Above it is related to olfactory tract and anterior cerebral, anterior communicating artery and inferior surface of frontal lobe of brain. Inferiomedially, it is related to posterior ethmoid and sphenoidal sinuses. Laterally, it is related to internal carotid artery. Intracranial portion is supplied by paraxial system and pial plexus.

VARIATIONS IN THE ARRANGEMENT OF FIBERS IN THE DISTAL AND PROXIMAL PORTIONS OF OPTIC NERVE

Optic nerve fibers arising from various quadrants of retina do not exactly follow the same position and arrangement in the distal and proximal portions of optic nerve, especially macular fibers.

In the distal portion (ocular side) of optic nerve (Fig. 6).

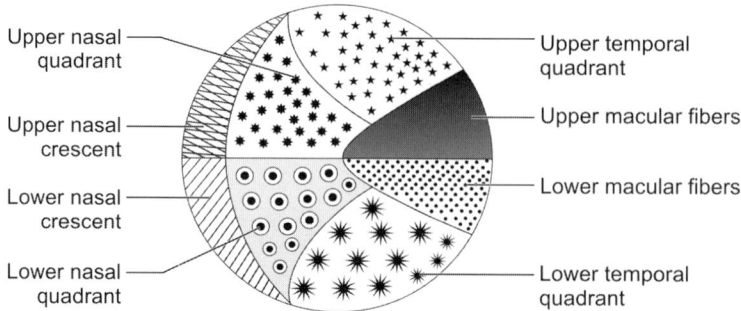

Fig. 6: Distal portion of optic nerve.

Temporal Fibers

- The fibers from upper temporal quadrant of retina (representing lower nasal quadrant of binocular visual field) occupy the upper temporal quadrant of optic nerve.
- The fibers from lower temporal retinal quadrant (representing upper nasal quadrant of binocular field) occupy the lower temporal quadrant of optic nerve.

Nasal Fibers

- The fibers from upper nasal retinal quadrant (contributing lower temporal visual field) stay in the upper nasal quadrant of optic nerve.
- Retinal fibers arising from lower nasal retinal quadrant (representing upper temporal visual field) stay in the lower nasal quadrant of optic nerve.

Macular Fibers

Macular fibers (upper and lower macular fibers) occupy the temporal aspect of optic nerve.

Nasal or Medial Crescent

Nasal or medial crescent: The fibers contributing the temporal uniocular visual field form a nasal or medial crescent in optic nerve.

IN THE PROXIMAL PORTION (CHIASMAL) OF OPTIC NERVE (FIG. 7)

Temporal Fibers

- The fibers from upper temporal quadrant of retina representing lower nasal peripheral field occupy upper temporal segment of optic nerve.

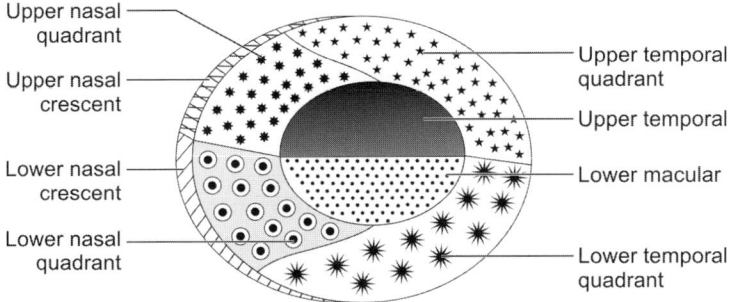

Fig. 7: Proximal portion of optic nerve.

- The fibers arising from lower temporal quadrant of retina contributing upper nasal peripheral field are situated in the lower temporal segment of optic nerve.

Nasal Fibers

- The retinal fibers of upper nasal retinal quadrant representing lower temporal visual field occupy the upper medial part of optic nerve.
- The fibers from the lower nasal retinal quadrant representing upper temporal visual filed occupy the lower medial part of optic nerve.

Macular Fibers

In the proximal part of optic nerve, the macular fibers which were occupying the temporal aspect of optic nerve in its distal portions slowly shift towards the central part. As they approach the chiasma macular fibers come and occupy its medial and distal part.

Temporal crescent fibers representing the temporal uniocular fibers occupy the medial edge of optic nerve.

FUNCTIONS OF OPTIC NERVE

- **Conduction of visual impulses** as action potentials from retina to brain. Visual signals travel faster through thicker and myelinated nerve *fibers at a velocity of about 20 meter per second*. It is less; *about 1 meter per second* in unmyelinated fibers of retinal portion of optic nerve. Functionally optic nerve contains following *types of fibers:*
    - Visual fibers concerned with Vision. Damage to these fibers results in visual loss
    - Pupillary fibers—concerned with pupillary reaction. A conduction block of these fibers due to inflammation, compression and trauma can produce an abnormal pupillary reaction—usually afferent pupillary defect
    - Retinomotor fibers from brain to retina
    - Inter-retinal fibers—commissural fibers between retinae
    - Trophic fibers.
- **Axoplasmic transport:** Axons transport intracellular chemicals, proteins and organelles (mitochondria) along them form cell body to terminal end of axons forwards (orthograde from eye to brain) and backwards (retrograde transport of lysosomes and mitochondria from brain to eye). Forward transport has a slow component carrying proteins and enzymes at a rate of 0.5–3 mm/day, intermediate rate transport of mitochondria and a rapid transport of organelle at a rate of 200–1000 mm/day.

Though the basic mechanism (pathogenesis) of papilledema is controversial it is now considered as mainly due to a blockage and consequent slowing of axoplasmic transport due to elevated CSF pressure resulting in swelling of optic disk and vascular changes on its surface.

SUMMARY OF MEASUREMENTS OF OPTIC NERVE

- *Length*
  - Total length   : 50 mm
  - Intraocular portion   : 0.7–1 mm
  - Intraorbital portion   : 33 mm
  - Intracanalicular portion : 7–10 mm
  - Intracranial portion   : 10 mm

  The intraorbital portion is 8 mm longer than the distance between eyeball and optic canal.

  Central retinal vessels pierce the sheath of optic nerve 12–15 mm behind eyeball.

- *Thickness*
  - Intraocular portion   : 1.5 mm
  - Portion behind eyeball : 3 mm

- *Optic nerve fibers*
  - Optical nerve is made of 1.2 million axons approximately
  - Fibers form about 1000 bundles
  - Each bundles carries 2000 fibers
  - 90% of fibers are 1 mm diameter
  - 10% of fibers are of 2–10 mm diameter
  - Impulses pass about 20 meter per second along myelinated nerve fibers
  - Impulses pass about 1 meter per second along unmyelinated nerve fibers.

CHAPTER 14

Measurements of Optic Chiasma

The intracranial portion of optic nerve of both eyes join together in the shape of a cross (x and hence the name), at the middle cranial fossa to form the optic chiasma. The purpose of this arrangement may be for the hemidecussation of optic nerve fibers that occur in this region result in certain visual advantages. In the chiasma, there is partial decussation fibers from each half of retina—fibers of the nasal half of retina cross over to opposite side (like other crossing tracts of central nervous system) but the fibers from temporal half of retina do not cross. Crossed and uncrossed fibers pass into optic tract. *Thus each optic tract contains optic nerve fibers from ipsilateral temporal retina and contralateral nasal retina producing contralateral hemified of vision* (Fig. 1). This crossing over contributes the following **visual advantages**.
- There is an overlapping of visual fields of both eyes which provide a large area of binocular vision.

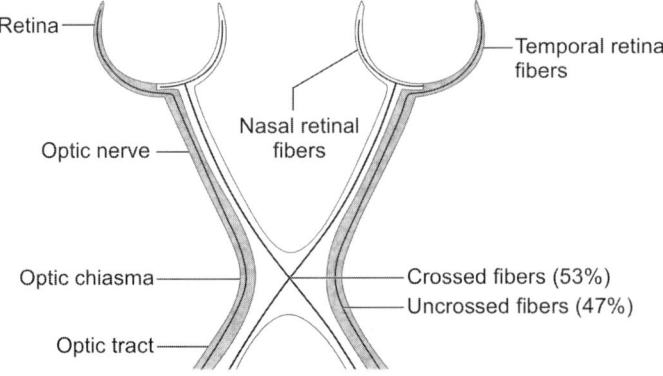

Fig. 1: Course and direction of temporal and nasal retinal fibers in optic chiasma.

- Representation of homonymous retinal halves together in the same cerebral hemisphere.

DIMENSIONS OF OPTIC CHIASMA (FIG. 2)

- *Length of chiasma (in anteroposterior direction) is about 8 mm.*
- *Width (transverse diameter) is 12 mm.*
- *Thickness (vertically) is about 4 mm.*

POSITION OF OPTIC CHIASMA IN THE CRANIAL CAVITY (FIG. 3)

Optic chiasma is situated in the middle cranial fossa. It overlies the diaphragma sellae, *which is a circular fold of dura (8 mm long and 11 mm wide)* that forms the roof of sella tursica (a concavity or cavern over the body of sphenoid in which pituitary gland is situated). The diaphragm separates pituitary gland

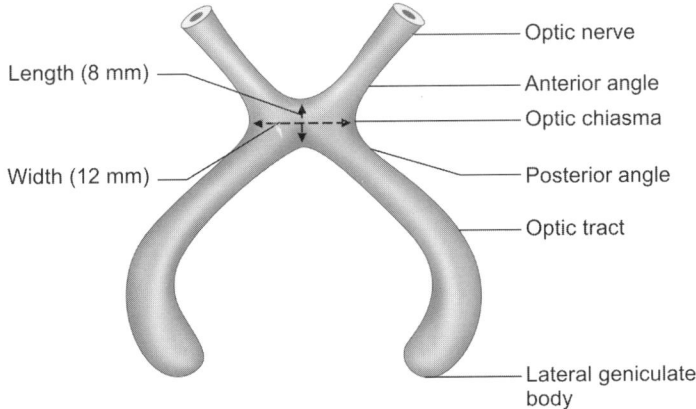

Fig. 2: Portions and dimensions of optic chiasma.

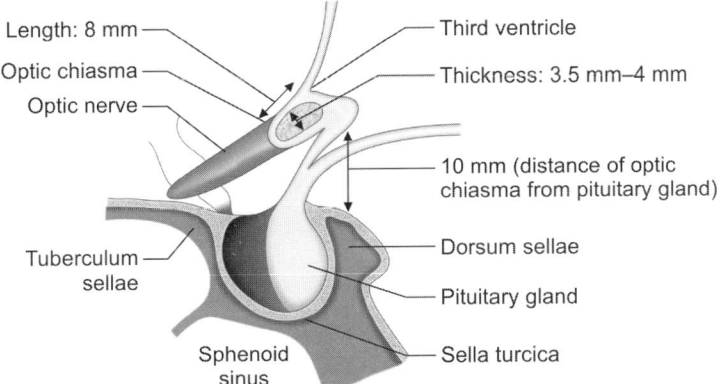

Fig. 3: Position, direction and angulation of optic chiasma in relation to pituitary gland and sella.

from suprasellar cistern and is penetrated by pituitary stalk. *Optic chiasma is not in contact with diaphragm, but lies in the basal cistern of subarachnoid space containing CSF and is separated from diaphragma sellae by 4 mm and from body of sphenoid by a variable distance of 0–10 mm.*

Optic chiasma is directed 45° obliquely from horizontal level in the direction of inclination of optic nerve. It is thus, concave anteriorly and directed downwards, forwards and towards the anterior clinoid process.

Optic chiasma is situated about *10 mm above pituitary gland.* Hence, only lesions large enough to fill this space (the inferior chiasmatic cistern) only can press on chiasma and produce visual field defects.

RELATIONS OF OPTIC CHIASMA

Structures under the chiasma (inferiorly) are:
- Diaphragma sellae—interpeduncular cistern separates the chiasma from diaphragma sellea by about 4 mm
- Pituitary body
- Sella turcica—anterior part of cavernous sinus and oculomotor nerve
- Sphenoidal air sinus in the body sphenoid bone is anterior and inferior to chiasma. Sphenoidal sinuses form the inferior relation only when they sufficiently extend posteriorly into the body of sphenoid.

On either side of chiasma (Fig. 4)
- Anterior perforated substance
- Internal carotid arteries

Anteriorly: Optic chiasma forms part of anterior and inferior wall of third ventricle between two thalami. Chiasma projects into 3rd ventricle and is in direct contact with cerebrospinal fluid (CSF) (chiasmatic cistern). Anteriorly chiasma is related to anterior cerebral and anterior communicating arteries. Aneurysms arising from them can press on the chiasma or one or both optic nerves.

Posteriorly: It is related to interpeduncular fossa and cerebral peduncles. Tuber cinereum to which infundibulum of pituitary gland is attached, is

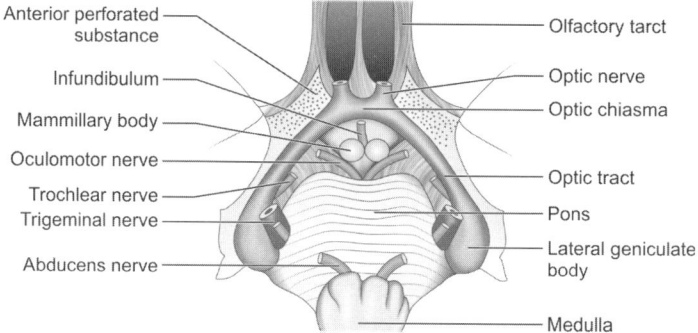

Fig. 4: Optic chiasma and its relationship with structures of inferior surface of brain.

immediately behind optic chiasma. It is also related to infundibular recesses of third ventricle.

Superiorly (Fig. 5): Above the chiasma is the third ventricle into which it projects. Thus, it is related to thalamus (supraoptic recess of third ventricle) and hypothalamus. So chiasma is very liable to get compressed or stretched by tumors of third ventricle or raised intraventricular pressure of internal hydrocephalus.

Middle Cranial Fossa

Middle cranial fossa (Fig. 6) is bordered anteriorly by the posterior border of lesser wing of sphenoid, anterior clinoid process and anterior margins of sulcus chiasmaticus. Posteriorly, it is bounded by superior borders of petrous part of temporal bones and dorsum sellae of sphenoid bone.

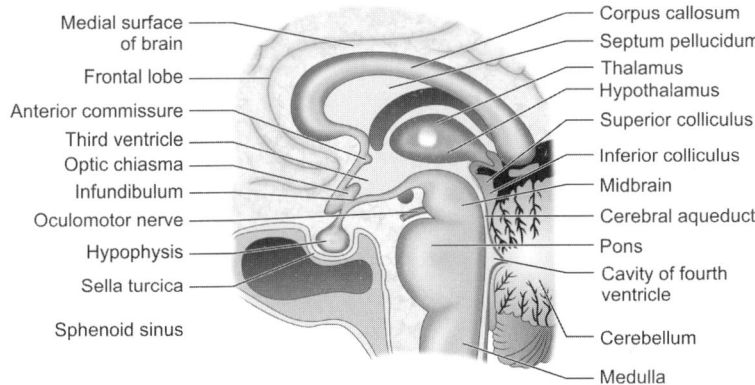

Fig. 5: Relations of optic chiasma (sagittal section of brain).

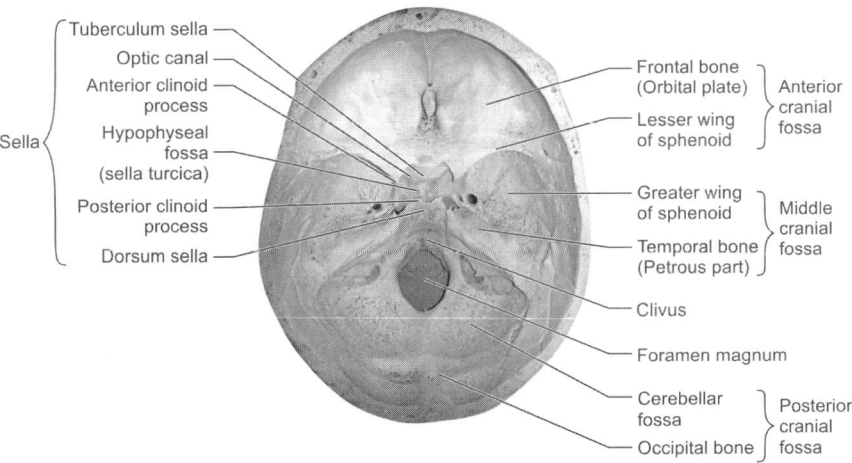

Fig. 6: Cranial fossae and sella. (*For color version, see Plate 5*)

Lateral borders of middle cranial fossa are formed by squamous part of temporal bone, frontal angles of parietal bones and greater wings of sphenoid.

The center of the floor of middle cranial fossa is narrower and is formed by the body of sphenoid. Anteriorly, this part is bordered by the groove formed by optic chiasma—*sulcus chiasmaticus*. This sulcus does not lodge optic chiasma and the latter lies above and behind it.

Sella Turcica, Pituitary Gland and Optic Chiasma (Fig. 7)

Behind the sulcus chiasmaticus, the upper surface of body of sphenoid is shaped like a Turkish Saddle—*Sella Turcica* which carries the pituitary gland. There is a prominence on the anterosuperior wall of sella—*Tuberculum sellae*. The groove for optic chiasma, sulcus chiasmaticus lies just anterior to tuberculum sellae. Optic foraminae are situated on either side of it. The posterior border of the lesser wing of sphenoid is prolonged medially on either side as anterior clinoid processes.

Behind tuberculum sellae, the surface of sella is hollowed to form the hypophyseal fossa which lodges the *hypophysis cerebri (pituitary gland)*. The floor of hypophyseal fossa forms the roof of sphenoid sinus. Cavernous sinus lies lateral to the fossa. Posterior to hypophyseal fossa is a square-shaped plate of bone which projects upwards and forwards—*dorsum sellae*.

On either side, the superolateral angle of dorsum sellae expands to form the *posterior clinoid process* which projects laterally and upwards. Radiologically, this segment of bone is about *1 mm thick*. It is posterior concavity merges with clivus. *An abnormal erosion of dorsum sellae is of great pathological significance.*

Lateral to sella turcica, the body of sphenoid has a shallow groove for internal carotid artery as it runs forwards from foramen lacerum. There is a small elevation on the anterior part of medial edge of carotid groove—middle clinoid process.

Thus, the portions of sella are:
- Tuberculum sellae ⎫ anteriorly
- Anterior clinoid process ⎭

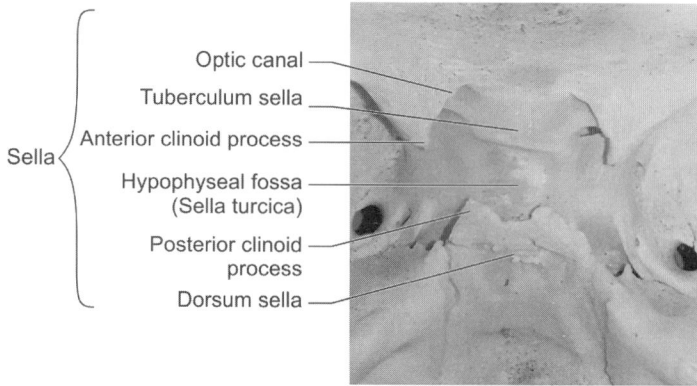

Fig. 7: Portions of sella. (*For color version, see Plate 6*)

- Pituitary fossa   Centrally
- Dorsum sellae   ⎫
- Posterior clinoid process ⎬ Posteriorly

MEASUREMENTS OF SELLA

Measurements of sella (Fig. 8) may help in:
- Diagnosis and assessment of intrasellar expanding lesions
- Determination of direct effect and erosion of sella from lesions of neighboring structures.

Diameter of sella: Anteroposterior diameter of sella is the distance between tuberculum sellae and dorsum sellae. The average diameter is 10 mm. Normally, the distance between anterior clinoid processes is greater than the distance between post clinoid processes.

Depth of sella: Is the greatest distance between floor of hypophyseal fossa and a line drawn between top of tuberculum sellae and dorsum sellae. It is about 8 mm.
- *Area of sella* is 843 mm^2
- *Volume of sella* is 594 mm^3

Pituitary gland occupies about 75% of the volume of sella. Considerable enlargement of pituitary gland can only produce recognizable ophthalmic and imageological signs.

VARIATIONS IN THE RELATIONSHIP OF OPTIC CHIASMA TO SELLA TURCICA AND PITUITARY GLAND

The optic chiasma lies directly above pituitary gland and diaphragma sellae in most patients. However, it may be located more posteriorly or anteriorly. This variability in position helps to explain the range of visual field defects seen in patients with tumors in this area.
- *Normal:* In 80% of persons the chiasma is above the pituitary gland and projects back on dorsum sella. This is the normal position (Fig. 9).
- *Prefixed:* In 15% of cases intracranial portion of optic nerve is short and chiasma lies anteriorly over the tuberculum sellae. Then chiasma is prefixed (Fig. 10).

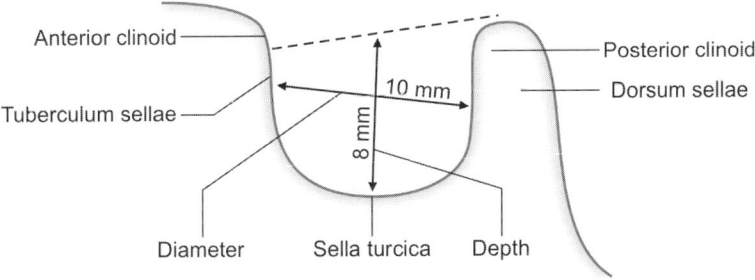

Fig. 8: Dimensions of sella.

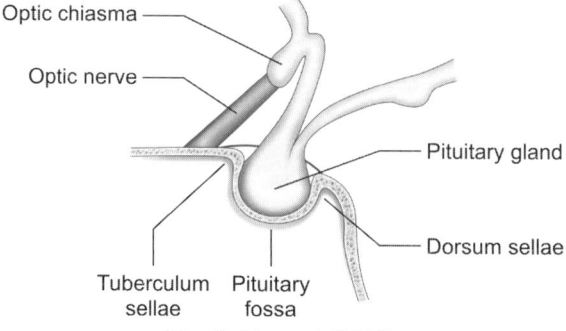

Fig. 9: Normal (80%).

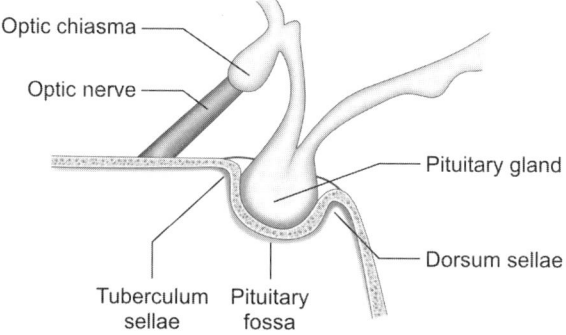

Fig. 10: Prefixed (15%).

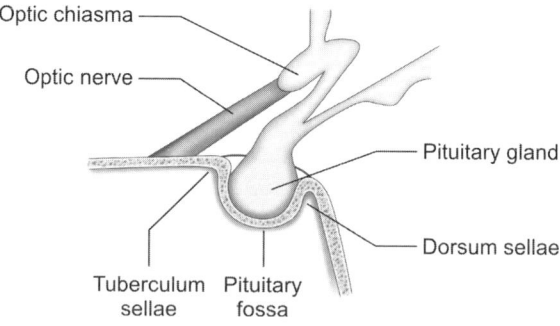

Fig. 11: Postfixed (5%).

- *Postfixed:* In 5% of individual intracranial portion of the optic nerve is longer and so the chiasma is placed far back over the dorsum sellae and posterior clinoids posterior to fossa. This chiasma is postfixed. Then distance between tuberculum sellae and anterior margin of chiasma increases to about 7 mm (Fig. 11).

  In compression of chiasma, pre and postfixed chiasma can lead to bizarre type of field defects. This can be misleading. These changes in positions of chiasma are also important in the surgical approach to this region.

ARRANGEMENT OF FIBERS IN OPTIC CHIASMA (FIG. 12)

Peculiar arrangement of fibers in chiasma produce characteristic visual field defects in lesions in and around it. Involvement of neighborhood structures induce characteristic symptoms also.

About **55% of the optic nerve fibers cross at the chiasma**, as the nasal retina contains more ganglion cells than temporal retina. *The ratio of crossed to uncrossed fibers is about 53:47.* This high percentage of crossed fibers contribute a large temporal crecent in the visual field. Therefore, *the temporal visual field is 60–70% larger than nasal visual field.* This is a result of the *monocular crescent*, representing extreme nasal retina which has no counterpart in the temporal retina of the other eye.

The crossing and uncrossing fibers of optic nerve fibers begins to separate from each other at the termination optic nerve with chiasma (anterior angle of chiasma).

Temporal (Uncrossed) Fibers

The optic nerve fibers from superior and inferior retinal quadrants of temporal retina (temporal hemiretina) run backwards through optic nerve to optic chiasma along its lateral part as a flattened band *without crossing to the optic tract of same side.*

Nasal (Crossed) Fibers

However, fibers from nasal half of retina cross over to opposite side. But this is not in a straight way. Again, the fibers from superior nasal quadrant of retina behave differently from those of inferior nasal quadrant, before they cross over to opposite optic tract in the following fashion.

- **Fibers from inferior nasal retinal quadrant** run in the anterior part of chiasma and the most anterior of these instead of entering optic tract of opposite side straight, *loop anteriorly to the proximal part of contralateral optic nerve for a distance of about 3 mms* [lower opposite anterior (LOA)], then run backwards to chiasma and cross over to the medial part of

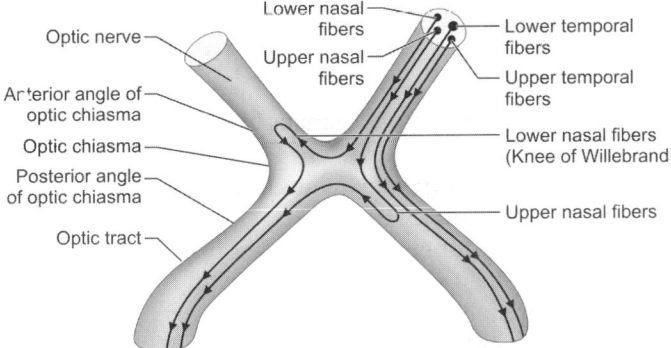

Fig. 12: Arrangement of fibers in optic chiasma.

contralateral optic tract. These fibers which loop anteriorly mingle with optic nerve fibers, parallel to the nerve axis form a characteristic interlacing network called **knee of Willebrand**. These fibers usually cross in the lower part of chiasma.

In compressive lesions of proximal part of optic nerve (as pituitary adenoma) these anterior loop of fibers from contralateral optic nerve are also involved resulting in involvement of the temporal and nasal halves of visual fields of same eye and upper temporal quadrant portion of visual field of opposite eye (Traquair junctional scotoma).

- **Fibers from superonasal retinal quadrant,** first run backwards into lateral aspect of chiasma. The most lateral of them instead of crossing directly to optic tract of opposite eye, *loop backwards (posterior loop) into the optic tract of same side, for about 1–2 mm come back to chiasma and then cross over to contralateral (superomedial aspect) optic tract* [(Upper-posterior same side (UPS)]. A lesion in optic tract at this level can produce incongruous, homonymnous hemianopia.

The crossing nasal optic nerve fibers from macula separate from non-crossing temporal fibers running upwards and backwards decussate in the posterior part of chiasma (a little chiasma within chiasma—Traquair). This portion of chiasma is related to supraoptic recess. A lesion in this portion of chiasma can produce a **central bitemporal hemianopic scotoma.**

COMMON LESIONS AFFECTING OPTIC CHIASMA

- Tumors: 25% of all intracranial tumors occur in chiasmal regions and half of them produce visual loss as the first symptom. Common tumors are:
  - Pituitary tumors : 50%
  - Craniopharyngioma : 25%
  - Meningioma : 10%
  - Gliomas : 7%
- Inflammations : Chiasmal arachnoiditis
- Demyelination
- Vascular lesions : Especially aneurisms
- Injuries

VISUAL FIELD DEFECTS IN CHIASMAL LESIONS

The causes and nature of visual field changes in lesions of various portions of chiasma are as follows:
- **Lesions primarily effecting anterior angle of chiasma (at the optic nerve chiasmal junction)** produce (Figs. 13A to C):
  - Extensive field defects or total blindness of ipsilateral (homolateral) eye
  - Upper temporal field defect of contralateral eye (superior quadrantanopia or Traquair junctional scotoma) due to involvement of crossed, ventral fibers of contralateral eye or
  - Contralateral hemianopia

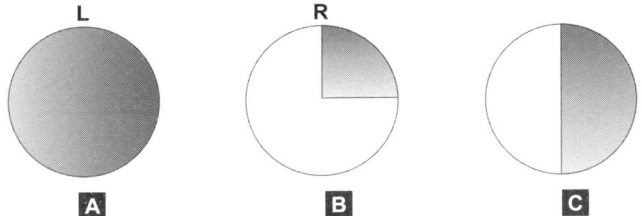

Figs. 13A to C: Field defects in lesions at optic nerve chiasmal junction (R). (A) Ipsilateral blindness; (B) Contralateral superior quadrantanopia (Traquair junctional scotoma); (C) Hemianopia.

- **Central (medial) part of optic chiasma** is involved (sagittal lesions) in (Fig. 14):
  - Pituitary adenoma
  - Craniopharyngiomas
  - Aneurysms
  - Meningiomas
  - Dysgerminomas (ectopic pinealomas)
  - Trauma

Lesions at this level producing damage of midline fibers of chiasma result in bitemporal field defect. It may be peripheral, central or both with or without macular splitting.

The field defect usually starts in the upper outer quadrant in pituitary adenoma (Fig. 15). If pressure continues, it damages the inferior nasal quadrant of chiasma, then superior nasal quadrant. The field loss then crosses midline. In right eye field defect progresses clockwise and in left eye counterclockwise. This is called *Walkers field loss*. Field defects resulting from tumors may be asymmetric and relative in tumors but absolute in those due to trauma.

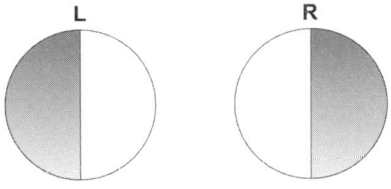

Bitemporal hemianopia

Fig. 14: Field defects in lesions affecting the central (medial) part of chiasma.

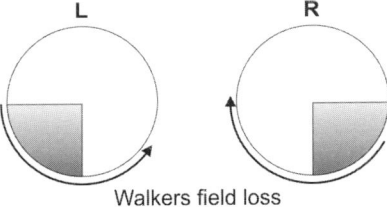

Walkers field loss

Fig. 15: Walkers cycle in progressive pituitary adenoma.

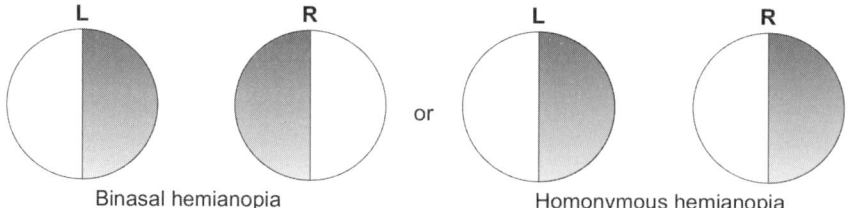

Fig. 16: Field defect in lesions affecting lateral aspects of chiasma or tract chiasmal junction.

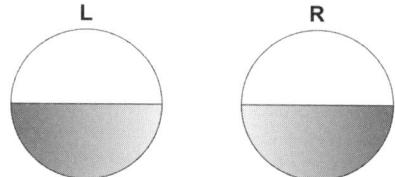

Fig. 17: Inferior altitudinal hemianopia.

- **Lesions of lateral aspects chiasma or tract chiasmal junction or posterior angle of chiasma (Fig. 16)** is usually caused by:
  - Tumors
  - Sclerotic carotid arteries.

  They press on the uncrossed temporal fibers and produce binasal hemianopia or homonymous hemianopia like lesions.

- **Pressure on chiasma from above or below can produce altitudinal hemianopia (Fig. 17).**

  Superior part of chiasma is affected (suprachiasmatic) by:
  - Meningioma of olfactory groove. It involves one eye completely producing ipsilateral blindness and affects crossed fibers of fellow eye leading to loss of temporal field of that eye.
  - Meningioma of tuberculum sellae damage the anterior angle of chiasma leading to junctional scotoma.
  - Meningioma of lesser wing of sphenoid produces irregular and asymmetric field defects.
  - Aneurism of anterior cerebral and anterior communicating artery produce bitemporal hemianopia.
  - Carniopharyngioma and dilatation of third ventricle from posterior cranial fossa tumors affect the posterior superior aspect of chiasma and produce bitemporal hemianopia.

- Meningitis and optochiasmatic arachnoiditis are perichiasmatic lesions enveloping chiasma leading to bitemporal or binasal or homonymous hemianopia.

  Aneurysms of internal carotid artery may be subclinoid aneurisms occurring within the cavernous sinus or supraclinoid aneurysms occurring above cavernous sinus lead to field loss, oculomotor and trigeminal nerve palsies.

- Glioma of chiasma and infections affecting the interior of chiasma (**intrachiasmatic lesions**) and produce bizarre type of bitemporal hemianopia.

CLUES FOR CLINICAL SUSPICION OF CHIASMAL LESIONS

- Any unexplained visual loss without obvious changes in the eye or its media can be due to chiasmal lesion. Loss of visual acuity is a common sign of pituitary tumors.
- Chiasmal lesion usually involves both the eyes.
- Field loss: Monocular or bitemporal or binasal hemianopia. Bitemporal hemianopia is the most common field defect in chiasmal involvement.
- Any type of visual loss with endocrine dysfunction—amenorrhea, galactorrhea, impotence, infertility, Cushing syndrome, acromegaly.
- Assoiciated ocular nerve palsies.

CHAPTER 15

Measurements of Eyebrows

Eyebrows are thick elevations of skin covered with bushy hairs supported by muscles and aponeurosis, and situated at the junction of upper eyelids and forehead. It is considered as the upper boundary where "Clinical Eye" starts.

DIMENSIONS OF EYEBROWS (FIG. 1)

Position and shape of eyebrow must be assessed before oculoplastic surgeries on eyebrows like correction of brow ptosis and blepharoplasty.
- *Shape:* Eyebrows of both eyes together make the shape of a bow. Medial end of each eyebrow is below the level of upper orbital margin. Then it follows the orbital margin. Laterally, it again curves upwards and outwards above the orbital margin.
- *Length:* Average length of eyebrow is about *6.7 cm*. There is no difference in length between right and left eyebrows. Males and females have almost the same eyebrow length.
- *Breadth:* Breadth of medial end of eyebrow is about *1.4 cm;* middle portion *1.2 cm;* lateral end *0.2 cm*.

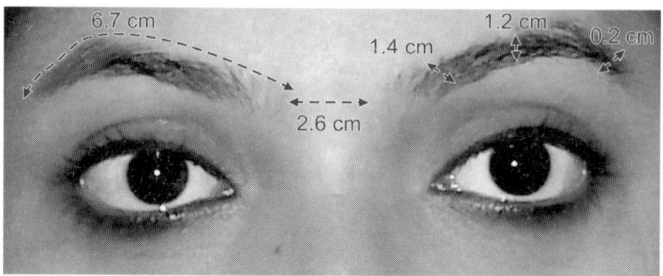

Fig. 1: Shape, length, breadth and the distance between two eyebrows.

- *Distance between eyebrows* of two eyes is about *2.6 cm*.
  Between two eyebrows there is a prominence which is smooth and hairless —glabella (glaber means hairless)
- The distance between the middle of the lower margin of eyebrow and the middle of the upper margin of upper lid is about *1.5 cm*, when eye is open and *2.5 cm* when eye is closed. This measurement has to be considered during correction of ptosis and lid reconstruction surgeries to attain good cosmetic acceptance.

LAYERS OR STRUCTURE OF EYEBROWS (FIG. 2)

Anatomically and morphologically eyebrows are considered as part of scalp. Eyebrows have the following layers:
- *Skin:* As different from skin of eyelids (very thin), the skin of eyebrows is *thick* and rich in sebaceous and sweat glands.
- *Subcutaneous fibrous tissue layer:* This layer of eyebrow is almost free of fat. At this level skin and muscles of eyebrows fuse and so move together as one layer.
- *Muscle layer:* The muscles of eyebrows are:
  - *Frontalis:* Anterior end of frontalis muscle shares in the formation of eyebrows which become continuous upwards to the forehead. It is inserted into the skin of eyebrow. There is no bony attachment. Frontalis is supplied by facial nerve. *It elevates the eyebrow directly and eyelid indirectly (synergist of levator palpebrae superioris). This function of frontalis is utilized in the correction of ptosis when there is no levator action (frontalis sling surgery).*
  - *Orbicularis oculi:* The upper portion of this muscle (muscular superciliaris) also forms the part of eyebrow.
  - *Corrugator supercilii:* It is deep to frontalis and orbicularis. It arises from the medial end of superciliary ridge and inserted into deep surface of skin of medial part of eyebrow. It pulls the medial end of eyebrow to the root of nose producing a vertical furrow (frown).

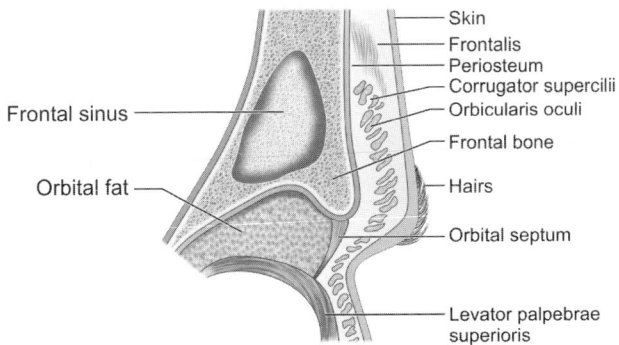

Fig. 2: Structure (layers) of eyebrow.

Procerus muscle: When it contracts, along with orbicularis oculi and corrugator supercilii it depress the eyebrow. It also produces horizontal creases at the root of nose and glabellar lines.

- *Submuscular areolar tissue layer:* It is between muscles of eyebrow and galea aponeurotica. Since there is no attachment of orbicularis to orbital margin free movement of eyebrow is possible.

There is a pad of fat under eyebrow. It is situated above the superior orbital margin. It facilitates the eyebrow movements. This fat layer can be send into the upper lid due to ageing and hereditary factors giving a fullness of the eyelid.

FUNCTIONS OF EYEBROWS

- Eyebrows prevent the flow of sweat from forehead to eyes.
- In very bright light which produces glare, eyebrows protect the eyes from excess light entering the eye by drawing the brows down and depressing the upper lid.
- In diffuse illumination, eyebrow allows more light to enter the eye by elevating the eyebrow and upper lid by contraction of frontalis.
- Muscles of eyebrows are sometimes considered as "secondary muscles of accommodation" since they act when vision is strained and control the amount of light entering the eye from above.
- Eyebrows contribute to facial expressions. The muscles of eyebrows are used for expression of mood and feeling.

CLINICAL SITUATIONS INVOLVING EYEBROWS

- Eye strain, frontal and occipital headaches are sometimes due to excessive contraction of frontalis (including the region of eyebrow) and occipitalis in persons who perform prolonged near work without correcting refractive error and muscle in balance.
- *Loss of eyebrow hairs (madarosis)*
  Eye brows are lost in:
  - Leprosy (Fig. 3)
  - Tuberculosis of the skin of eyelids
  - Hypothyroidism
  - Injuries
- *Brow ptosis (Eyebrow descent):* It is drooping of eyebrows. It usually occurs in old age and is probably due to involutional loss of underlying elastic tissues of eyebrow and skin changes of forehead. It can follow dermatochalasis also. Browptosis produce not only cosmetic problem (looking older than actual age) but also chronic blepharitis, dry eye, lateral hooding of skin and lash ptosis leading to deffective vision, feild effect and decrease contrast sensitivity. Treatment is surgical correction by browplasty or upper lid blepharoplasty.

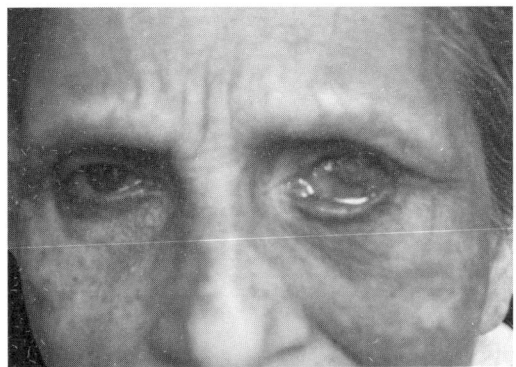

Fig. 3: Loss of eyebrow hairs in leprosy. (*For color version, see Plate 6*)

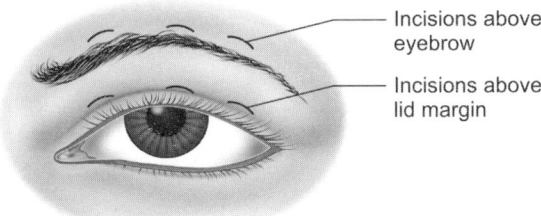

Fig. 4: Ptosis correction by frontalis (brow) suspension.

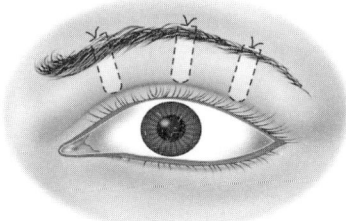

Fig. 5: Double-armed sutures are passed from tarsal plate to frontalis.

- *Ptosis surgery:*
    - Ptosis correction by frontalis (Brow) suspension
    - Double armed sutures are passed from tarsal plate to frontalis
    - Frontalis muscle portion of eyebrow is often utilized (when there is poor or no levator action) in elevating upper lid in ptosis correction by anchoring tarsal plate to frontalis muscle—**Brow suspension (Figs. 4 to 10).**

Steps of Frontalis Sling (Brow Suspension) Surgery for Correction of Ptosis

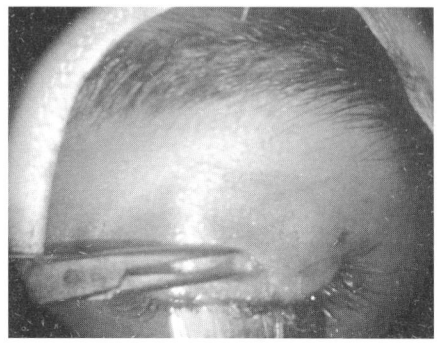
Fig. 6: Incisions above lid margin (muscle deep).

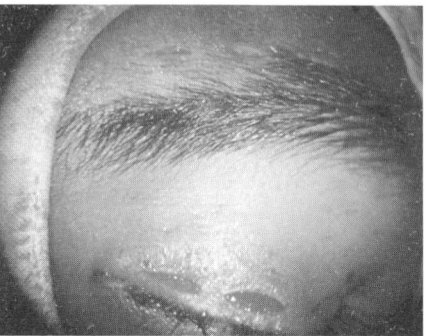
Fig. 7: Incisions above eyebrow (muscle deep).

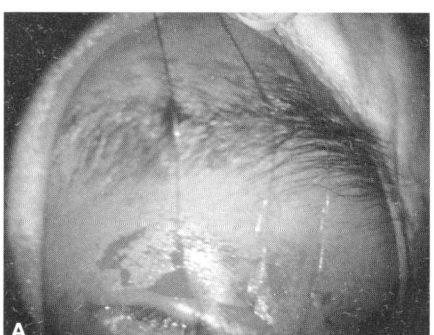
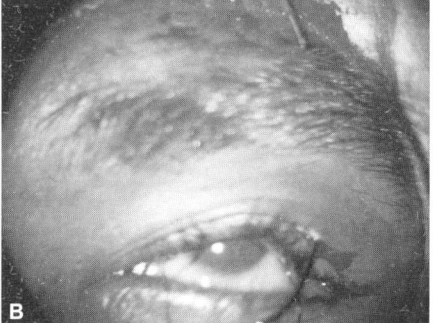
Figs. 8A and B: Three double-armed sutures passed from tarsal plate through submuscular space and anchored to fontalis muscle.

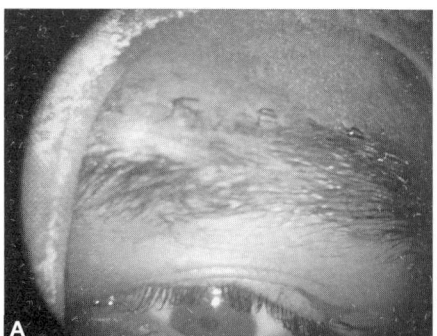
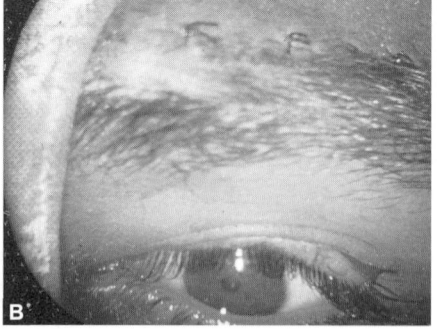
Figs. 9A and B: Sutures tied to frontalis muscle and skin closed at completion of surgery (ptosis corrected).

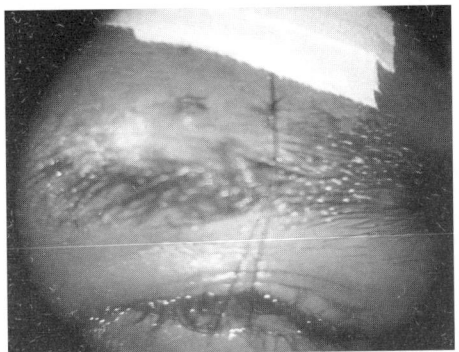

Fig. 10: Frost suture to protect cornea.

CHAPTER 16

Measurements of Eyelids

Eyelids—"the protective curtains" of eyeballs are mucocutaneous folds enclosing muscles, nerves, blood vessels, glands, etc. The upper and lower lids slightly differ in their measurements, structure and functions.

GROSS MEASUREMENTS OF UPPER LID

Upper lid probably starts near the lower margin of eyebrow.
Length of upper lid is about 3.8 cm. Breadth is around 2.4 cm, when eye is closed and 1.5 cm when open (Figs. 1 and 2). Thickness of lid is approximately 1.5 mm. The lid margin is broader about 2 mm in breadth.

STRUCTURE OF UPPER LID

Structural components of upper lid are to a great extent continuation of those of forehead and upper part of orbit. A good awareness and understanding of these structures and their measurements is important in management of disorders of upper lid. Clinically, the upper eye lid is considered to have two portion; the upper *preseptal* (orbital) portion and the lower *pretarsal* portion.

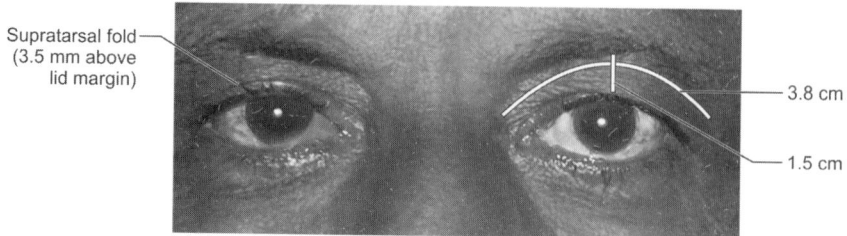

Fig. 1: Length and breadth of upper lid (eye open).

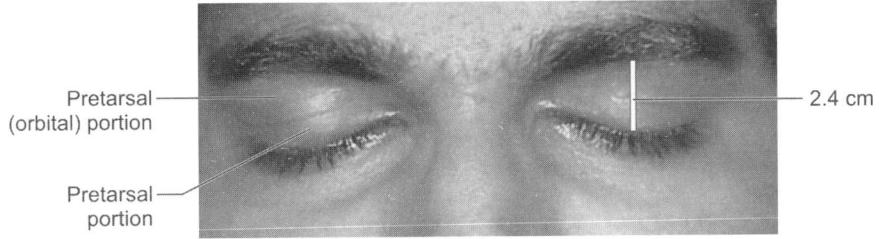

Fig. 2: Breadth of upper lid (eye closed).

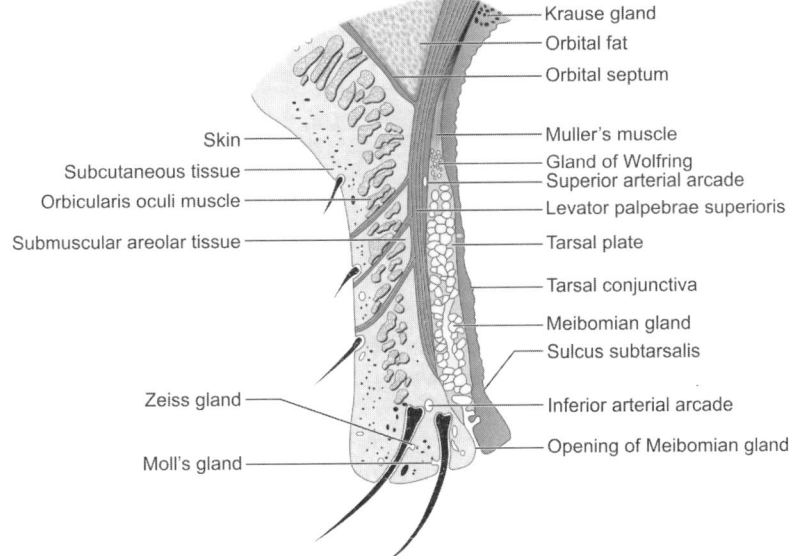

Fig. 3: Structure of upper lid.

The component tissues are arranged loosely preseptal portion. So fluid can collect in its potential space leading to lid edema. In the pretarsal portion, the tissues are almost attached to underlying tarsus.

There are about *10 component* structures in eyelid from surface to depth (Fig. 3).

- *Skin:* Skin of upper lid extends from eyebrow to anterior margin of lid. The skin of upper eyelid is thinnest compared to other parts of body, due to the thin dermis and the absence of fat in subcutaneous tissue. It becomes slowly thicker towards eyebrow. Skin is loose but firmly attached to the underlying structures at lid margin and eyebrow. One or more attachments of levator aponeurosis to the skin produce horizontal folds, most prominent of which is situated *5–7 mm* above lid margin. In ptotic eyelids, their presence indicate some levator muscle function. Absence of lid fold in oriental races is due to the lower attachment of levator aponeurosis.

The skin of eyelid has fine hairs, sebaceous glands and sweat glands. But at the lid margin the hairs of the skin become long, thick, curved outwards

and arranged in two rows as eyelashes. *Upper eyelid has about 100–150 eyelashes and lower lid has about 50–75.* The glands in relation to the eyelashes are also larger compared with other parts of eyelid. The large sebaceous glands of eyelashes are called Zeiss glands and sweet glands are called Moll's glands. The functions of eyelashes are as follows:
- To protect eye from large airborne particles
- They are very sensitive to touch which induces sudden blink reflex.
- **Subcutaneous areolar tissue layer:** This layer is fat free and is loosely adherent to the underlying orbicularis oculi muscle.
- **Orbicularis oculi (Fig. 4):** This striated sphincter muscle of eyelid has an orbital and palpebral portion.
  - **Orbital portion:** Cover the rim of orbit and is used for forced closure of eyelid in certain facial expressions.
  - **Palpebral portion:** It has three smaller parts:
    - Preseptal part: Overlies the orbital septum. It originates from fascia overlying lacrimal sac (lacrimal fascia) and runs back to posterior lacrimal crest.
    - Pretarsal part: Lies over tarsal plate, it arises from posterior lacrimal crest and anterior limb of medial canthal tendon, runs laterally to join the lateral palpebral raphe and insert into the periorbital of lateral orbital tubercle.
    - Muscle of Riolan: It is the smallest striated muscle of our body, a part of orbicularis oculi, is situated in lid margin.

The terminal fibers of levator aponeurosis pass between the orbicularis muscle fibers at the junction of preseptal and pretarsal portions and is inserted into the skin to produce the skin folds of upper lid.
- **Submuscular areolar tissue:** This layer is a sheet of tissue between orbicularis oculi and tarsal plate. Nerves and blood vessels of eyelid run in this layer. A local anesthetic is injected into this layer to produces analgesia and akinesia of lids, during lids surgeries. This layer produces a gray line in lid margin between eyelashes and openings of Meibomian glands. Lid can be split into an anterior musculocutaneous layer and a posterior tarsoconjunctival layer during plastic reconstructive surgeries of lids and tarsorrhaphies.

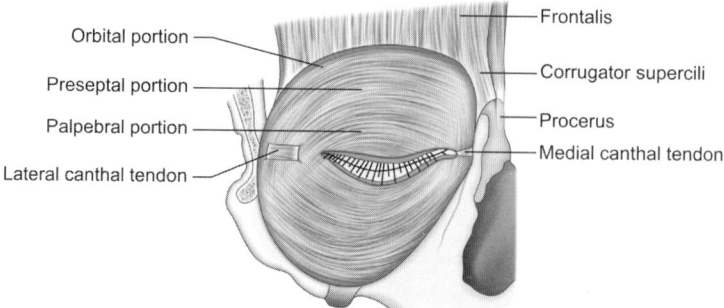

Fig. 4: Orbicularis oculi muscle and related muscles of facial expression.

- **Orbital septum:** It is a thin fibrous tissue sheet stretched across orbital margins and forms a barrier between orbit and anterior structures of eyelid. It retains orbital fat and prevent its prolapse into eyelid. The septum originates peripherally from the orbital margins at the junction of periosteum and periorbita. Centrally, it gets attached to many palpebral, orbital and lacrimal structures; mainly to the upper border of upper tarsus and lower border of lower tarsus. In the upper lid it forms a sheet behind the posterior surface of preseptal portion of orbicularis oculi. *It fuses with the aponeurosis of levator muscle about 10–12 mm above the level of upper border of tarsus,* where it ends and can be identified as a white roll of tissue, *superior transverse ligament of Whitnall* situated approximately at the level of equator of globe. This is an important guide to identify levator muscle from other structures during *ptosis surgery* (Fig. 5).
- **Preaponeurotic pad of fat:** Orbital fat forms a layer in the upper part of eyelid. This is a wedge-shaped portion of orbital fat which extends forwards and downwards between levator and orbital septum. *It is an important landmark for identification of levator muscle during its resection by skin approach.* This pad of fat has a yellow colored central portion and white colored nasal portion. During surgery this central yellow portion has to be distinguish from the adjacent prolapsed lacrimal gland. Then latter is firm, pink and glandular in appearance.
- **Levator palpebrae superioris muscle:** This muscle elevates the upper lid. The muscle originates from the periorbita of lesser wing of spheniod above annulus of Zinn and runs forwards under roof of orbit above superior rectus. It enters the lid just anterior to the level of superior rectus insertion. Once it passes the level of superior rectus tendon, it bends down and descends posterior to orbital fat wedge. After that it become less muscular,

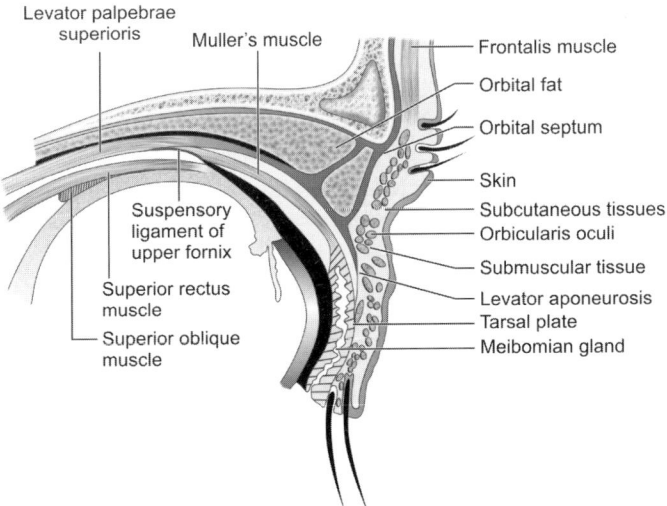

Fig. 5: Structure of upper eyelid and related structures of upper portion of orbit and face.

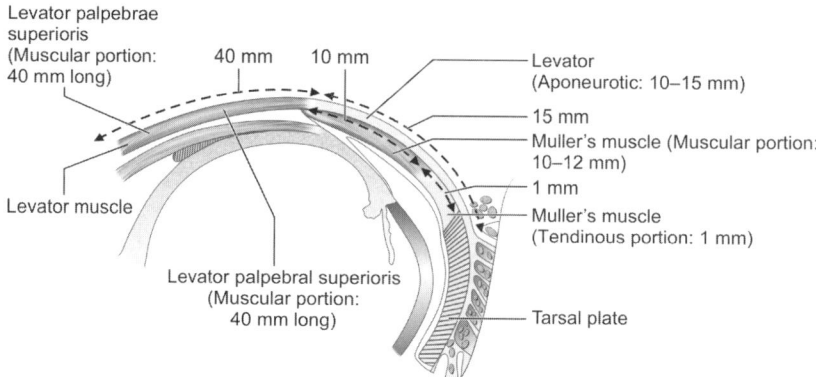

Fig. 6: Dimensions of levator and Muller's muscle.

then tendinous—the levator aponeurosis. As the muscle enters the lid a small ligament extends from its inferior surface to upper conjunctival fornix and suspends it. This is called the suspensory ligament of upper fornix. Levator palpebrae superioris has two portions mainly (Fig. 6):
- *The muscular (Striated portion) of levator is about 40 mm long*
- *Tendinous (aponeurotic portion) is about 10-15 mm* long and has a width of 30-35 mm.

In levator resection we are mainly concerned with the terminal portion of striated muscle and the central portion of aponeurosis. The aponeurotic portion runs downwards and forwards and divides above the level of upper border of tarsus into several portions and get attached to the following five structures.
- *Attachment to skin:* The anterior thin fibers of aponeurosis pass between prespetal and pretarsal portions of orbicularis muscle to get attached to skin and produce the superior lid skin folds of upper lid.
- *Attachment to anterior surface of tarsus:* The posterior thicker portion of LPS aponeurosis runs down and gets inserted into anterior surface of *tarsal plate 3-4 mm below its upper border.*

The tendon then fans into medial and lateral horns.
- *Medial horn gets attached to upper border of posterior limb of the medial canthal tendon.*
- *Lateral horn, thicker than medial gets attached to the superior edge of the lateral canthal tendon.*
- **Conjunctival fornix:** Connective tissue fibers from the sheath of levator muscle and superior rectus muscle are attached to the superior conjunctival fornix.
- **Muller's muscle:** It is a small thin strip of muscle made of nonstriated muscle fibers. Muller's muscle *arises from the under surface of the muscular (striated) portion of levator from the level of about 40 mm* from its origin and become aponeurotic. About *10-12 mm above superior border of tarses,* Muller's muscle leave the posterior surface of levator aponeurosis, run

downwards behind it (loosely adherent to it) and gets inserted into upper border of tarsus by a *tendon of 1 mm* length. The levator aponeurosis is anterior to Muller's muscle and conjunctiva behind it. Muller's muscle is supplied by sympathetic nerve fibers from cervical sympathetic chain reaching the muscle around its blood vessels. *Though the upper lid elevation is mainly by the levator action, the height of lid margin is adjusted by Muller's muscle. It contributes about 2-3 mm of elevation of upper lid.*
- Length of Muller's muscle : 10–12 mm
- Thickness of Muller's muscle : 0.5 mm
- Length of Muller's muscle tendon : 1 mm

- **Fibrous layer of eyelids (Fig. 7):** It provides structural framework to the eyelids. The fibrous layer extends almost to the entire length and breadth of eyelids. Its thickness varies in different portions. The component structures of fibrous layer are:
  - **Tarsal plates:** It form the thickest central portion
  - **Orbital septum:** It forms the thinnest peripheral portion between tarsal plates and orbital margins
  - **Medial and lateral canthal tendons** (Palpebral ligaments)—by which tarsal plates are anchored almost near the middle of medial lateral orbital margins.
  - **Tarsal plates:** They give shape and strength to eyelids. They are stiff plates of dense fibrous tissue and contain the Meibomian glands almost in their middle depth.
- Tarsal plate of upper lid (Fig. 8): Tarsal plate of upper lid is shaped and like an inverted boat, upper border is convex and lower border almost straight. *The length of upper tarsal is about 25–29 mm. Width is about 9–10 mm at the middle which is the widest part. Thickness is 1 mm.*
  - **Upper border** is thin. The structures attached to the upper border are:
    - Orbital septum: Tarsal plate becomes continuous with the orbital septum except where it is pierced by levator.
    - Mullers muscle

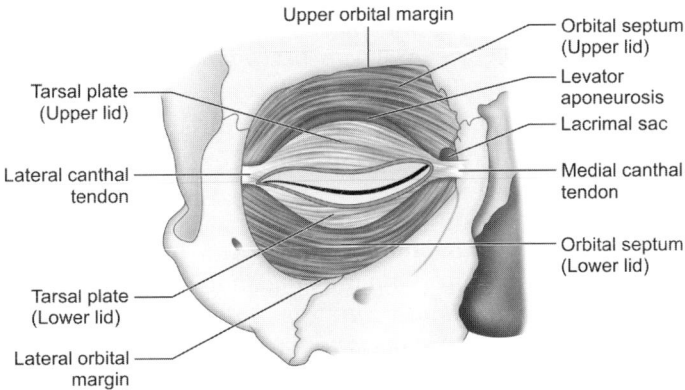

Fig. 7: Fibrous layer of eyelids.

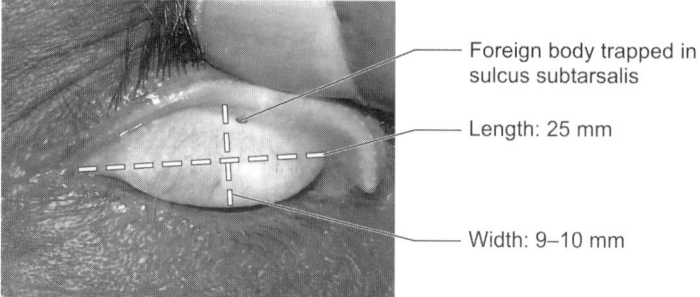

Fig. 8: Length and breadth of tarsal plate of upper lid (everted).

- *Lower border*: Lower border of tarsal plate is thicker than upper and becomes part of cilary portion of eyelid margin.
- *Anterior surface*: Anterior surface of tarsal plate is convex. The major portion of LPS aponeurosis gets attached to anterior surface of tarsal plate starting about *3–4 mm* from its upper border. Areolar tissue separates the anterior surface from orbicularis occuli to facilitate movement of tarsal plate. Between upper *3–4 mm* of tarsal plate and levator aponeurosis is the *pretarsal space*. This is a useful surgical landmark. It is occupied by the peripheral arterial arcade.
- *Posterior surface*: Posterior surface is concave conforming to the convexity of apex of eyeball. *Just above the lid margin, the posterior surface of tarsal plate is more concave and has a horizontal groove, sulcus subtarsalis in which foreign bodies may get trapped.*
- **Tarsal plate of lower lid (Figs. 9 and 10)** is smaller and thinner than upper lid. Its shape is also slightly different from that of upper lid. *While upper tarsus is D shaped; lower is bean shaped. The lower border of lower tarsus is less convex than upper border of upper tarsus. The length of lower tarsus is 25 mm (upper lid 29 mm) and width or height of lower tarsus is 4–5 mm (upper lid 10 mm). Thickness is 0.75 mm. Laterally tarsal plate is attached to the lateral orbital tubercle of orbit by lateral canthal tendon. Medially tarsal plate is attached to anterior and posterior lacrimal crests through anterior and posterior portions of medial palpebral ligament. Structures attached to the lower border of tarsal plate of lower lid are:*
  - Orbital septum
  - Inferior palpebral (Tarsal) muscle
  - Capsulopalpebral fascia
- **Orbital septum - refer back**
- **Medial and lateral canthal tendons (Palpebral ligaments):** *Tarsal plates start laterally from a point 7 mm from the middle of lateral orbital margin and end at the level of about 9 mm from anterior lacrimal crest medially (almost at the level of lacrimal puncta). Then the medial and lateral extremities of tarsal plates get attached to (join) the orbital margin by means of medial and lateral palpebral ligaments respectively.*

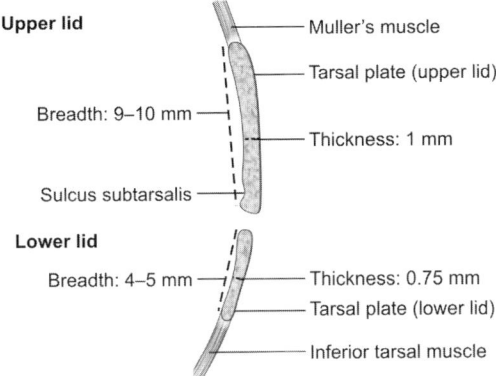

Fig. 9: Dimensions of tarsal plates.

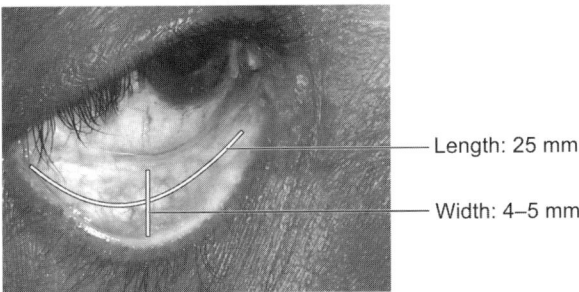

Fig. 10: Length and breadth of tarsal plate of lower lid.

- **Medial palpebral ligament** is attached to the maxilla between anterior lacrimal crest and the suture between frontal process of maxilla and nasal bone. The ligament is triangular in shape. Its base is at the anterior lacrimal crest where divides into:
    - Posterior portion becoming continuous with the lacrimal fascia covering the upper portion of lacrimal sac.
    - Anterior portion divides into two bands (Y-shaped) at medial canthus, cross lacrimal fascia and join the medial end of tarsal plates. A vertical incision made *2 mm* from medial canthus in this structure can thus expose the lacrimal sac. Above it is continuous with periosteum and below pass some fibers of orbicularis. Clinical significance of medial canthal tendon are:
        - In surgeries of lacrimal sac (dacryocystectomy and dacryocystorhinostomy) the MPL form an important landmark for skin incision and for the identification of the sac.
        - Fracture and lateral displacement of medial wall of orbit can result in traumatic telecanthus, rounding and disfigurement of medial canthus which may require surgical reconstruction and reattachment of medial canthal tendon.

- **Lateral palpebral ligament:** It is about *7 mm* long and *2.5 mm* broad, less thicker and less prominent than medial palpebral ligament. Its medial end becomes continuous with the lateral extremities of tarsal plates and the lateral end is attached to the lateral orbital margin (orbital tubercle). Clinical importance of lateral palpebral ligament (LPL) are as follows:
  - *Lateral cantholysis:* During reconstructive procedures of large defects of eyelids, relaxation and mobilization of lateral aspect of lid may necessitate cutting (lysing) of the crus of lateral canthal ligaments. *This will facilitate almost 5 mm mobilization of lateral aspect of lid medially helping the closure of the lid defect.*
  - *Fracture of lateral wall of orbit* (zygomatic fracture) can result in downward displacement of lateral canthus and globe and will require surgical reduction of zygomatic fracture for its correction.
- **Palpebral conjunctiva:** This is the most posterior layer of upper lid. The lower portion of palpebral conjunctiva is attached firmly to posterior surface of tarsal plate. But the upper portion is loosely attached to the Mullers muscle.

PALPEBRAL FISSURE (FIG. 11)

Palpebral fissure is the space between margins of upper and lower lid. It has the shape of a flattened 's'; Curve being concave upwards in its central part. Palpebral fissure is widest and more curved at the junction of its medial and central third.

Length: Length of palpebral fissure is about *30 mm (25–30 mm)*.

Width (height): It is around *9–10 mm* at its widest portion in primary position of gaze (Males 7–10 mm: females 8–12 mm).

In blepharophimosis, the length of palpebral fissure is reduced to a variable extent from *8–22 mm* and width *2–5 mm*.

Free margin of lids are about *25–30 mm* long and *2 mm* broad. The lacrimal punctum is situated on an elevation (lacrimal papilla) at the junction medial 1/6th and lateral 5/6th of lid margin.

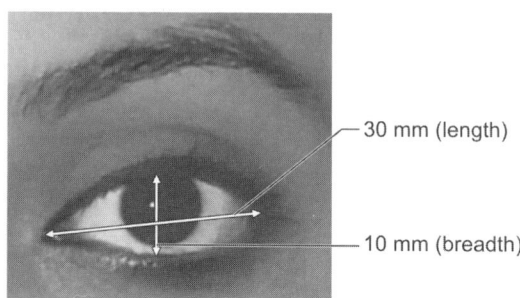

Fig. 11: Dimensions of palpebral fissure.

RELATIVE LEVELS OF MEDIAL AND LATERAL CANTHI (FIG. 12)

The extreme ends of palpebral fissure are called canthi (angles). *Lateral canthus is normally 1-2 mm above the level of medial canthus* and this measurement must be kept in mind during ptosis correction. In Mongolian races lateral canthus is even more at a higher level than normal. A relative lower level of lateral canthus in normal persons is often considered as a sign of beauty.

Canthal Angle

Normal canthal angle is about 60°. It becomes abnormal in most of the diseases which produces ptosis or lagophthalmos.

Normal Intercanthal Distance, Telecanthus (Fig. 13)

Normal distance of medial canthus from midline is about *15 mm*. Thus, the normal distance between two medial canthi (intercanthal distance) is *30 mm*. The normal interpupillary distance is *60 cm*. An increased distance between two medial canthi *(wide intercanthal distance) with normal interpupillary distance is called telecanthus (Fig. 14)*. This may be associated with epicanthus and is usually bilateral. This condition can occur in:
- Craniofacial syndromes such as Waardenburg syndrome
- Trauma: Leading to severe fracture of medial wall of orbit. Traumatic telecanthus is usually unilateral. When it becomes symptomatic it may require surgical correction.

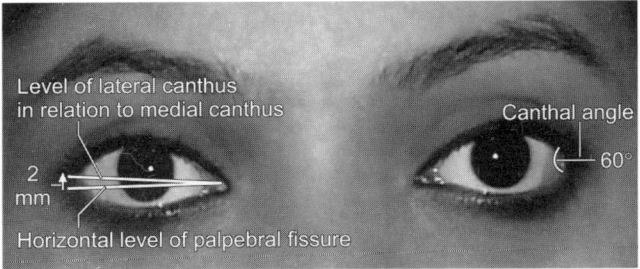

Fig. 12: Relative levels of medial and lateral canthi.

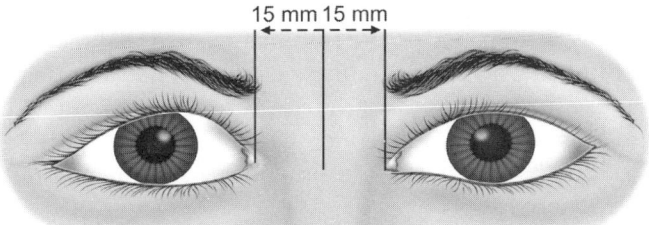

Fig. 13: Distance of medial canthus from midline.

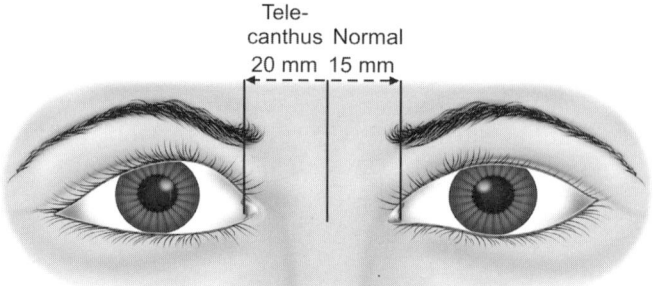

Fig. 14: Unilateral (right) telecanthus (Traumatic).

Muscles Involved in Upper Lid Elevation

The main elevators of upper lid are levator palpebrae superioris and Muller's muscle. But there is some assistance from frontalis, superior rectus, and suspensory ligament of Whitnall. *The normal range of excursion of upper lid from extreme down to upgaze is about 15-20 mm.* Of this:
- Levator palpebrae superioris (LPS) contributes about *15 mm;* but variable of this 2 mm is due to the help from superior rectus muscle to which it is attached posteriorly.
- Muller's provides about *2 mm* of elevation which adjusts the height of upper lid and width of palpebral fissure.
  - Frontalis helps around *5 mm* of lid elevation by lifting eyebrow in extreme upgaze.

Measurement of Levator Action and Upper Lid Excursion

- The normal width of palpebral fissure is about *15 mm* at its widest portion
- If the width is at least *6-8 mm* on looking from down to up (after elimination of action of frontails), the levator action is good
- The LPS action is weak if it is less than *5 mm.*

The specific contribution of levator in the excursion of upper lid (levator action) is assessed only after elimination of action of frontalis muscle (Fig. 15). Patient is asked to look down and keep the head steady without any movement. The examiner fixes the frontalis muscle of patient by applying the thumb of one hand horizontally over the eyebrow pressing it firmly. Then patient is asked to look upwards slowly to the maximum. The range of excursion of lid margin from down to upgaze is measured with a mm ruler held on the other hand. This measurement will give the amount of levator action and function.
- Levator action is good if the lid excursion is *8 mm* or more.
- Levator action is fair if the lid excursion is about *5-7 mm.*
- Levator action is poor if the lid excursion is *4 mm* or less.

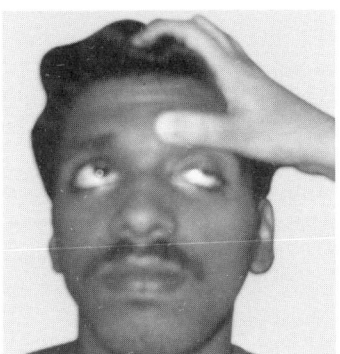

Fig. 15: Assessment of levator action.

MEASUREMENTS OF PTOSIS

Normally upper lid margin covers (at the level) the superior *1.5–2 mm* portion of cornea in straight gaze. In this position of eye, if upper lid covers more than *2 mm* of superior cornea the lid is ptotic.

The severity of ptosis can be measured in two ways.
- *From the difference in the width of palpebral fissure* between normal and ptotic eye (in unilateral ptosis cases)(Figs. 16 A to C)
  - Mild ptosis: : The difference is only *2–4 mm*
  - Moderate ptosis : The difference is *4–7 mm*
  - Severe ptosis   : The difference is more than *7 mm*.
- *From the difference between marginal reflex distance (MRD)* of two eyes in unilateral ptosis and from the difference between MRD measurement and normal values in bilateral ptosis (Fig. 17).

The upper lid margin is normally at the level of about midway between upper border of pupil and upper limbus. MRD is the distance between the middle of lid margin and the central corneal (light) reflex on throwing light into eye when the eyes are in primary position of gaze. MRD can be measured from upper lid margin (MRD1) and lower lid margin (MRD2) to the central corneal reflex. Total of the two MRDs in mm will give the height of palpebral fissure.

Measurement of MRD is important in grading the severity of ptosis and for guiding and planning of ptosis surgery.

Patient is asked to look straight to a distant object; surgeon sitting with his (her) eye at patient's eye level and shows a lighted torch to the center of cornea and measures the distance between central lid margin and central corneal light reflex with a mm ruler.

MRD 1 is the distance between the middle of upper lid margin and central corneal light reflex. It is normally about *4–4.5 mm*. In unilateral ptosis, the degree of ptosis is the difference between the MRD 1 in ptotic eye and normal eye. In bilateral ptosis the measurement of ptosis is the difference between MRD measurements in ptotic eyes and normal value.
- If the difference is about *2 mm* ptosis is mild.
- If the difference is around *3 mm* ptosis is moderate
- If the difference is more than *4 mm* ptosis is severe.

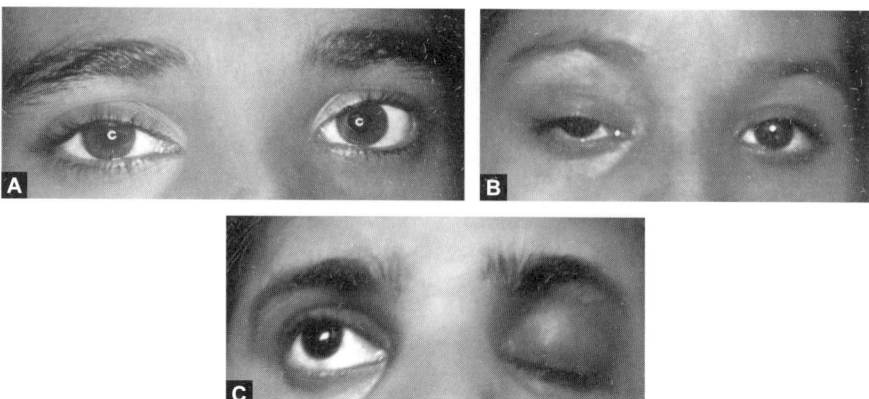

Figs. 16A to C: (A) Mild ptosis right upper lid; (B) Moderate ptosis right upper lid; (C) Severe ptosis left upper lid.

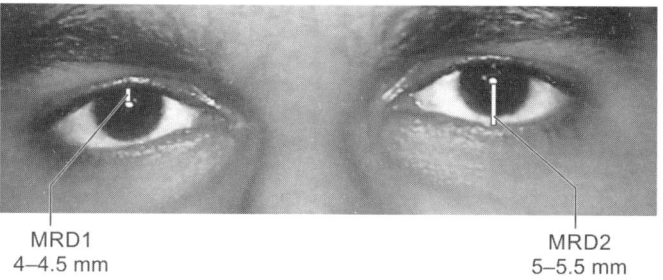

MRD1
4–4.5 mm

MRD2
5–5.5 mm

Fig. 17: Marginal reflex distance (MRD).

MRD 2 is the difference between central corneal reflex and the middle of lower lid margin. Normally, it is about *5–5.5 mm*.

General guidelines regarding the length of levator resection to be done in surgical correction of ptosis
- Surgery on levator palpebrae superioris for correction of ptosis is considered only if there is some levator action and function.
- *Fasanella-Servat* operation (partial resection of LPS) is done for correction of mild ptosis of about **2 mm**.
- Conjunctiva: *Mullerectomy* (Putterman) a modification of Fasanella-Servat procedure (after preoperative testing with phenylephrine eye drops) for mild ptosis (2–3 mm) with good levator action (10 mm) has advantage of lack of skin incision (scar), early healing and predictable results. This surgery can be done for mild ptosis of Horner's syndrome.
- Pleating of LPS is preferred surgery for ptosis of about *4 mm* especially senile ptosis which shows variation with fatigue.
- Levator resection (Blascovics or Everbush's technique) is done for moderate to severe ptosis especially congenital ptosis. *As a general rule:*
    - Resection of 3–4 mm of LPS is expected to raise the upper lid for about 1 mm. At least 10 mm resection should be done in congenital ptosis to get a good result.

- *Resection of about 15–22 mm of LPS is expected to correct the ptosis of 4–7 mm.*
- *Mild congenital ptosis* with fair levator action of about *8 mm or more* and intact aponeurosis, may get corrected by *10 mm* levator resection.
- *Moderate ptosis* with medium levator action requires *12–15 mm* levator resection.
- *Severe ptosis* with poor levator action and function of about *4–5 mm* may get corrected with *18–24 mm* of levator resection.

MEASUREMENTS OF LOWER LID

The structure, function and measurements of lower lid are slightly different from those of upper lid. Anatomically, the lower lid starts probably from the level of inferior palpebral furrow which is about *20–30 mm* below lower lid margin.

Gross Measurements of Lower Lid (Figs. 18A and B)

- *Length* of lower lid is about *38 mm* in males and *35 mm* in females.
- *Width or height* of lower lid is about *20 mm* when eye is closed and *18 mm* when open in both males and females.
- *Thickness* of lower lid is *1.5 mm* and breadth of lid margin is *2 mm*
- *The relationship of lower lid margin to the lower limbus*—normally lower lid margin is at the level of lower limbus, when eye is open and in primary position of gaze. Rarely, it may reach *1 mm* above or below this level.

Structure of Lower Lid (Fig. 19)

Though lower eyelid also has the basic seven-layered structure from skin to palpebral conjunctiva, some layers are different from those of upper lid. Just as few layers of upper lid continue to forehead some structures of lower lid continue to those of midface. Clinically, it is useful to group the component structures of lower lid into three lamellae:
1. Anterior lamella—consisting of skin and orbicularis
2. Middle lamella of orbital septum
3. Posterior lamella of tarsus, lower lid retractors and palpebral conjunctiva.

Layer-by-layer, lower lid structures have the following special features:
- Though *the skin and subcutaneous areolar tissue* of upper and lower lid have almost similar structure as that of upper lid, skin of lower lid become thicker in its lower portions.

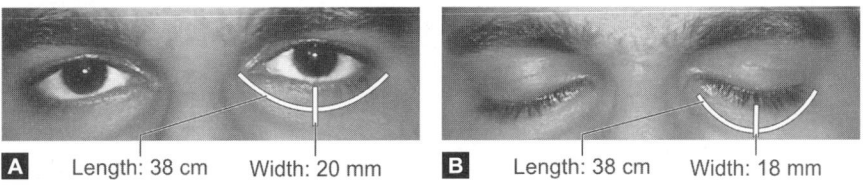

A Length: 38 cm   Width: 20 mm   **B** Length: 38 cm   Width: 18 mm

Figs. 18A and B: Gross measurements of lower lid.

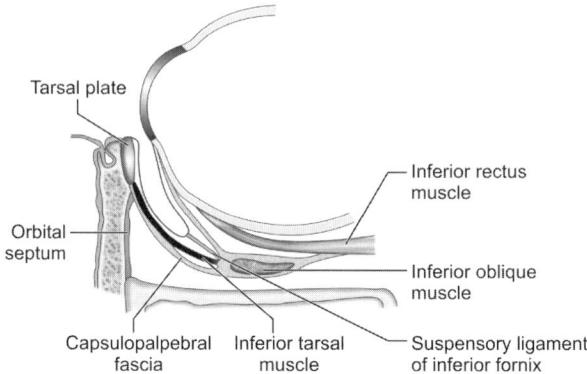

Fig. 19: Structure of lower lid.

- Beneath *the orbital portion of orbicularis oculi muscle* of lower lid is the suborbicularis oculi fat (SOOF) of midface which in turn continues as buccal and malar pad of fat.
- *Tarsal plate of lower lid* is smaller and thinner than upper lid.
- *Lower lid retractors* pull the lower lid downwards during opening of eyes and in down gaze. They form a structural combination which originates from anterior and inferior surface of inferior rectus muscle. They consist of:
  - *Inferior tarsal muscle:* This muscle is a poorly developed smooth muscle corresponding the Muller's muscle of upper lid. The muscle originates from the sheath of inferior rectus muscle. It is inserted into inferior border of tarsus. The activity of this muscle is to pull lower lid down leading to widening of the palpebral fissure.
  - *Capsulopalpebral fascia:* It is the most anterior portion of the fibrous tissue sheet extending from the sheath of inferior rectus muscle. This sheet splits and enclose the inferior oblique muscle as it runs horizontally through the orbit joining on the way to the inferior suspensory ligament (Lockwoods) of globe. It then carries the inferior tarsal muscle slips and finally gets attached to lower border of tarsus. This fibrous sheet is anatomically similar to the aponeurosis of levator of upper lid.
  - *Inferior suspensory ligament of lower conjunctival fornix:* It is another portion of the lower lid retractors. It is the most posterior portion of the fibrous sheath which originates from the anterior surface of inferior rectus muscle and extends anteriorly to get attached to the lower conjunctival fornix.
- *Tarsal conjunctiva* is the most posterior layer of lower lid and is adherent to tarsal plate. It continues inferiorly as inferior fornix and is attached to lower lid retractors.

Lower Lid Movement

Lower lid moves normally about 4–7 mm during opening and closure of eye. Movement of lower lid *precedes upper lid by about 0.2 seconds.*

Lower Lid Retraction

In lower lid retraction, the position of lower lid margin reaches variable distances below the lower limbus. The position of lower lid margin in relation to the limbus is measured from the center of the lower lid margin to the center of pupil (inferior lid margin to pupillary light reflex distance).

The weakness and laxity of lower lid retractors produce lowering and entropion of lower lid (e.g. involutional), which is almost similar to ptosis of upper lid. When the lower lid becomes lax lateral canthal angle become lower than the level of medial canthus.

In lower lid retraction, the lower lid margin will be lower and away from limbus exposing limbus and sclera (scleral show). The MR2 becomes longer. Such lower lid retractions require horizontal shortening of lower lid to avoid lagophthalmos and exposure. This may be done as an isolated procedure or along with ptosis surgery of upper lid.

Steatoblepharon: It is convex bulging of lower lid resulting from attenuation of orbital septum and herniation of lower eyelid pad of fat. Orbicularis oculi weakness and laxity also can produce similar bulging of lower lid.

Surgical Importance of Tarsal Plate

Tarsal plate is the skeleton of eyelids providing it structure, strength and integrity especially lid margins. Thus, tarsal plate becomes the central structure in many surgical procedures of eyelids.

- *Chalazion surgery (Figs. 20A to C):* Chalazion, the chronic inflammatory granuloma of Meibomian gland (situated almost in the center of tarsal plate) often require removal by incision and curettage by opening the tarsal plate. For this a vertical incision is made on the conjunctival aspect of tarsal plate to reach, expose, curette and remove the granuloma, situated within the tarsal plate which is only about *0.75–1 mm* thick.
- *Full thickness lid tear (Fig. 21):* It is surgically repaired by the "three suture technique" using 6-0 silk to attain a good anatomical approximation, to safeguard the structural integrity of lid margin and avoid notching. The three sutures are:
  1. First anchoring suture is applied to lid margin at gray linear tarsal plate using 6-0 black silk.
  2. Second or posterior suture is done near of the posterior lid margin using 6-0 black silk.

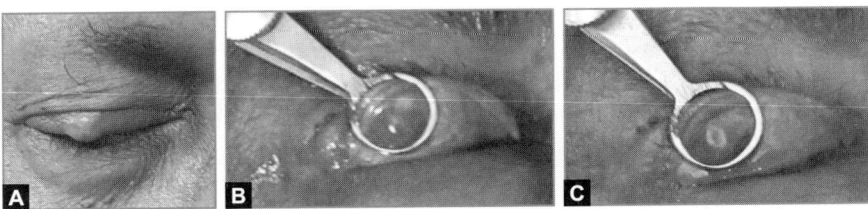

Figs. 20A to C: (A) Chalazion; (B) Lid everted with chalazion clamp to expose the granuloma; (C) Tarsal plate opened for removal of granuloma.
(*For color version, see Plate 6*)

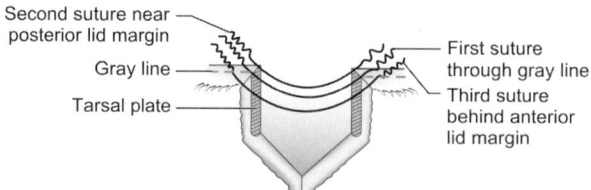

Fig. 21: Repair of full thickness lid tear.

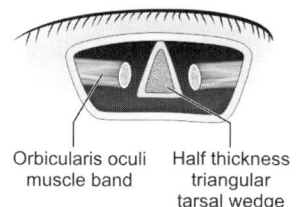

Fig. 22: Correction of entropion lower lid.

3. Third or anterior suture is put just behind the anterior lid margin. Torn margins of tarsal plate are sutured using 6-0 chromic catgat. Torn orbicularis of either side is further joined and strengthened by using interrupted 6-0 plain catgut sutures. Skin wound is closed using 6-0 interrupted black silk switches.

- *Entropion surgery (modified Wheelers operation) (Fig. 22)*
  - In the procedure of surgical correction of entropion especially the involutional type, involving lower lid, a partial thickness resection and removal of a portion of tarsal plate and approximation of the edges by suturing is an important step for strengthening of the lax, long and inturned eyelid.
  - A skin incision is made *3 mm* below and parallel to lower lid margin. By blunt dissection, separation of a *4 mm* broad orbicularis oculi band overlying tarsal plate and orbital septum is carried out to expose tarsal plate. A triangular incision is made on the anterior surface of tarsal plate involving half of its thickness. The base of the triangle is towards the inferior margin of tarsal plate and apex to the lid margin. *The length of the base is assessed from the severity of entropion; usually a 5-7 mm based incision is made. A superficial, half thickness lamellar portion of tarsal plate is dissected and removed.* The margins of the defects in the tarsal plate are approximated and sutured using 6-0 catgut. Over this the orbicularis oculi bands are overlapped, sutured (mattress sutures) and anchored to the lower border of tarsus and orbital septum. Skin incision is closed interrupted 5-0 silk sutures.
- *Ectropion correction surgeries like modified Kuhunt Szymanowski procedure* require removal of a *full-thickness wedge of lower lid in a pentagonal shape* and suturing of defects layer-by-layer including tarsal plate.

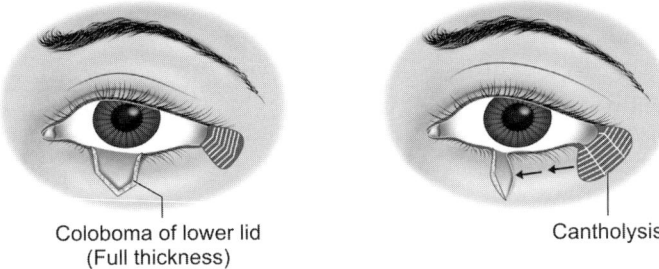

Coloboma of lower lid (Full thickness)   Cantholysis

Fig. 23: Reconstruction of lower lid coloboma after lateral cantholysis.

- *Reconstructions of eyelid colobomas (Fig. 23)*—congenital, traumatic and those following excision of tumors also necessitate the approximation and suturing of *full thickness of tarsal plate*.

FUNCTIONS OF EYELIDS

- Eyelid protects eyeball from injuries, infections and dryness.
- Blinking (frequent momentary closure of eyelids, about 15 times a minute, each lasting for *0.32 seconds*) helps in spread of tears and uniform moistening the ocular surface.
- Lid separation permits vision.
- Lid closure protect eye from excessive light.
- Blinking helps in sucking of tear fluid over ocular surface into lacrimal sac and further emptying into nose (lacrimal pump). 60% of tears enter the lower punctum and canaliculus.

MEASUREMENT OF UPPER LID (GROSS)

- Length : 3.8 cm
- Height (breadth) : 2.4 cm (eye closed)
  : 1.5 cm (eye open)
- Thickness : 1.5 mm
- Breadth of lid margin : 2 mm
- Level of most prominent skin fold : 5–7 mm above the lid margin

MEASUREMENTS OF INDIVIDUAL EYELID STRUCTURES

- *Levator palpebrae superioris muscle*
  - Length of muscular (striated) portion : 40 mm
  - Length of tendinous (aponeurotic) portion : 10–15 mm
- Attachment to tarsal plate: 3–4 mm below upper border of tarsus.
- *Muller's muscle*
  - Length : 10–12 mm
  - Breadth : 10 mm

- Thickness : 0.5 mm
- Tendon : 1 mm long
- Tarsal plate (upper lid)
  - Length : 25–29 mm
  - Width : 9–12 mm (10 mm) at the widest point
  - Thickness : 1 mm
- Tarsal plate (lower lid)
  - Length : 25 mm
  - Width : 5 mm
  - Thickness : 0.75 mm

Measurements of Lacrimal Apparatus

Lacrimal apparatus, the external secretory and drainage system of eye has the following components.

Lacrimal glands which produce 'tear proper' or the aqueous portion of precorneal tear film. They are as follows:
- Main lacrimal gland—has two portions (Fig. 1)
  - Orbital lobe
  - Palpebral lobe
- Accessory lacrimal glands
  - Glands of Krause
  - Glands of Wolfring

Lacrimal passages: Carry whatever excess amount of tears left in conjunctival sac to nose after use for the physiological functions of eye especially eyelids, conjunctiva and cornea. Main parts of lacrimal passages are:
- Lacrimal puncta
- Lacrimal canaliculi/ampullae/common canaliculus

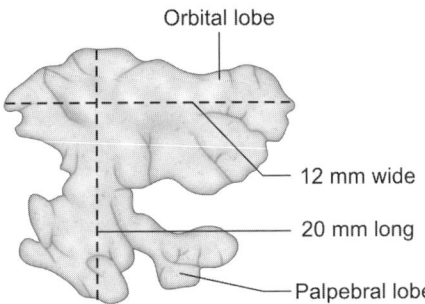

Fig. 1: Dimensions of main lacrimal gland.

- Lacrimal sac
- Nasolacrimal duct.

MAIN LACRIMAL GLAND AND ITS MEASUREMENTS

Main lacrimal gland is situated under the roof of orbit at its anterior and outer corner. *The gland is about 20 mm long, 12 mm wide and 5 mm thick.* It has the shape of a bean, flattened from above.

Lateral edge (horn) of levator palpebrae superioris muscle runs across the anterior surface of the gland, grooving it deeply into an orbital and palpebral portion (lobes) connected by a glandular bridge.

Orbital Lobe

Orbital lobe is situated under the periorbita of anterior and lateral portion of orbital plate of frontal bone, where the bone is smooth, little concave and is called fossa *glandulae lacrimalis*. This portion of gland extends to the lateral most part of orbit up to the frontozygomatic suture and is attached to the fossa by multiple ligaments. Its anterior border is almost sharp, parallel to orbital margin but within it.

- Anterior relations (Fig. 2) of the gland from surface to depth are skin, orbicularis oculi, orbital septum and outer horn of levator muscle.
- Posteriorly, the gland is round and in close relation to orbital fat.
- Superiorly, it is related to periorbita of orbital plate of frontal bone.
- The inferior relation is to the sheath of levator. The under surface of the gland is in close relation to the eyeball.
- Medial end of gland lies on the levator muscle
- Laterally, it extends to the lateral rectus muscle and tied down to periorbita.

Palpebral Lobe

Palpebral lobe is situated under the aponeurosis of levator palpebrae superioris muscle and project beyond orbital margin into the upper and outer part of superior conjunctival fornix. This is the only portion of lacrimal gland which

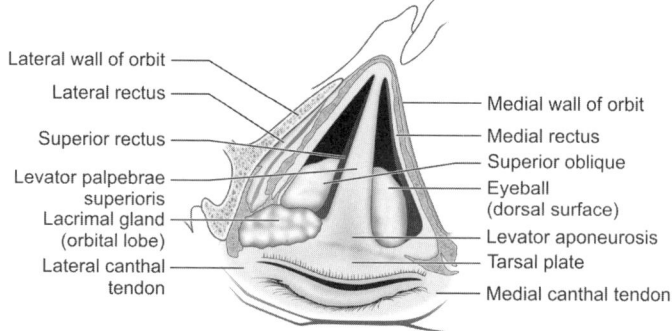

Fig. 2: Relation of orbital portion of lacrimal gland.

can be seen outside as a small swelling in this region in normal persons (Fig. 3). *Palpebral lobe has only half the size of orbital lobe and consists only of a few lobules situated along the duct of orbital portion.*

Lacrimal secretion from lacrimal gland is drained by about *12–14 ducts, 2–5 of them from orbital lobe and 6–8 from palpebral lobe.* The small tear collecting ducts are first intralobular then become extralobular. These then join to form a *dozen of ducts* which run close together and open separately into the upper and outer *conjunctival fornix about 4–5 mm above upper border of upper tarsus.*

ACCESSORY LACRIMAL GLANDS

The tears are not produced entirely by main lacrimal gland but by accessory lacrimal glands also. Thus, even if the main lacrimal gland is diseased, absent congenitally or removed surgically as for lacrimal gland tumors, accessory lacrimal glands secretion can still maintain the physiological functions of tears to a certain extent. Accessory lacrimal glands are:

- *Glands of Krause:* Which are situated in the deeper layers (adenoid layer) of conjunctival fornices. There are about *20 glands in upper lid and 8 glands in lower lid.* They drain their secretions by ducts into the fornices.
- *Glands of Wolfring:* They are small glands situated just above the border upper of tarsus.

Plica and caruncle also have a few rudiments of accessory lacrimal glands.

Functions of Tears

- Tears provide oxygen and nutrition to cornea
- It lubricates ocular surface facilitating movements of lids and globe
- Tears keep eye moist and wet
- It creates a smooth anterior surface for light transmission and refraction for the eye.
- Tear fluid protect eye from injuries and infections due to the bacteriostatic activity of lysozyme present in it.
- Washes away the dust and irritants from ocular surface.

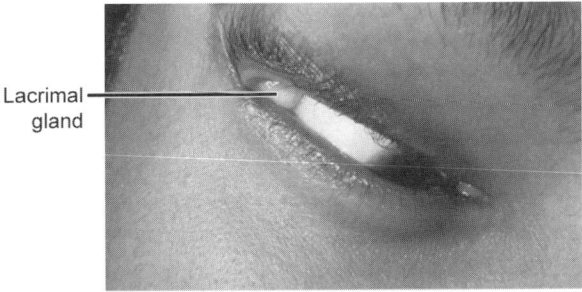

Fig. 3: Palpebral lobe of normal lacrimal gland visible in the upper and outer conjunctival fornix. (*For color version, see Plate 6*)

LACRIMAL PASSAGES AND THEIR MEASUREMENTS

Lacrimal passages carry tears from conjunctival sac to nose. The passages have following portions.

Lacrimal Puncta (Fig. 4)

The lacrimal passages start from oval or round openings called lacrimal puncta situated on *posterior surface of each lid margins about 6 mm* from the medial canthi. *The punctum is about 0.25–0.3 mm in diameter. It can be dilated three times of this size using punctum dialator for surgical purposes,* due to the presence of a ring of elastic tissue around it. The punctum is situated on a pale elevation called lacrimal papilla. Upper punctum is more nearer to the medial canthus than lower. Both face towards bulbar conjunctiva. Diseases which produce their eversion can cause epiphora. *During closure of eye, puncta are drawn 2–3 mm towards medial canthus due to contraction of orbicularis oculi.*

Lacrimal Canaliculi (Fig. 5)

Lacrimal puncta leads to lacrimal canaliculi which form the second portion of lacrimal passages. They carry tears from puncta to lacrimal sac. Each canaliculus has three smaller portions:

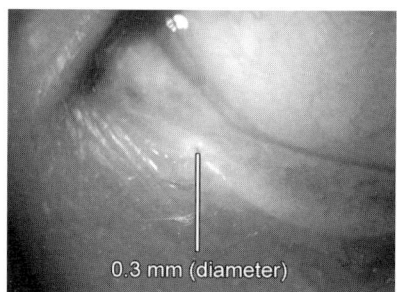

Fig. 4: Lacrimal punctum.

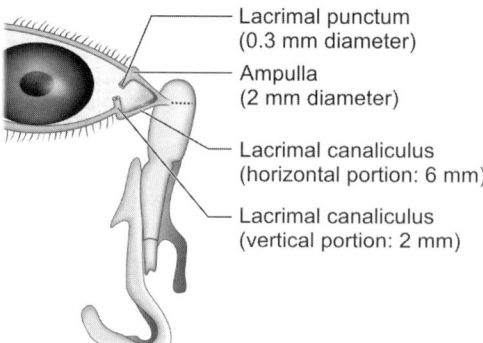

Fig. 5: Dimensions of lacrimal passages (from punctum of canaliculus).

1. *Vertical portion:* It is about *1.5–2 mm in length.* This part of canaliculus is surrounded by a portion of orbicularis oculi (Horner's muscle) and acts as a sphincter.
2. *Ampulla:* The vertical portion leads to a slight dilated portion called ampulla before canaliculus become horizontal. *The ampulla is about 2–3 mm in its longest diameter. It participates in the pumping of tears.*
3. *Horizontal portion:* is directed medially and is about *6–7 mm long.* Lower is slightly longer than upper.

   Vertical portion makes almost *90° angulation* with the horizontal portion. The first 3–4 mm of the horizontal canaliculus is very superficial (lying just under the palpebral conjunctiva). The upper canaliculus lies about 2 mm above posterior margin of upper lid. The lower canaliculus is situated about 2 mm below the posterior margin of lower lid. The last 3 mm of the horizontal portion lie deep in the tissues of lid. They pass through lacrimal fascia before they make entry into the sac. *The points of entry are about 2–5 mm below the fundus of the sac on its posterior lateral aspect.* In 90% of cases, the upper and lower canaliculi join to each other to from *common canaliculus of about 1 mm length* and open into the sac by a single punctum. In some persons, before the sac entry the common canaliculus may slightly dilate to form the *sinus of Maier.*

Lacrimal Sac (Fig. 6)

Lacrimal canaliculi carry the tears to the lacrimal sac, the widest portion of the lacrimal passages. It is situated in the lacrimal fossa. Lacrimal sac is about *15 mm long and 5–6 mm wide when distended.* The potential space in the sac has *a capacity of about 20 cumm* but can enlarge even to *120 cumm* in pathological conditions (dacryocystitis).

The lacrimal sac has three portions, which are only faintly demarcated from one another.

- *Head (Fundus)* is the broader round upper *3–5 mm portion* of the sac above the level of medial palpebral ligament. It is slightly flattened from side to side.

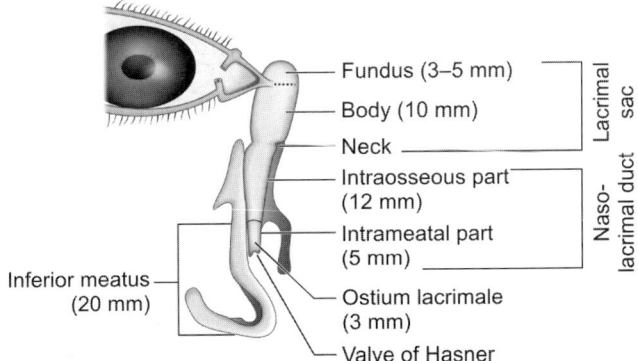

Fig. 6: Dimensions of lacrimal passages (from sac to inferior meatus).

- *Body* is the rest of the less broader portion of about *10 mm long*.
- *Neck* is the last slight constriction where sac joins the nasolacrimal duct.

Relations of lacrimal sac are slightly different in its upper and lower portions
Upper portion of the sac is covered *anteriorly* (laterally) by:
- Skin
- Fascia
- Orbicularis oculi
- Medial palpebral ligament (thinner portion)
- Lacrimal fascia

Lacrimal fascia is the periosteum of lacrimal fossa which extends across the sac from anterior lacrimal crest to posterior lacrimal crest.

Upper portion of sac is covered *posteriorly* by:
- Reflected tendon of MPS
- Horners muscle

Lower portion of the sac is covered anteriorly by:
- Skin
- Fascia
- Orbicularis oculi
- Orbital septum
- Lacrimal fascia

Lowermost portion of sac is related anteriorly to orbital septum and origin of inferior oblique muscle and posteriorly to orbital fat.

Lacrimal Fossa (Fig. 7)

Lacrimal fossa is a concavity on the medial wall of orbit adjacent to the lower 2/3rd of its anterior border. It is occupied by lacrimal sac. The fossa is formed by two bones:
1. Frontal portion of maxilla anteriorly, forming anterior half of the fossa (strong).
2. Lacrimal bone posteriorly, forming the posterior half of the fossa (thin and fragile).

Lacrimal fossa is bounded anteriorly by anterior lacrimal crest (frontal process of maxilla) is ill-defined above but well defined below and becomes

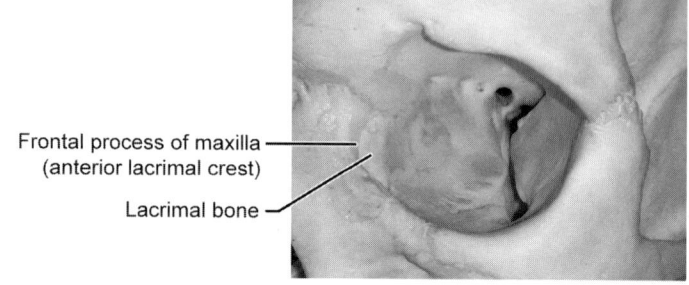

Fig. 7: Bones forming lacrimal fossa.

continuous with lower orbital margin where there is often a lacrimal tubercle. The fossa is bordered posteriorly by posterior lacrimal crest (lacrimal bone). There is no definite boundary above but lower portion become continuous with the osseous nasolacrimal duct.

Dimensions of Lacrimal Fossa (Fig. 8)

The vertical length of lacrimal fossa is about 16.5 mm (average 12 mm), the transverse width about 6.5 mm (average 5 mm). It is almost 5 mm deep in the lower part, but becomes shallow in the upper part. Lacrimal bone has a thickness of only 106 μm. So it is very fragile and can be easily penetrated when we make the ostium for dacryocystorhinostomy. Rarely, the fossa may become less broader in the middle or upper portion. Anterior lacrimal crest is the most important landmark by which we locate and separate the lacrimal sac from fossa during lacrimal sac surgeries. Upper half of the fossa lies over the anterior ethmoidal cells. Lower half is adjacent to the middle meatus of nose, just anterior to the attachment of middle turbinate bone. Ideally, the ostium for DCR is made in this lower half and avoid injury to ethmoid bone and its cribriform plate, which can lead to cerebrospinal fluid (CSI) leak.

Clinical Localization of Swellings produced by Lacrimal Sac Disorders (Figs. 9A to C)

Clinically, lacrimal sac disorders like dacryocystitis, tumors of sac, etc. produce a swelling of face below the level of medial canthus (medial palpebral ligament). But diseases of frontal sinus produce swelling above the medial canthus.

NASOLACRIMAL DUCT

Nasolacrimal duct carries tear fluid from lacrimal sac to inferior meatus of nose. Most of the portions of the duct pass through a bony canal—nasolacrimal canal. This canal is a groove or canal which occupies maxilla mainly. Medial wall of the canal is formed by:

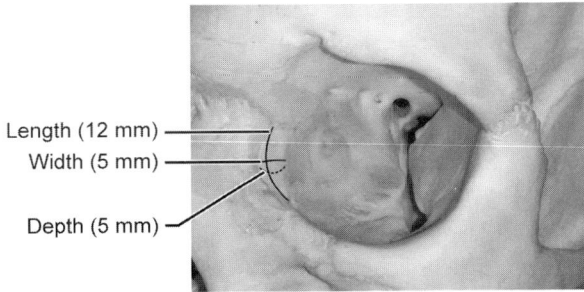

Fig. 8: Dimensions of lacrimal fossa as marked on left orbit.

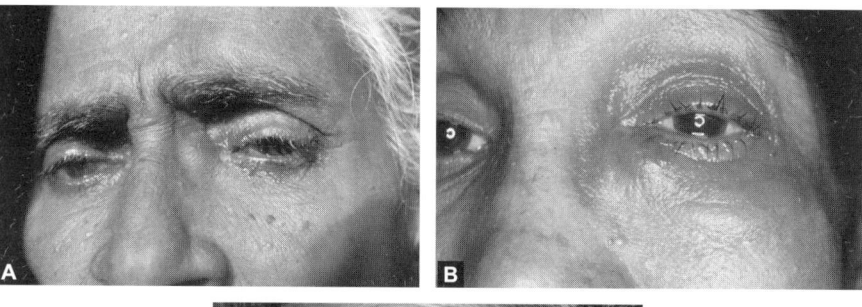
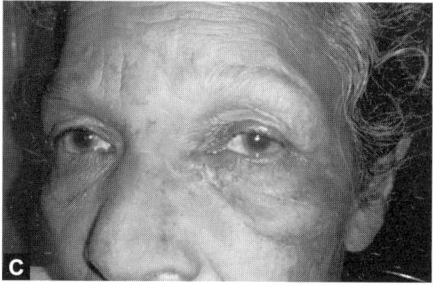

Figs. 9A to C: (A) Chronic dacryocystitis; (B) Acute dacryocystitis; (C) Lacrimal fistula.

- Small portion of lacrimal bone (upper part)
- Lacrimal process of inferior turbinate bone (lower part)

Laterally, it is related to:
- Middle meatus
- Maxillary antrum.

The canal produces a groove on the anteromedial wall of maxillary sinus. Hence, a maxillary sinusitis can produce an obstruction of nasolacrimal duct. *The direction of the canal is downwards, backwards and outwards. The canal is about 12-18 mm long and 3 mm wide. It opens into the inferior meatus of nose by a circular opening.*

The nasolacrimal duct has two portions.

1. *An upper intraosseous part occupying the nasolacrimal canal for about 12 mm long and 3 mm wide.*
2. *Lower intrameatal part which extends beyond the bony canal as a membranous tube which is only 5 mm long.*

This portion lies within the mucous membrane of lateral wall of nose which ends almost *20 mm above nostrils.*

The lower portion usually opens on the anterior part of the lateral wall of inferior meatus of nose (rarely middle meatus) by an opening, the ostium lacrimale. *The shape of the opening may be circular, oval or slit like. It has a valve called valve of Hasner. The size of the opening is around 3-4 mm when it is open.* The valve can prevent reflux of tears into the canal. Probably, it may also prevent the entry of air into the sac during blowing of nose.

The lacrimal sac and NLD lumens are only clefts under normal conditions and can allow the passage of a probe of even 3 mm diameter.

Congenital Nasolacrimal Duct Obstruction

Lacrimal passages develop at the 10-12 mm stage of embryo along with the development of face from an ectodermal thickening lying in the groove between lateral nasal and maxillary processes, which later get detached from surface ectoderm and become burried into maxillary mesoderm. This chord of cells get canalized and develop into the various portions of lacrimal passages.
- Upper portion develops into canaliculi
- Middle portion develops into lacrimal sac
- Lower portion develops into nasolacrimal duct.

Congenital nasolacrimal duct obstruction is due to an incomplete or noncanalization or membranous obstruction of the lower end of canal, mostly at valve of Hasner. It affects about 20% of infants and is the most common cause of unilateral or bilateral watering and discharge from eyes in children. *Of these 1/3rd of cases have bilateral obstruction.* Spontaneous resolution occurs in many cases by one year of age. The condition is managed by:
- *Sac massage: The direction of lacrimal passages can be marked on the surface of face by an imaginary line connecting a point from the medial canthus, to the groove between ala of nose and cheek [almost at the level of first upper molar tooth (Fig. 10)]. Massaging for relief of congenital nasolacrimal duct obstruction has to be performed in this area and direction (Fig. 11).*

After applying gentle, but firm pressure over lacrimal sac area, with the thumb or index finger of mother massaging performed and continued from medial canthus downwards to the level of ala of nose of infant. It is done for about 5 times morning and 5 times evening until the symptoms are relieved. Relief usually occurs in 75% of cases by this method by about one year.
- *Probing* surgery under GA without or with silicone tube intubation/balloon catheterization is attempted when the symptoms are not relieved in the first

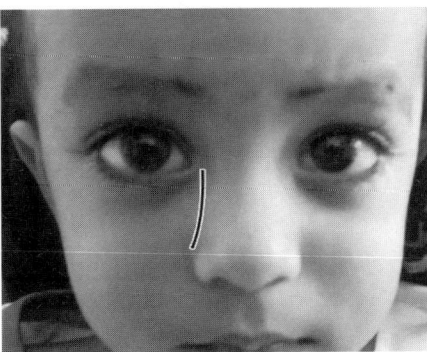

Fig. 10: Surface marking of lacrimal passages.

year by massaging. Probing is successful in NLD block in 75% of cases and success rate decreases when attempted in children above 3 years of age.
- *Dacrocystorhinostomy* (DCR) is advised only in elder children (above 3 years of age) in whom massaging and probing were unsuccessful and also in complex cases following injuries and craniofacial anomalies.

LACRIMAL SAC SURGERY MEASUREMENTS

Dacryocystectomy and dacryocystorhinostomy (external, endonasal or laser) are the two most common surgeries done for lacrimal sac disorders. Angular vein crosses the medial palpebral ligament about 8 mm medial to medial canthus and forms an important anterior relation of sac (Fig. 12). Therefore, incision for lacrimal surgeries is generally made 3 mm away (medial) from medial canthus to avoid injury to angular vein. The incision for these surgeries starts about 2 mm above and 3 mm medial (nasal) to medial canthus and extends vertically downwards for about 4 mm. Then it is curved outwards along the level of anterior lacrimal crest to a point 2 mm below inferior orbital margin (Figs. 13A to E).

In excision of rhynosporidial sac or tumors of sac, a slight deviation from this classical incision may be necessary. It is better to make incision a little nearer to the nose (medial) to leave provision for excision of affected skin and mobilization of skin for primary closure of wound in case of loss of affected skin.

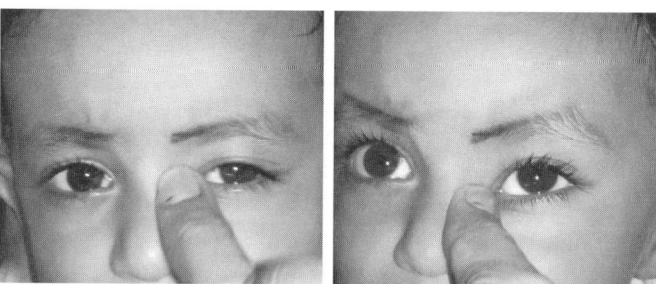

Fig. 11: Sac massaging.

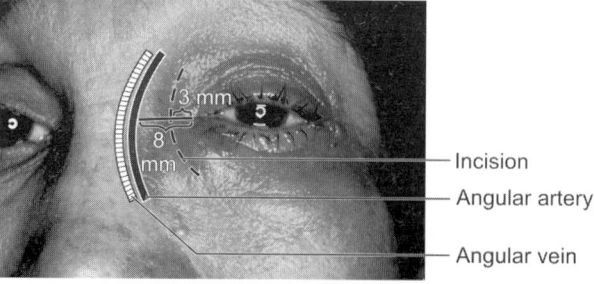

Fig. 12: Position of incision for lacrimal sac surgeries and angular vessels.

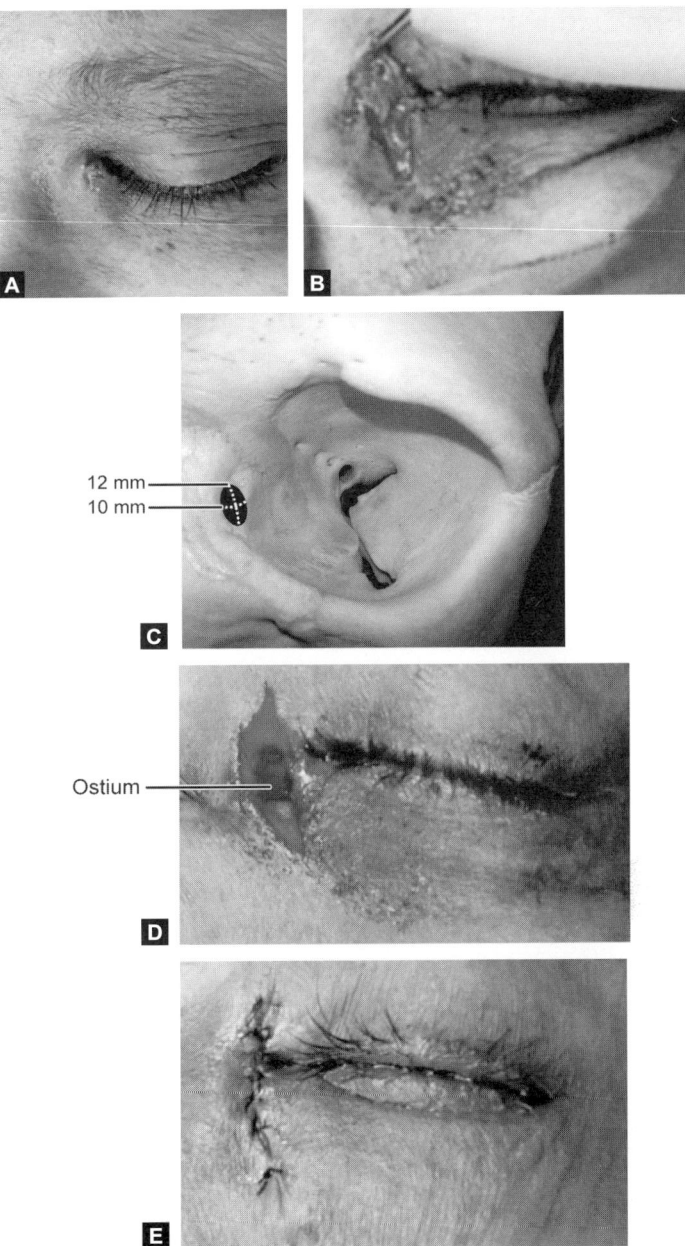

Figs. 13A to E: DCR steps: (A) Dacryocystitis; (B) DCR incision; (C) Dimensions of DCR ostium on lacrimal fossa, (D) DCR ostium; (E) DCR incision closed. (*For color version, see Plate 7 for A and D*)

Ideal Bony Ostium in Dacryocystorhinostomy

During DCR, an ostium of sufficient size has to be made in (in the lower part of) lacrimal fossa to allow gravitational drainage of tear into middle meatus of nose and prevent postoperative block of anastomosis between sac and nasal mucosal flaps. An ideal DCR ostium made is a round or oval window roughly 1 cm in size (12 mm long and 10 mm wide) having a smooth corners and extending from anterior to posterior lacrimal crest down to the beginning of NLD.

CHAPTER 18

Measurements of Orbit

Orbits are two bony sockets in craniofacial skeleton protecting eyeballs, allowing them good mobility in all directions facilitating binocular vision. (Fig. 1).

Each orbit is shaped almost like a four-sided pyramid. Base is directed forwards, laterally and slightly downwards opening in face. Apex is probably at or between optic foramen and superior orbital fissure and directed backwards communicating with middle cranial fossa. Orbit acquires a triangular configuration at its apex.

DIMENSION OF ORBITS (FIG. 2)

Orbits attain adult dimensions by the age of 12 years. Difference in size of orbits of two sides of more than 2 mm (measurements) is significant.
- *The facial opening (base) of orbit has a height of 35 mm and a width of 40 mm in adults; height and width are same in children.*
- *The orbit is widest immediately (1.5 mm) behind its rim.*
- *The **depth** of orbit is around 45 mm.*

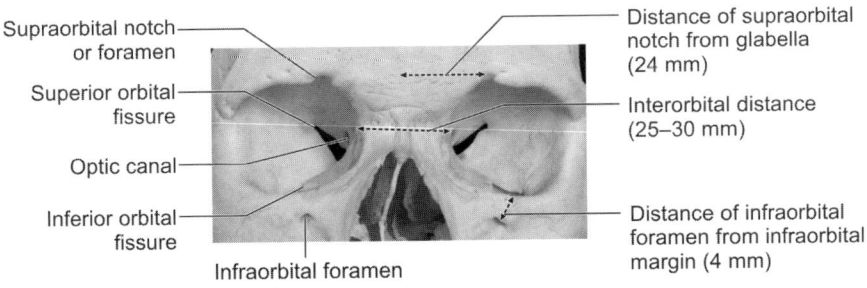

Fig. 1: Orbits.

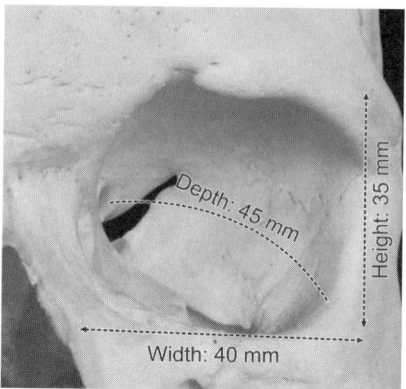

Fig. 2: Dimensions of orbit.

- The **volume** is 30 mL. (Fig. 2)
- The relationship of height and width of orbit is represented by the **orbital index** (of Broca) = $\dfrac{\text{Orbital height} \times 100}{\text{Orbital width}}$
  - Orbital index is high in children
  - In black races orbit is rectangular in shape, smaller (microseme) and orbital index is less than 84.
  - European races have medium sized orbits (mesoseme) and orbital index is about 88.
  - Yellow races have round larger orbits (megaseme) and orbital index is greater than 89.
- Distance between two orbits is 25 to 30 mm in adults. Interorbital distance is small in children and so eyes appear more closer giving a false appearance of squint which disappears as child grows.

Hypertelorism

Hypertelorism is *an increase in interorbital distance of more than 33 mm in adults (little less in children).* ***It can occur as an*** inherited autosomal recessive or dominant trait or as an isolated defect. Hypertelorism can produce an apparent appearance of divergent squint and is one of the causes of pseudosquint. This condition is associated with broadening and depression of bridge of nose, prominent forehead, optic atrophy, astigmatism, displacement of lacrimal puncta laterally, ptosis and inverse epicanthus. Hypertelorism is common in Cruzon's disease and Apert syndrome and may not require treatment always.

Hypotelorism

Hypotelorism is a decrease in the interorbital distance than normal. So, eyes are nearer than normal. This condition is seen in Down syndrome, trigonocephally and craniofacial anomalies.

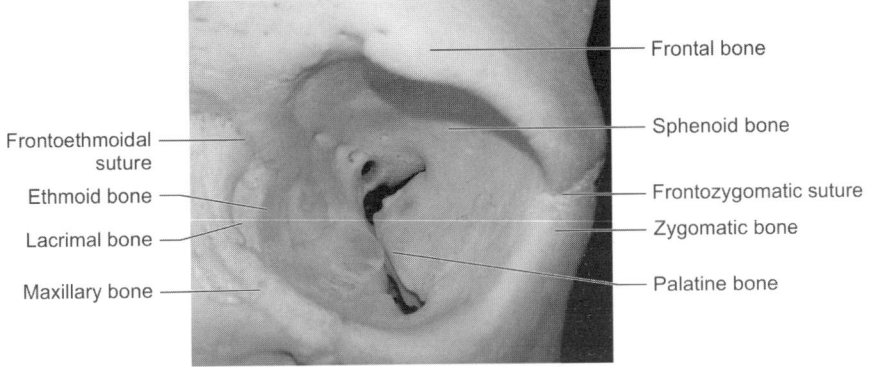

Fig. 3: Bones of orbit.

BONES AND WALLS OF ORBIT

Of the 22 skull bones, 7 take part in the formation of orbit, 6 partially and 1 completely framing the roof, lateral wall, floor and medial walls of orbits (Fig. 3). They are as follows:
- *Frontal bone:* The frontal bone takes part in the formation of roof
- *Zygomatic bone*: Participate in lateral wall and floor
- *Sphenoid bone*: Shares roof, lateral wall and medial wall
- *Maxillary bone*: Contributes to the floor and medial wall
- *Ethmoid bone*: Forms part of medial wall
- *Palatine bone:* Gives a small contribution to the floor.
- *Lacrimal bone*: The smallest bone of body and fully forms part of medial wall.

Walls of Orbit (Fig. 4)

Orbit is walled by a roof, lateral wall, floor and medial wall.
- *Roof* is formed by orbital plate of frontal bone and lesser wing of sphenoid
- *Lateral wall* is constituted by orbital surface of zygomatic bone and greater wing of sphenoid.
- *Floor* is contributed by orbital processes of maxilla, orbital surface of zygomatic and orbital processes of palatine bone.
- *Medial wall* is formed by frontal processes of maxilla, lacrimal bone, orbital plate of ethmoid and a small portion of body os sphenoid.

The roof, floor and lateral wall are almost triangular in shape, but medial wall is oblong and quadrangular in shape.

Roof is 45 mm long, lateral wall 50 mm (longest), floor 35–40 mm (shortest) and medial wall 45–50 mm.

Orbital Margins (Fig. 5)

- *Superior orbital margin:* It is made entirely of frontal bone
- *Lateral orbital margin:* It is formed of zygomatic process of frontal bone above and zygomatic bone below.

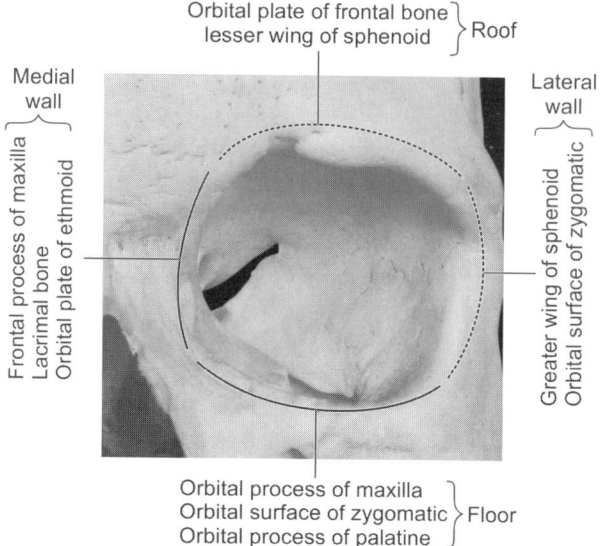

Fig. 4: Walls of orbit.

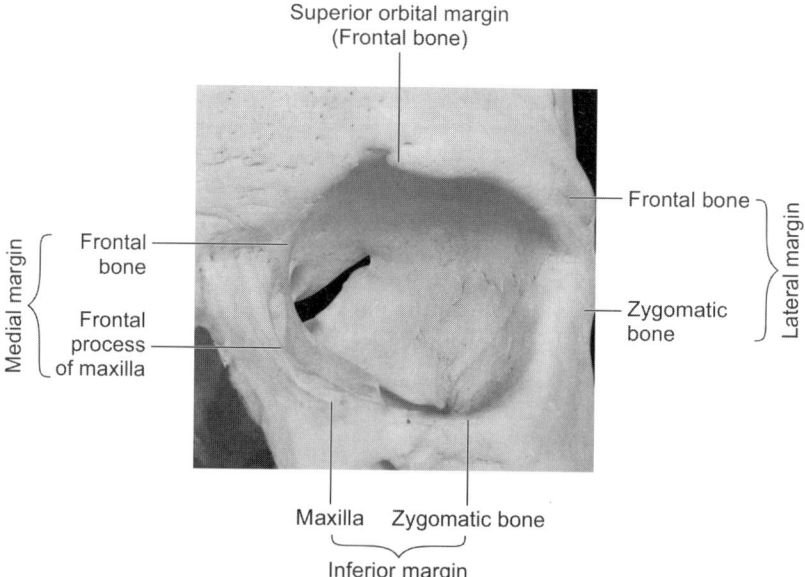

Fig. 5: Bones of orbital margins.

- *Inferior orbital margin:* It is constituted by zygomatic bone laterally and maxilla medially.
- *Medial orbital margin:* It is formed of frontal bone above and frontal process of maxilla below (Fig. 5).

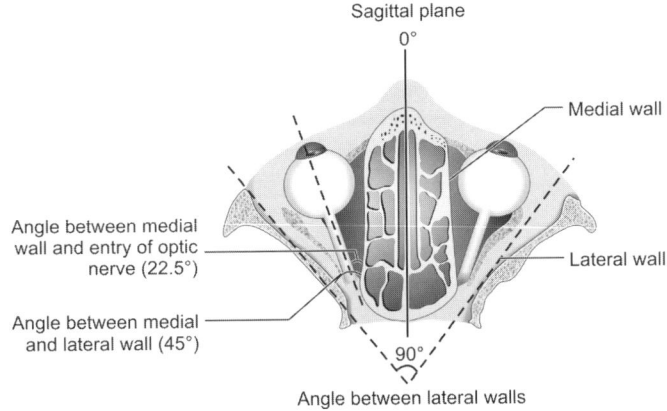

Fig. 6: Configuration of orbits.

Configuration of Orbit (Fig. 6)

Each orbit is pyramidal in shape. Medial walls of two orbits are parallel to each other. Lateral wall of each orbit make an *angle of 45° with the medial wall*. Lateral wall of one orbit subtend an *angle of 90° with the lateral wall of other orbit*. Optic nerve enters the orbit making an *angle of 22.5° with the medial wall* (Fig. 6).

ORBIT-EYEBALL RELATIONSHIP—NORMAL AND ABNORMAL

Normal

The volume of orbit is 30 mL and that of eyeball is about 7 mL. Thus, globe occupy only 25% of orbital space. Eyeball is situated in the anterior half of orbit. It is not placed in the center of orbit, but more near lateral wall and roof than medial wall and floor. This position can vary slightly according to the movement of eyeball. Closed lids over the apex of cornea will almost be at the level of middle of superior and inferior orbital margins. But eyeball normally project about 16 mm (12–18 mm) beyond lateral orbital margin (Fig. 7).

Proptosis/Exophthalmos

Orbital cavity is almost a closed space, surrounded posteriorly and on the sides by bony orbital walls and anteriorly by the weak orbital septum fusing with tarsal plates and opened only through the front gap of palpebral fissure through which eyeball is exposed. Any increase in intraorbital pressure can push eyeball forwards from normal position from orbit (Fig. 8).

Ptosis is a passive abnormal forward movement (protrusion) of the eyeball from orbit, by a retrobulbar mass. Protrusion of eyeball from orbit can be measured conveniently from the level of lateral orbital margin using different exophthalmometers. Normal protuberance is between 14 mm to 20 mm. An

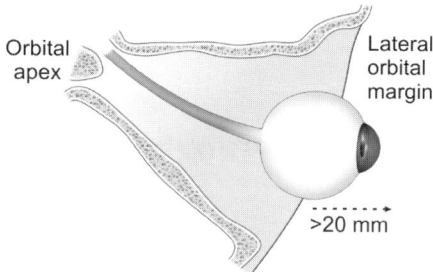

Fig. 7: Proptosis—measurement

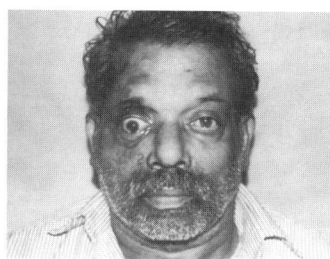

Fig. 8: Proptosis—right eye.

abnormal protrusion of one eyeball 2 mm more than the other eyeball (normal position) is relative proptosis. Exophthalmometric measurements of one or both eyeballs more than 21 mm is absolute proptosis.

An active abnormal prominence of eyeball due to thyroid eye disease (especially hyperthyroidism) is exophthalmos and is the most common cause of bilateral proptosis.

Enophthalmos

Abnormal retraction of eyeball in relation to orbit leading to an exophthalmometric measurement of less than 10 mm is called enophthalmos. (Figs. 9 and 10). Common causes are:
- Blowout fracture of orbit (usually floor) leading to orbital expansion or increasing space of the orbit and sinking of orbital contents into the maxillary sinus.
- Fibrous contraction of orbital tissues following orbital cellulitis or secondaries from scirrhous carcinoma breast.
- Duane's retraction syndrome
- Horner's syndrome
- Destruction of orbital wall following an orbital or periorbital tumor
- Following radical maxillectomy.

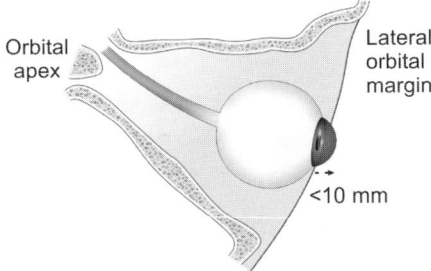

Fig. 9: Enophthalmos—measurements

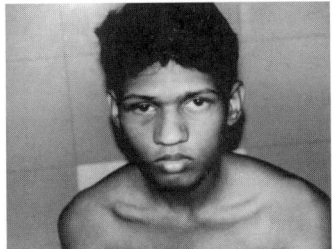

Fig. 10: Enophthalmos—right eye.

WALLS OF ORBIT

Roof of Orbit (Fig. 11)

Orbital roof is the strongest of orbital walls. It can resist a force of about 800–2200 pounds. This wall is triangular in shape with its base forwards and facing slightly downwards and forwards; anterior portion concave and posterior portion relatively flat.
- *The breadth of superior orbital rim is about 40 mm.*
- *The length of orbital roof is about 45 mm.*

Bones of Orbital Roof

Two bones contribute the formation of roof:
1. *Orbital plate of frontal bone:* It forms the major anterior part of roof. It is thick anteriorly but become thin, fragile posteriorly. So, its posterior portion can break easily by trauma and can be penetrated by sharp objects. The sulci and gyri of cerebral side of frontal lobe of brain produce ridges and depressions on it. It extends laterally up to the suture between it and zygomatic bone (zygomaticofrontal suture), in front of greater wing of sphenoid. Medially, it forms a suture with lacrimal bone in front and ethmoid bone behind (frontoethmoidal suture). This suture is at the junction of roof and medial wall and has the foramina for anterior and posterior ethmoidal vessels and nerves.

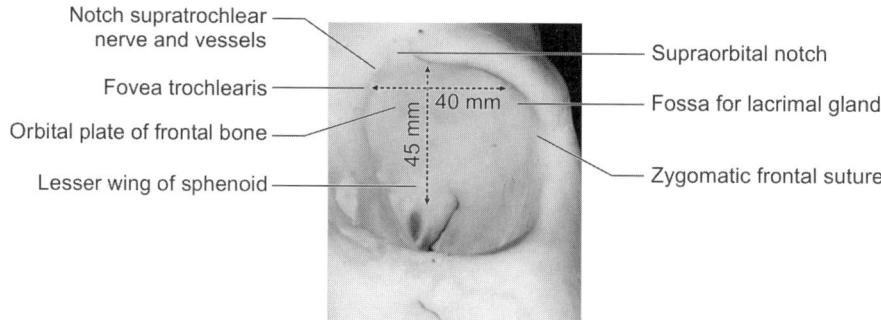

Fig. 11: Roof of orbit.

2. *Lesser wing of sphenoid:* It is the thickest part of roof (3 mm thick) and contributes to the small posterior portion of roof forming part of orbital apex. This portion is separated from lateral wall by the superior orbital fissure.

Landmarks

- Superior orbital margin and Supraorbital notch: *At the junction of the medial 1/3rd and lateral 2/3rd of supraorbital margin (about 24 mm lateral to glabella), is the supraorbital notch (foramen in 25% of individuals), which transmit supraorbital nerves and vessels.* A supraorbital nerve block is given almost at this site.
- Supratrochlear nerve and vessels may pass through another notch 10 mm medial to supraorbital notch.
- Zygomaticofrontal suture is between roof and lateral wall anteriorly.
- Frontoethmoidal suture is between roof and medial wall posteriorly
- Fossa for lacrimal gland is a smooth concavity situated anteriorly and laterally under the orbital plate of frontal bone.
- Fovea trochlearis (trochlear fossa) is *a small depression situated 3–5 mm behind the supraorbital rim anteromedially,* provide attachment of trochlea (pulley) for passage of superior oblique muscle tendon.
- *Anterior and posterior ethmoidal canals (about 15 mm long)* and foramina lie in the suture between orbital plate of frontal bone and ethmoid bone, which conduct the anterior and posterior ethmoidal vessels and nerves.
- Tuberculum musculare of Kiss is the bony tubercle on sphenoid for origin of extraocular muscles and is situated just below the optic canal.

Relations of Orbital Roof

- Frontal and ethmoidal sinuses invade roof anteromedially. Frontal sinus may reach even the middle of roof.
- Anterior cranial fossa: Orbital plate of frontal bone separates orbit from frontal lobe of brain with its meningeal coverings in anterior cranial fossa. Thus, an *'Orbital blow in fracture'* from the cranial cavity can injure frontal and parietal lobe of brain of that side and also orbital and ocular tissues

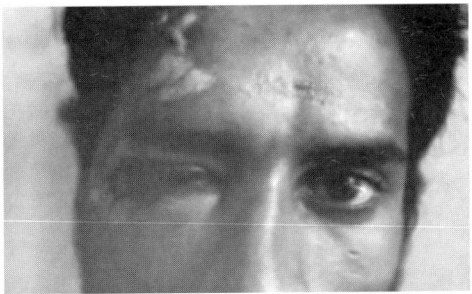

Fig. 12: Roof and lateral orbital wall injury.

of that side leading to proptosis, optic nerve and ocular motor palsies. Infections, tumors and other disorders can spread between orbit and cranial cavity.
- Frontal nerve and supraorbital artery are just under periorbita of roof.
- Levator palpebrae superioris and superior rectus muscles are under them.
- Trochlear nerve lies in the medial part of roof on its course to superior oblique muscle.
- Lacrimal gland is in the anteromedial corner of roof
- Superior oblique muscle is at the junction of roof and medial wall.

Orbital Roof Fracture

Orbital roof fracture can be caused by road traffic accidents (RTA), blunt trauma missile injuries, etc.

Eye signs of is orbital roof injury are: (Fig. 12)
- *Ptosis* due to damage of LPS muscle or its nerve supply
- *Proptosis* resulting from orbital hemorrhage or emphysema
- *Diplopia* caused by injury to extraocular muscles, trochlea or entrapment of muscles.
- *Visual loss* contributed by optic nerve injury, displacement of sella or chronic arachnoiditis.

LATERAL WALL OF ORBIT

This wall is the thickest of all walls of orbit; but thickness is not uniform. It is thick in the anterior part, then become thin, thick again and becomes thin posteriorly. Anterior thin portion separates orbit from muscular temporal fossa and posterior thin portion forms middle cranial fossa. *This portion is only 1 mm thick.*

Lateral wall is about 50 mm long anteroposteriorly and has a height of 35 mm. In relation to the eyeball, lateral orbital rim is placed about 12–18 mm behind cornea exposing the lateral aspect of eyeball up to equator (Fig. 13).

Lateral wall is triangular in shape; base directed anteriorly. It is slightly concave anteriorly, flat centrally and convex posteriorly. It makes an angle of 45° with median sagittal plane.

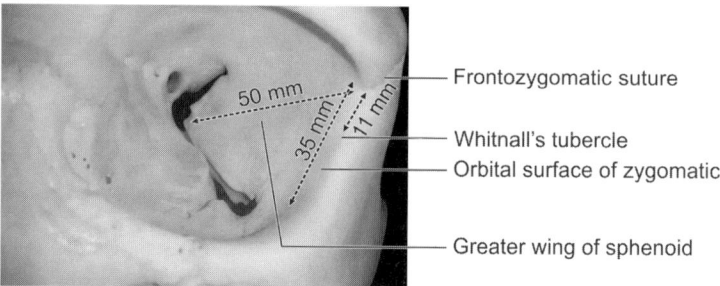

Fig. 13: Lateral wall.

Bones of Lateral Wall

Two bones take part in the formation of lateral wall.
1. *Orbital surface of zygomatic (malar) bone:* It constitutes the anterior third of lateral wall (upper portion of zygoma). Zygoma is continued below as anterolateral part of floor of orbit.
2. *Greater wing of sphenoid:* It make the posterior two-third of lateral wall. Superior orbital fissure separates this portion from roof and inferior orbital fissure from floor.

Landmarks of Lateral Wall and their Clinical Significance

- *Frontozygomatic suture* separates greater wing of sphenoid form orbital plate of frontal bone near *upper third of lateral wall.*
- *Zygomaticosphenoid suture* is vertically oriented and is the thinnest portion of lateral wall. *This is a convenient breaking point in lateral orbitotomy.*
- *Frontozygomatic suture* is the boundary between lateral wall and roof. Some persons have a meningeal foramen just above this suture transmitting a recurrent artery (external carotid system) anastomosing with lacrimal artery (internal carotid system). *This collateral system is important when primary internal carotid vascular supply is compromised.*
- *Zygomatic foramen,* near orbital rim for transmission of zygomaticofacial nerve and vessels as they leave orbit.
- *Foramen for zygomaticotemporal nerve.*
- *Whitnall's tubercle* (Lateral orbital tubercle): *It is small round prominence of zygomatic bone of lateral wall about 11 mm below the frontozygomatic suture and 3-4 mm inside lateral orbital margin and can be felt just within the middle of lateral orbital margin.* It gives attachment to:
  - Lateral canthal tendon
  - Lateral horn of levator aponeurosis
  - Check ligament of lateral rectus and support ligament of globe—ligament of Lockwood
  - Check-ligament of levator palpebrae superioris—Whitnall's ligament
  - Deep pretarsal aponeurosis
  - Expansion of superior rectus muscle sheath.

Relations of Lateral Wall

- Outer surface of anterior portion of lateral wall is related to temporal fossa and posterior portion to middle cranial fossa and temporal lobe of cerebrum
- Lateral rectus muscle is closely related to inner surface of lateral wall with orbital fat in between
- Lacrimal artery and lacrimal nerve are just above the lateral rectus
- Lacrimal gland: Inferior pole of orbital portion of main lacrimal gland reaches up to the lateral wall. Here the gland receives the parasympathetic contribution from zygomatic branch along with its vessels.

Fracture of Lateral Wall

Lateral orbital wall fracture is common and usually result from blunt trauma following a fall hitting the side of head as it occurs very often after a road transport accident. It involves the orbit rim and zygomatic bone (zygoma) more. Because of the multiple articulations, fractures of zygoma disrupt a wide area of face and attain the form of a zygomaticomaxillary complex fractures (ZMC fracture) leading to following *clinical signs* (Fig. 14).

- Check depression
- Inferior displacement of lateral canthal angle (lateral canthal dystopia)
- Trismus: Difficulty in opening mouth due to the spasm of muscles of mastication or impingement of coronoid process of mandible.
- Hypoesthesia of lateral midface due to a rupture of branches of zygomaticotemporal and zygomaticofacial nerves and vessels and infraorbital nerve.

FLOOR OF ORBIT

Orbital floor is the shortest of orbital walls, and is only 35–40 mm long (Fig. 15). It is also triangular in shape. It has slight slope downwards from medial to lateral aspect.

The length of inferior orbital margin is about 40 mm. The depth of orbit from inferior margin of orbit to optic foramen differs from, 35–40 mm in different individuals. The floor is strong laterally, but thins posteromedially

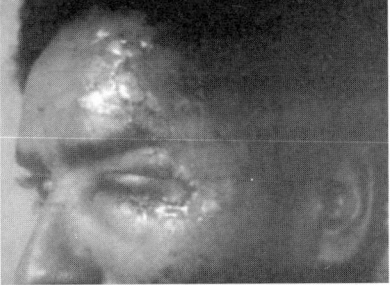

Fig. 14: Lateral orbital wall injury.

Basic Measurements in Ophthalmology

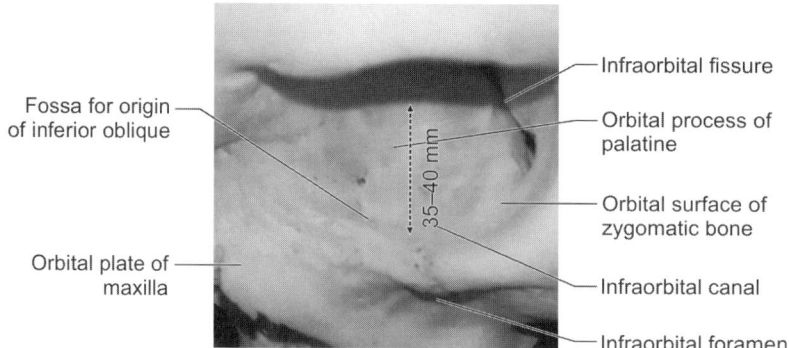

Fig. 15: Floor of orbit.

over maxillary sinus. *Thickness of floor slowly reduces behind orbital margin 1–0.5 mm posteromedially* where it can easily break due to trauma (blowout fracture). Thus, it is an ideal site for starting orbital decompression.

Bones of Orbital Floor

Floor of orbit is formed of portions of three bones.
1. *Orbital plate of maxilla* constituting medial and large central area of floor
2. *Orbital surface of zygomatic* bone forming the anterior and lateral portions of floor.
3. *Orbital process of palatine* bone filling a small triangular area of floor posteriorly.

Landmarks and Structures Passing Through Orbital Floor

- *Fossa for origin of inferior oblique* muscle: It is a shallow or rough area in the extreme anteromedial angle of orbital floor. This is just lateral to the opening of nasolacrimal duct.
- *Infraorbital groove*: It is a shallow gutter extending from inferior orbital fissure forwards and medially to the center of floor. Its posterior half is open. Anterior half is converted into a canal by a thin bone (lamina infraorbitalis). Anteriorly, this canal sinks deep into the maxilla and appear below infraorbital margin as infraorbital foramen. *The foramen is situated 4 mm below the center of inferior orbital margin.* This groove or canal transmits.
  - Infraorbital artery
  - Infraorbital vein
  - Infraorbital nerve: Which also have middle and anterior superior alveolar (dental) branches and pass through canals of same name, the middle superior alveolar nerve supplying bicuspid teeth of upper jaw and anterior superior alveolar nerve supplying the canine and incisors.
- *Nasolacrimal canal:* Starts from the anteromedial part of orbital floor, passes for 12 mm through maxillary bone vertically downwards and outwards to inferior meatus of nose.

- *Floor* is separated from medial wall by a fine suture.
- *Floor* is continuous with lateral wall anteriorly and separated from it posteriorly by inferior orbital fissure.

Relations

- Orbital floor is related to maxillary sinus below it for most of its portions. Tumors and infections of maxillary sinus can directly invade orbit through this wall.
- Most posterior portion of wall is related to palatine air cells.

Orbital Floor Fracture

Orbital floor fracture commonly follows blunt trauma and usually results in a blowout fracture producing following clinical features (Figs. 16 and 17).
- *Swelling and pain* of eyes and vomiting (due to traction on muscles leading to oculocardiac reflex)
- *Ecchymosis of lids*
- *Subconjunctival hemorrhage*
- *Surgical emphysema* due to communication of periorbital tissues with paranasal air sinuses.
- *Proptosis* In the early stage due to orbital hemorrhage.

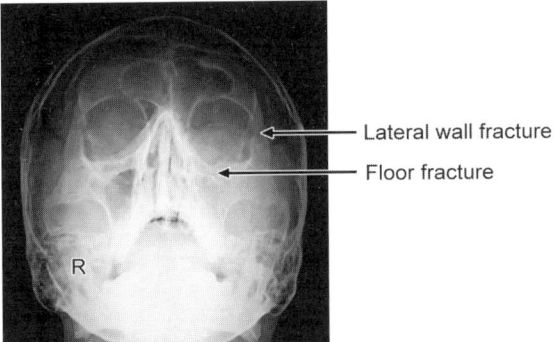

Fig. 16: X-ray skull (PNS) showing fracture of floor and lateral wall of orbit.

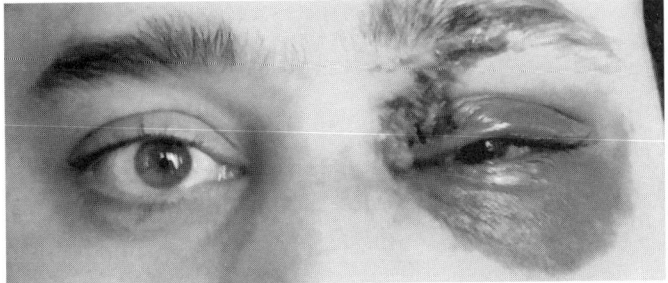

Fig. 17: Orbital floor injury (left). (*For color version, see Plate 7*)

- *Enophthalmos:* When orbital contents sink into the maxillary sinuses and orbital hemorrhage resolves.
- *Infraorbital hypoesthesia* due to injury of infraorbital nerve.
- *Limitation of ocular motility and diplopia*; limitation of vertical movements and vertical diplopia are more common than horizontal due to entrapment of subcutaneous tissue and extraocular muscles or hematoma or nerve injury of orbit.
- *Superior sulcus deformity* to lower displacement of eyeball.
- *Hypoglobus:* Considerable sinking of eyeball into maxillary antrum through a large floor dehiscence.

MEDIAL WALL OF ORBIT

Medial wall is almost *quadrangular in configuration*. Medial walls of two orbits are parallel to one another and to the sagittal plane of orbits. *The length of medial wall from anterior lacrimal crest to orbital apex is about 45–50 mm.*

Bones of Medial Wall (Fig. 18)

Medial orbital wall is framed by four bones united by vertical sutures. Anteroposteriorly, they are as follows:
- *Frontal process of maxilla* constitutes the thickest anterior portion
- *Lacrimal bone* is the thin next portion
- *Orbital plate (lamina papyracea) of ethmoid* is the *thinnest part of orbit* and make the major middle central region of medial wall. *It has a honey combed structure, papery thin and the thickness is only 0.2–0.3 mm.* Blunt injuries can easily fracture the bone—"blow out fracture". But medial wall blowout fracture are less common than that of floor because the former is more protected.
- *A small portion of Lateral aspect of body of sphenoid* makes the most posterior aspect of medial wall.

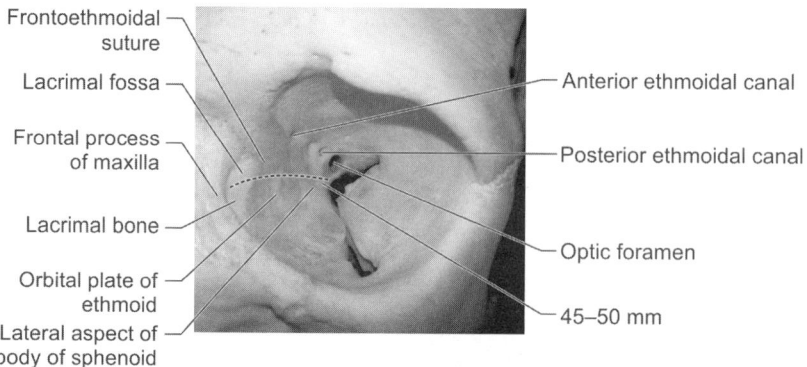

Fig. 18: Medial wall.

Landmarks

- *Lacrimal fossa:* At the lower and the anterior part of medial wall is the lacrimal fossa.
- *Anterior ethmoidal foramen is situated in the anterior part of the frontoethmoidal suture approximately 24 mm posterior to anterior lacrimal crest.* It transmits:
  - Anterior ethmoidal artery
  - Anterior ethmoidal branch of nasociliary nerve (internal nasal nerve)
  - Lymphatics
- *Posterior ethmoidal foramen is situated in the posterior part of frontoethmoidal suture about 36 mm behind medial orbital rim. The foramen transmits:*
  - Posterior ethmoidal artery
  - Sphenoethmoidal branch of nasociliary nerve
  - Lymphatics
- *Optic foramen: It is situated about 6 mm behind posterior ethmoidal foramen.*

Medial wall injury/fracture (Fig. 19) is caused by fall or blunt trauma and has following clinical features:
- Emphysema of lid and orbit
- Traumatic telecanthus
- Rounding of medial canthus
- Blowout fracture producing limitation of lateral movement and horizontal diplopia
- Trochlear injury leading to diplopia
- Damage to lacrimal passage resulting in dacryocystitis.

ORBITAL APEX (FIG. 20)

Which anatomical portion of orbit form the orbital apex—whether optic foramen or medial end of superior orbital fissure or the bony portion between them or all of them—is controversial. It may be a combination of:
- Optic canal
- Medial end of superior orbital fissure
- Posterior extremities of orbital walls (except floor)
- Neurovascular structures passing through them

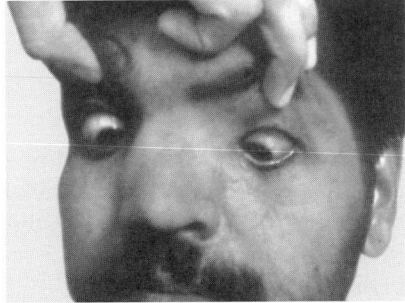

Fig. 19: Floor and medial orbital wall injury (left).

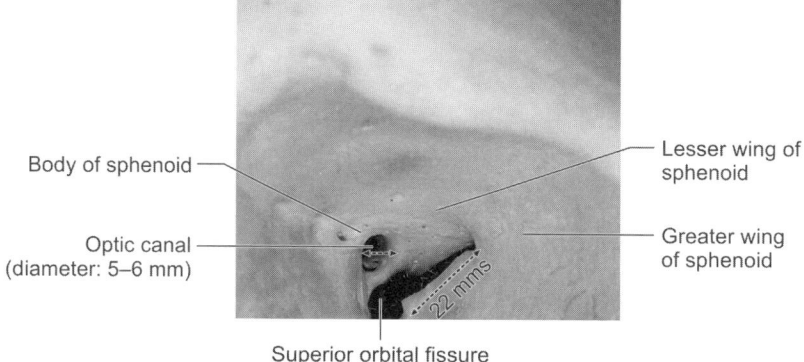

Fig. 20: Orbital apex.

- Annulus of Zinn
- Origins of extraocular muscles.

The position of apex structures in the orbit is crucial. Many diseases including inflammations, tumors and injuries of orbital apex can result in a variety of disorders particularly *orbital apex syndrome* and *superior orbital fissure syndrome* leading to visual loss and oculomotor and sensory abnormalities. Also diseases can spread to and fro between orbit and cranial cavity through orbital apex.

A knowledge of anatomy of measurements of orbit is important in mastering the art and science of ophthalmic anesthesia and diagnosis and management of orbital disorders.

Apex of orbit is in the same sagittal plane of orbit and optic foramen is situated posteriorly and medially in the orbit. Though the orbit has an outline of a four-sided pyramid in its anterior portion, it acquires a triangular configuration at the apex. This is probably because the orbital floor is shortest of orbital walls (35–40 mm only) and is not taking part in the apex formation and ends before orbital apex at pterygopalatine fossa.

Annulus of Zinn is a fibrous ring attached to the sphenoid at the orbital apex from which recti muscles originate. The ring encircles the optic foramen and medial end of superior orbital fissure. Annulus is situated at the apex of intracoronal space (the base of the space is the Tenon's capsule covering the posterior surface of globe). *Most of the extraocular muscle originate from this ring and get inserted in the sclera at variable distance behind the limbus.*

Orbital Apex Syndrome

Orbital apex syndrome is a complex orbital and ocular disorder due to involvement of the structures of orbital apex and neighborhood leading to paralysis of IInd, IIIrd, IVth and Vth cranial nerves. Common causes are:
- Inflammations (e.g. orbital periostitis)
- Injuries (e.g. hemorrhages and fractures)
- Tumors (e.g. sphenoids wing meningioma)

Orbital apex syndrome has following symptoms and signs:
- Neuralgic pain in forehead, orbit and eyes (in the area of distribution of ophthalmic division of trigeminal nerve)
- Considerable loss of vision due to optic nerve damage (amaurosis)
- Sensory abnormalities: Anesthesia of upper lid, sides of nose, forehead, temple, conjunctiva and cornea due to involvement of ophthalmic and sometimes maxillary division of trigeminal nerve
- Ptosis and lid edema
- Chemosis
- Axial proptosis
- Total restriction or absence of ocular movement in all directions due to paralysis of oculomotor nerves
- Keratitis due to loss of corneal sensation
- Absolute pupillary paralysis (internal ophthalmoplegia) resulting from third nerve paralysis
- Optic neuritis or papilledema leading to postneuritic optic atrophy

The resultant blindness (Amaurosis) due to optic atrophy, ocular motor nerve paralysis and trigeminal anesthesia are together called *Jacod's triad*.

COMMUNICATIONS OF ORBIT

Orbit communicates to the surrounding structures through the following canals and fissures:
- Optic canal
- Superior orbital fissure
- Inferior orbital fissure
- Anterior ethmoid canal
- Posterior ethmoid canal
- Nasolacrimal canal.

OPTIC CANAL

Optic canal is located in the apex of the orbit at the junction of its roof and medial wall and is superomedial to superior orbital fissure. This canal transmits optic nerve with its meningeal coverings, ophthalmic artery and its sympathetic plexus. The canal is situated almost within the lesser wing of sphenoid and is formed by its two roots and a small contribution from the body of sphenoid inferomedially. Medial wall of the canal is thinner than lateral. The canal is directed forwards laterally and slightly downwards from orbital apex. Its anteroposterior axis makes an angle of 35° with midline.

Dimensions (Figs. 21 and 22)
- *Optic canal reaches its adult dimension by the age of about 3 years.*
- *The canal has an average length of 8–10 mm*

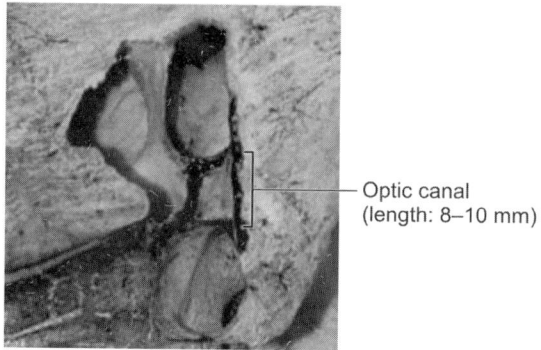

Fig. 21: Optic canal (after removal of its roof in a skull bone).

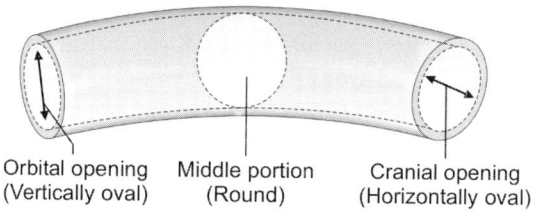

Fig. 22: Dimensions of optical canal.

- *Diameter of optic canal is 4 mm in neonates, 5 mm in 6 month and is 5 to 6 mm in adults.*
- *The canal is funnel-shaped*
- *On the orbital side canal is vertically oval in cross-section, circular in the middle portion and horizontally oval on the cranial side.*
- *The distance between orbital openings of two canals is 30 mm and intracranial openings is 25 mm.*
- *The size of the orbital openings are 4.5 mm horizontally and 6-6.5 mm vertically.*
- *Distance from posterior surface of eyeball to optic foramen is about 18 mm.*

   A difference in diameter of canal of two sides more than 1 mm is considered as abnormal. Optic nerve tumors like glioma produce uniform enlargement and meningioma. An irregular enlargement of optic canal is produced by meningioma usually unilateral. All can be demonstrated radiologically.

Configuration (Normal and Abnormal)

- Normally optic canals of two sides have the same configuration.
  - A key hole anomaly is often unilateral and can occur in 4% of individuals.
  - *A figure of 8 shaped optic canal occur in 1.2% of persons.* In these ophthalmic artery passes between the posterior and anterior portions.
  - Duplicate optic canal.

Enlargement of Optic Canal

Widening of optic canal of 2 mm more than normal is clinically significant.

- Enlargement of optic canal is seen in:
  - Optic nerve gliomas
  - Optic nerve sheath meningioma
  - Raised intracranial tension
  - Aneurism of ophthalmic artery and internal carotid artery

- Narrowing of optic canal is seen in:
  - Fibrous dysplasia
  - Meningioma
  - Paget's disease
  - Enucleation.

SUPERIOR ORBITAL FISSURE

Superior orbital fissure is situated in the orbital apex between posterior portions of roof and lateral wall of orbit. It is bound by greater and lesser wings of sphenoid, closed laterally by frontal bone, and is the largest communication between orbit and middle cranial fossa allowing the passage of important vessels and nerves between them. *It is just lateral to the optic canal. This fissure is comma shaped, lateral and superior part narrower than medial and inferior part.* At the junction of the two is the spina recti lateralis from which lateral rectus muscle originate. Common tendinous ring is attached between medial and lateral part of superior orbital fissure. *The fissure is about 22 mm long and its lateral end (tip) is about 30–40 mm behind frontozygomatic suture.*

Common tendinous ring of Zinn divides the fissure into three compartments and transmit various structures (Fig. 23).

1. Part of the fissure above the ring transmits the following nerves and vessels from above downwards, in order:
   - Lacrimal nerve
   - Frontal nerve

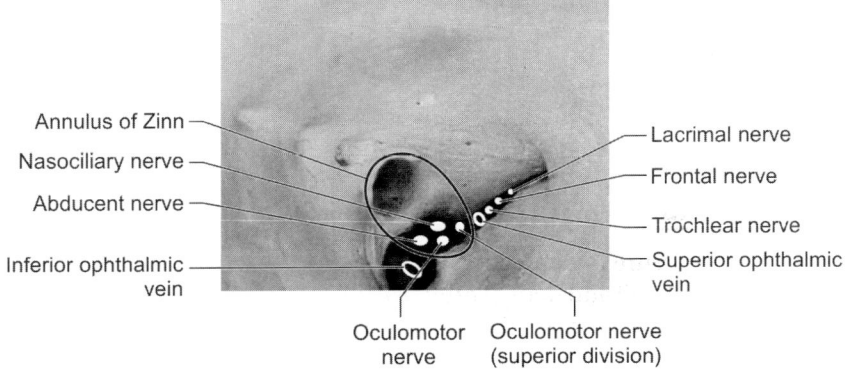

Fig. 23: Structures passing (inferior division) through superior orbital fissure.

- Trochlear nerve
- Superior ophthalmic vein
- Recurrent branch of ophthalmic artery and some sympathetic fibers from cavernous sinus
2. Intermediate portion of fissure transmits:
   - Superior division of oculomotor nerve
   - Nasociliary nerve
   - Inferior division of oculomotor nerve
   - Abducent nerve
3. Part of fissure below ring transmit
   - Inferior ophthalmic vein.

Superior Orbital Fissure Syndrome

This is the clinical presentation of involvement of structures passing through superior orbital fissure due to various causes. Condition was first reported by Rochon-Duvigneaud (1896) Djaean (1927) Rojur and Athez (1935).

Causes

- Inflammations: Especially following periostitis and pansinusitis
- Neoplastic—primary tumor of sphenoid bone (meningioma of sphenoid ridge of superior orbital fissure) and secondaries
- Trauma—leading to fracture or hematoma in the region
- Aneurism of internal carotid artery
- Occlusion of superior ophthalmic vein
- Allergy.

Clinical Features

Clinically superior orbital fissure syndrome differs from orbital apex syndrome mainly in the absence of optic nerve involvement in the former. Rarely, optic nerve may get secondarily affected in the later stages. Symptoms and signs are:
- Pain in forehead and eye
- Anesthesia of eyelids and forehead resulting from involvement ophthalmic division of trigeminal nerve.
- Lid edema and ptosis
- Proptosis
- Paralysis of 3rd, 4th and 6th nerve leading to total ophthalmoplegia
- Sympathetic disturbances.

INFERIOR ORBITAL FISSURE (FIG. 24)

Inferior orbital fissure is located near the orbital apex between the posterior portions of lateral wall and floor of orbit. *It is below and lateral to optic foramen and close to medial end of superior orbital fissure. This fissure is about 20 mm long and runs forwards and laterally. The anterior end of this canal is 20 mm behind inferior orbital margin.* It is narrow in the center and wide anteriorly.

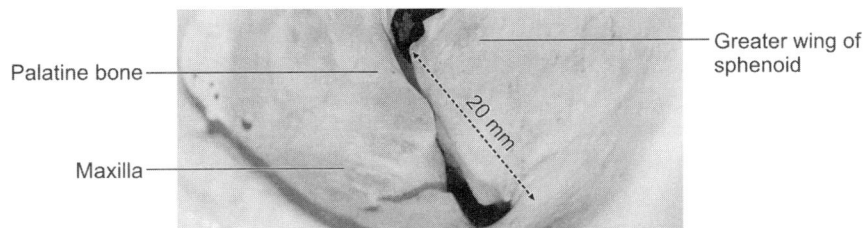

Fig. 24: Boundaries and dimensions of inferior orbital fissure.

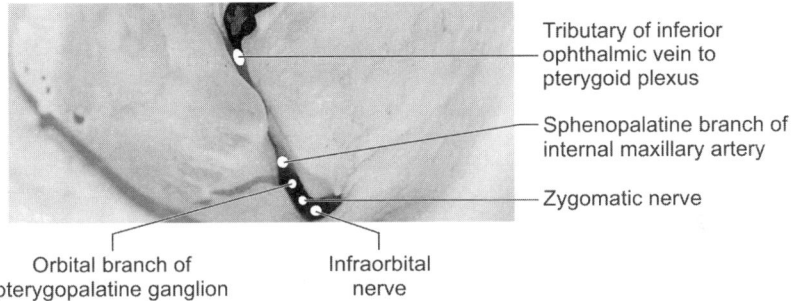

Fig. 25: Structures passing through inferior orbital fissure.

Fissure is close to foramen rotundum and sphenopalatine foramen. The boundaries are:
- Anteromedially: Maxilla and orbital process of palatine bone
- Posterolaterally: Margin of orbital surface of greater wing of sphenoid

Anterior aspect is closed by zygomatic bone. The lower margin of fissure is notched by the infraorbital groove which becomes canal and opens as the infraorbital foramen which transmits infraorbital nerve (a contribution of maxillary nerve) and vessels.

Through the fissure orbit *communicates* with infratemporal and pterygopalatine fossa, and *transmit (Fig. 25)*.
- Tributaries of inferior ophthalmic vein which carry venous drainage from inferior portion of orbit to the veins of pterygoid plexus in the infratemporal fossa (communication between inferior ophthalmic vein and pterygoid plexus)
- Sphenopalatine branch of internal maxillary artery
- Orbital branch of pterygopalatine ganglion
- Zygomatic nerve
- Infraorbital nerve.

Measurements of Extraocular Muscles

Six extraocular muscles, 4 recti and 2 obliques rotate the eyeball in all directions. They originate from orbital apex except inferior oblique and inserted into the sclera at variable distance from the limbus. *The muscles have an average length* of 40–45 mm. Recti muscles are inserted anterior to the equator of the globe and oblique muscles insert posterior to the equator and so the actions of recti and obliques are opposite to one another.

Medial Rectus Muscle

Medial rectus is the largest and most fleshy extraocular muscle. *It is about 40.8 mm long.* The muscle *originates* from the medial part of annulus of Zinn, runs forwards and medially adjacent to the medial wall of orbit. *Its belly is large but tendon is short and has 3.7 mm length. The muscle get inserted into the sclera in a vertical line of 10.3 mm, in the horizontal meridian of globe, anterior to the equator, 5.5 mm behind the medial limbus.* It is supplied by a branch of oculomotor nerve which enters ocular surface of muscle 15 mm behind its origin.

Medial rectus has only one *action*; adduction of eyeball.

Lateral Rectus Muscle (Fig. 26)

Lateral rectus muscle is 40.6 mm long. It *originates* by two tendons from the lateral end of superior and inferior aspects of annulus of Zinn, runs forward adjacent to the lateral wall of orbit and over the inferior oblique muscle and get *inserted* on the sclera in the horizontal meridian, *in front of the equator 6.9 mm behind lateral limbus. Length of the tendon is 8.8 mm and the breadth of insertion is 9.2 mm and the insertion is almost vertical.* The muscle is supplied by abducens nerve which enters the inner (ocular surface) of muscle about 15 mm behind its origin.

The lateral rectus has also only one *action*; abduction.

Superior Rectus Muscle (Fig. 27)

Superior rectus muscle of the recti, superior rectus is the farthest inserted muscle from limbus and has the widest insertion. It only 41.8 mm long. The muscle

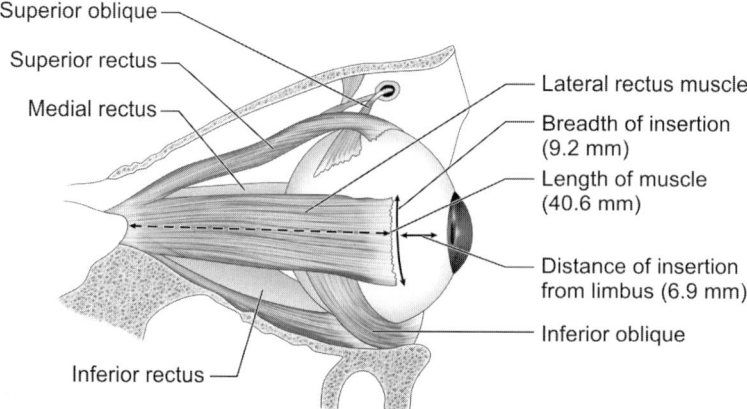

Fig. 26: Lateral rectus muscle.

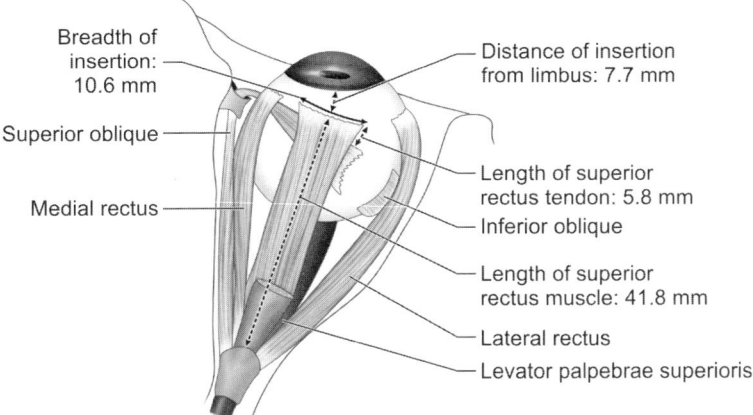

Fig. 27: Dimensions of superior rectus muscle.

originates from the upper part of annulus of Zinn just below the origin of Levator and the dural sheath of optic nerve. Unlike horizontal recti the direction of superior rectus is not straightforward, but slightly *upwards and outwards making an angle of 23° with the sagittal diameter of globe*. Before insertion it runs over the tendinous part of superior oblique muscle. *The tendon of superior rectus is 5.8 mm long and get inserted 7.7 mm behind upper limbus slightly nasal to the vertical meridian of globe in front of equator. The insertion is 10.6 mm long* but curved and oblique and the convexity of curve facing slightly backwards and medially. Thus, the lateral end of insertion is farther from limbus than medial end. Levator palpebrae superioris separates superior rectus from orbital roof and they are closely associated. The muscle is supplied by superior division of oculomotor nerve which enters from its inferior surface on its ocular surface. Since the muscle plane is not straight and the course is slightly oblique, its *action* is also complex.
- Primary action: It is elevation of globe, maximum in abducted position.
- Subsidiary action: Intorsion and adduction.

Inferior Rectus Muscle (Fig. 28)

Inferior rectus *originates* from the lower part of annulus of Zinn. *It is about 40 mm long*. This muscle also does not proceed straight to the insertion but runs slightly downwards and outwards at an angle of *23° with sagittal diameter of globe*. Its tendon is *5.5 mm long*. It gets inserted to the sclera in the inferior aspects of globe in the vertical meridian, about *6.6 mm behind limbus*. The insertion is not parallel to the limbus but slightly curved and oblique, lateral end being farther than medial and is *9.8 mm long*. The muscle is supplied by inferior division of oculomotor nerve which enters at the junction of posterior third and anterior two-third of its ocular surface. As the course of inferior rectus is not straight and 23° away from sagittal diameter of globe, it brings out multiple actions.

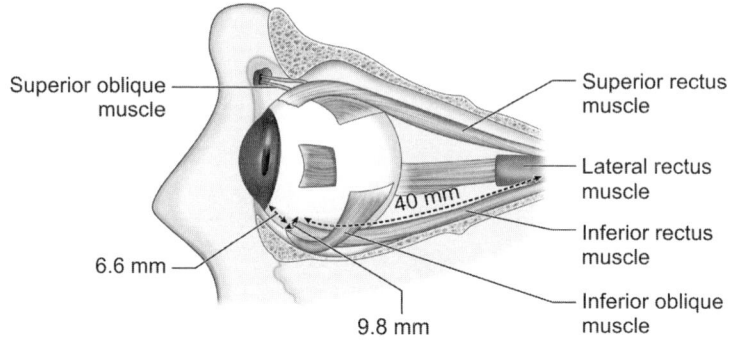

Fig. 28: Dimensions of inferior rectus muscle.

- Primary action: Depression of globe, maximum in abducted position
- Subsidiary action: Extortion and adduction.

GENERAL CONFIGURATION AND SURFACE MARKING OF RECTI MUSCLE INSERTIONS

Most of the surgical procedures of extraocular muscles are centered around their insertions. Their tendons in general have a glistening and silky appearance. The muscle fibers of superior and inferior rectus merge with their tendon in a V-shaped configuration and those of inferior rectus and medial recuts end in a dentate line.

The distance of insertion of recti muscles from limbus increase circumferentially, from medial rectus to superior rectus; *the inferior rectus is inserted 2.1 mm farther from limbus than insertion of medial rectus. The distance of insertion of lateral rectus from limbus is 0.3 mm more than the insertion of inferior rectus. Superior rectus is inserted 0.8 mm farther than that of lateral rectus from limbus.* Thus, superior rectus is the farthest inserted of the recti muscles from the limbus and medial rectus is the nearest inserted rectus muscle.

Again recti muscles insert approximately 1mm anterior or posterior to ora serrata.

Superior Oblique Muscle (Fig. 29)

- *Superior oblique is the longest extraocular muscle (60 mm long)*
- It is the thinnest also
- This is the only extraocular muscle in which the nerves supply enters the orbital surface of muscle *(trochlear nerve) entering 12 mm behind the origin of muscle.*

The muscle has two parts:
1. Direct part: It is *40 mm long* and start from its origin at the orbital apex and runs forwards to the anterior upper and medial part of orbit to trochlea. This portion of muscle is muscular untila point 10 mm behind trochlea.

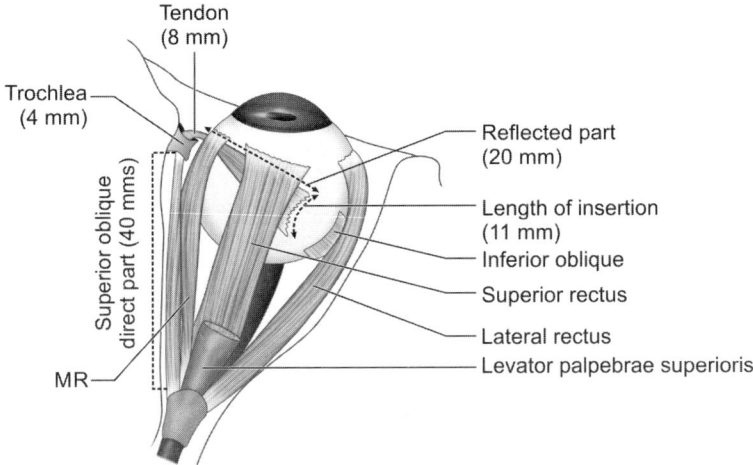

Fig. 29: Dimensions of superior oblique muscle.

2. Reflected part: It is *about 20 mm long* and runs in the reverse direction of direct part, from trochlea to insertion and is tendinous.

The **origin** of superior oblique is not from annulus of Zinn. The direct part of muscle originates from the periosteum of body of sphenoid at the orbital apex immediately above and medial to the optic foramen and slightly posterior and superior to origin of medial rectus. It then runs forwards between upper part of medial wall (parallel to it) and roof above medial recuts to the junction of anterior part of roof and medial wall. It then becomes tendinous approximately *10-15 mm behind orbital margin* and gets threaded through a cartilaginous pulley (trochlea) and *then runs almost in a reverse direction—backwards, downwards and laterally at an angle of about 54° to the axis of primary position (vertical plane) of eyeball to insertion*. In adduction the range of movement of the tendon through trochlea, between maximum elevation and depression is about 16 mm (8 mm anteriorly and 8 mm posteriorly). *The tendon is about 8 mm long and is relatively avascular.*

The *trochlea is a pulley shaped, curved, cartilaginous plate (6 mm × 4 mm) attached to the trochlear fossa of frontal bone 4 mm behind the orbital margin* tied down by fibrous tissue, situated in the anterior superior and medial corner of orbit, through which the tendon of superior oblique pass. It is 5.5 mm long, 4 mm broad and 4 mm deep. Its concave medial surface is directed towards the trochlear fossa.

The **insertion** of the muscle is to the sclera at the upper and lateral aspect of globe behind equator. In this portion of insertion of superior oblique is covered by superior rectus. It passes under and *2-3 mm behind the medial edge of insertion of superior rectus and emerges at its lateral edge, because of its oblique course. The length of insertion is about 11 mm.* The anterior end of insertion is about 0.5 mm in front of equator. Here it is 4.5 mm behind equator and beyond the lateral end of superior rectus insertion. Superior temporal vortex vein is also close to the superior oblique insertion. Except a small anterior portion all other portions are inserted behind equator. The insertion is convex posteriorly and laterally along a curved line in the upper part of posterolateral part of globe with concavity towards the trochlea and lying obliquely. *So the distance of anterior and posterior ends of insertions of muscle from the limbus is about 13.8 mm and 18.8 mm respectively.*

Since, the tendon of the muscle take a reverse course from that of muscle belly, the action is also in a reverse direction of what we expect from a superior muscle. The **actions** are as follows:
- Primary action: intorsion of globe
- Subsidiary action: Depression (maximum in adducted position) and abduction.

Inferior Oblique Muscle (Fig. 30)

Inferior oblique muscle differs from other extraocular muscles in many aspects.
- It is the only extraocular muscle which is not originating from apex of orbit but from anterior part of orbit
- Shortest extraocular muscle (only 37 mm long)
- Origin is short
- Almost whole length of muscle is muscular
- Tendon is very short and only 1–2 mm long

The muscle **originates** from a shallow depression in anterior, inferior and medial corner of orbit (orbital plate of maxilla). The origin is just lateral to the lower part of lacrimal fossa and some fibers may originate from facial covering of lacrimal sac. *It then runs backwards, upwards and laterally at angle of 51° with the visual axis (vertical plane)* of eyeball and under inferior rectus, then curves around lower part of eyeball below the lower border of lateral rectus.

It then gets **inserted** into sclera in the posterotemporal quadrant of eyeball below horizontal meridian behind the equator below its posterior pole. *The insertion of inferior oblique is a guide to macula externally from the posterior surface of eyeball. The macula is about 2.2 mm above and nasal to medial border of insertion of inferior oblique (Fig. 31). The length of insertion is about 9.5 mm and the angle is 15–20° to the horizontal plane.* Insertion is convex above and

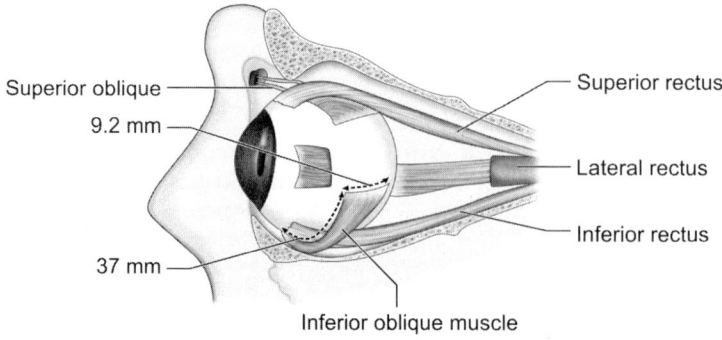

Fig. 30: Dimensions of inferior oblique.

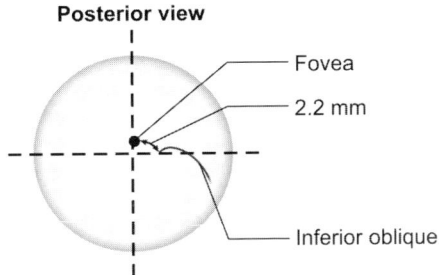

Fig. 31: Inferior oblique muscle insertion and mucula—(right eye)

laterally with its concavity towards origin. The line of insertion is oblique; anterior portion of insertion is more nearer limbus than posterior. Anterior limit of insertion in 9.5 mm behind and 2 mm above the lower limit of insertion of inferior rectus. *The posterior end of insertion of inferior oblique is 3-6 mm below the optic nerve and 1-2 mm lateral to macula.* The borders of insertion of muscle are related to superior and inferior vortex vein. Inferior temporal vortex vein is 7-8 mm below the insertion. *The distance between insertion of superior and inferior oblique muscle is about 15 mm.*

This muscle is supplied by inferior division of oculomotor nerve which contain the parasympathetic fibers to intraocular muscles also and its damage can result in internal ophthalmoplegia also. The nerve cross the posterior surface of the muscle and enter its ocular surface when it passes lateral to inferior rectus.

Since the muscle has an oblique course from medial and inferior part of orbit backwards, upwards and laterally making an angle of about 51° to vertical plane of eyeball and inserted behind its equator, the **action** is also reverse of what we expect from an inferiorly placed muscle. The actions are:
- Main action is: Extortion
- Subsidiary action: Elevation (maximum in adducted position) and abduction.

DIMENSIONS OF EXTRAOCULAR MUSCLES

Table 1 shows the dimensions of extraocular muscles.

TABLE 1: Dimensions of extraocular muscles.

	Length of muscle	Length of tendon	Length or breadth of insertion line	Distance of insertion from limbus
Medial rectus	40.8 mm	3.7 mm	10.3 mm	5.5 mm
Lateral rectus	40.6 mm	8.8 mm	9.2 mm	6.9 mm
Superior rectus	41.8 mm	5.8 mm	10.6 mm	7.7 mm
Inferior rectus	40 mm	5.5 mm	9.8 mm	6.6 mm
Superior oblique	60 mm	8 mm	11 mm	13.8–18.8 mm
Inferior oblique	37 mm	1–2 mm	9.5 mm	-

ANGLE OR MERIDIAN OF INSERTION OF EXTRAOCULAR MUSCLES

Table 2 shows the angle or meridian of insertion of extraocular muscles.

VISUAL AXIS, OPTIC AXIS, CENTRE OF ROTATION OF EYEBALL, ORBITAL PLANES AND ORBITAL AXIS

A good understanding and awareness of visual axis, optic axis, center of rotation of eyeball, orbital planes and orbital axis are important in ophthalmic (infiltration) anesthesia and diagnosis and management of orbital disorders.

Orbital Plane

Medial walls of orbits are parallel to each other and to the sagittal plane of head. lateral wall of each orbit makes an angle of 45° with its medial wall. Lateral of one orbit is at right angle (90°) with the lateral wall of other orbit. Optic canal (orbital apex) is in the same plane as the medial wall and both optic foramina are placed medially and posteriorly in the orbit.

Visual Axis (Fig. 32)

Visual axis is an imaginary line connecting object, nodal point and fovea of eye. In primary position of eyes visual axis are parallel to each other.

Optic Axis (Fig. 33)

Optic axis is an imaginary line which passes from object, 0.25 mm nasal to the center of cornea, approximately through the center of pupil, lens and center of rotation of eye. Intersecting visual axis and extent more nasally, posteriorly.

TABLE 2: Angle or meridian of insertion of extraocular muscles.

Medial rectus	Horizontal meridian of globe
Lateral rectus	Horizontal meridian of globe
Superior rectus	Makes an angle of 23° with the sagittal diameter of globe
Inferior rectus	Makes an angle of 23° with the sagittal diameter of globe
Superior oblique	Makes an angle of 54° to vertical plane (primary axis) of globe
Inferior oblique	Makes an angle of 54° to vertical plane (primary axis) of globe

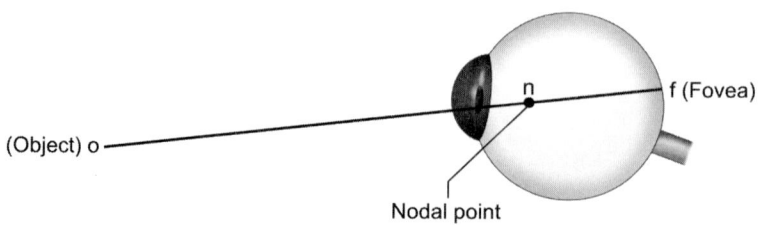

Fig. 32: Visual axis.

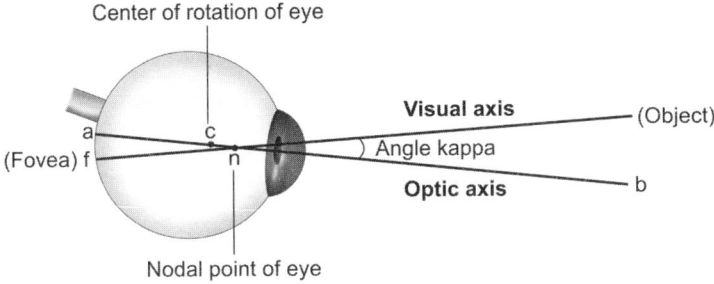

Fig. 33: Visual axis and optic axis.

The angle between visual axis and optic axis is called angle gamma. This angle is assessed clinically at pupillary plane and is named angle kappa.
- *Positive angle kappa:* In normal eyes (emmetropic) angle kappa is supposed to be positive since the optic axis pass inner to fovea. In hypermetropes the angle is more (larger) and positive than emmetropes and gives false appearance of divergent squint (pseudosquint).
- *Negative angle kappa:* In myopes the visual axis become parallel to optic axis or even pass outer to fovea making the angle negative or even absent giving a false appearance of convergent squint.

Thus, hypermetropia can produce a false divergent squint appearance due to large positive angle kappa and myopia can produce a false appearance of convergent squint due to negative angle kappa.

A false or apparent appearance of squint, pseudosquint can also occur in:
- Facial asymmetry (due to facial palsy) produces a false appearance of vertical squint
- Hypertelorism can give pseudo divergent squint appearance
- Epicanthal fold with flat bridge of nose can produce a false convergent squint appearance.

A false squint can be differentiated from true squint in the following ways.
In peseudosquint:
- Hirschberg test: The corneal reflex will be in the center of the cornea in both eyes
- Cover test: No deviation of eyes
- Pseudosquint may disappear with refractive correction or as the child grows but true squint may get masked due to compensatory head posture.

Orbital Axis (Fig. 34)

Orbital axis another imaginary line passing probably from the level of lateral limbus of eyeball anteriorly and then along the point where optic nerve enters globe (3 mm medial to posterior pole) and again parallel to the distal and middle portion of optic nerve to orbital apex.

Orbital axis makes an angle of 23° with the visual axis in primary position of eyes (Fig. 35).

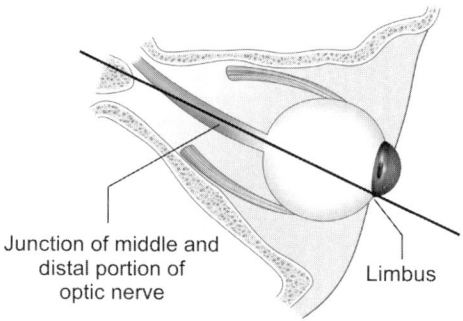

Fig. 34: Orbital axis.

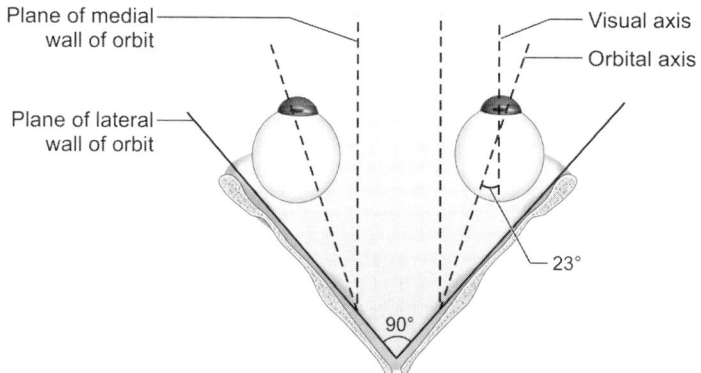

Fig. 35: Angle between orbital axis and visual axis.

CENTER OF ROTATION OF EYEBALL (FIG. 36)

Extraocular muscles rotate the eyeball around its center of rotation. Center of rotation lies about 12–13 mm behind the center of cornea in the horizontal plane.

The Relative Roles and Effectiveness of Vertically Acting Muscles in Vertical Movements and Torsions of Eyeball (Figs. 37A and B)

- The four vertically acting muscles: Superior and inferior recti and superior and inferior obliques are *maximum effective as vertical rotators when their muscle plane* become parallel to visual axis of eyeball.
- In this position their action is only in one direction: Upwards or downwards. *In primary position of eyeball 3/4th of the power of vertical rotators is utilized for vertical rotation and only 1/4th for torsion. Of the total vertical actions 2/3rd is contributed by the vertical recti and 1/3rd by obliques.*
- Once the visual axis deviates from the muscle plane they produce mainly torsions.
- *Superior and inferior recti are maximum (100%) effective as elevators or depressors of eyeball, when the eye is abducted 30° from muscle plane and*

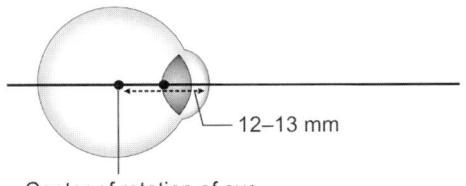

Fig. 36: Center of rotation of eyeball.

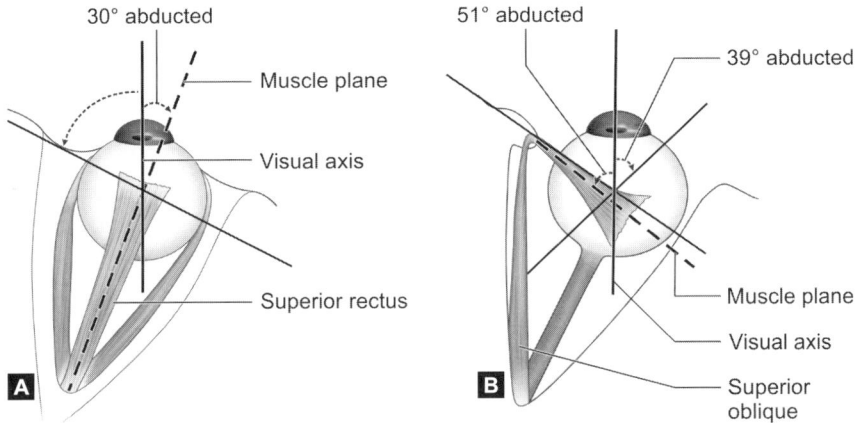

Figs. 37A and B: The relationship between visual axis and muscle plane in the effectiveness of vertical rotators. (A) Vertical recti; (B) Obliques

mainly act as intorters or extorters only when the eye is adducted 67° from primary position.
- *Thus, superior and inferior obliques are maximum (100%) effective as depressors or elevators when the eye is adducted 51° and act only as intorters or extorters when eyes are abducted 39° from primary position.*

Thus, superior and inferior recti act mainly as elevators or depressors when the eyes are in abducted position. In adducted position they mainly intort or extort the eyeballs. Superior and inferior obliques mainly act as depressors or elevators when the eyes are in adducted position. They only intort or extort eyeballs when the eyes are in abducted position.

GENERAL PRINCIPLES AND MEASUREMENTS IN SURGICAL CORRECTION OF SQUINTS

Horizontal Squints

Concomitant Squints
- In general, surgical treatment is considered for concomitant squint only in high degrees of phorias and tropias in children which squint had not got

corrected within a reasonable time (1-3 months) and does not shown any improvement after optical correction and orthoptic treatment.
- It is better to perform surgery at least by the age of 4 or 5; because at this stage child might cooperate for postoperative orthoptic treatment. If surgical intervention is delayed even later than 10 years of age, surgery can gain only cosmetic benefit and may not help in the development of binocular vision or prevention of amblyopia.
- In actual surgical procedure: The strong muscle which is the likely culprit producing deviation is made weak by recession and the weak muscle is strengthened by resection and advancement. Thus, in right divergent squint, excess power in right lateral rectus is reduced by recession and weak ipsilateral medial rectus is strengthened by resection and advancement.

  In recession surgery: The muscle is detached from its insertion and the disinserted end is sutured (reinserted) to sclera sufficient distance (according to the amount of squint) behind the original insertion.

  In resection surgery: The muscle is detached from its insertion and a sufficient length of muscle necessary for correction of squint is excised and the cut end of muscle is advanced and resutured to the site of original insertion.
- *The decision:* How much to recess or resect is a clinical and not mathematical and will determine the postoperative result. *A rough calculation is 1mm recession or resection is likely to correct 2.5° to 3° of squint. The maximum recession/resection allowed is 10 mm.* When the squint is small (less than 10°) recession of strong muscle alone is enough for correction. Along with recession, resection of its ipsilateral antagonist and even surgery of the fellow eye may become necessary for correction of larger degrees of deviations.
- Combined recession and resection in same eye in one sitting may be 25% more advantageous than two surgeries done in one eye separately at larger intervals.
- Recti should always be reinserted on sclera in front of equator of eyeball and obliques behinds its equator.

Paralytic Squint

In incomitant squint, surgery is considered only when the cause of paralysis has been treated and the cause is no more active and there is no chance of recovery of muscular activity by any other methods of treatment. The purpose of surgery is to regain comfortable binocular single vision as far as possible.

In a simple paralysis or palsy of one extraocular muscle of one eye alone, following surgical options may be considered: for example in right lateral rectus paralysis—options are:
- Overacting contralateral synergist (left medial rectus) may be weakened by recession.
- Paralyzed and weak muscle may be strengthen by resection.
- Overacting and contracted ipsilateral antagonist may be weakened by recession.

- Contralateral antagonist weakened by disuse palsy may be strengthened by resection.

Vertical Squint

- The amount of surgery in vertical squint is decided from the degree of squint in primary position.
- *An approximate 'rule of thumb' is, 1mm recession or resection of oblique muscle give 1 prism diopter of squint correction.*
- *Total recession of 4 mm or less give only little effect because of the effect in cutting and tying the muscle.*
- *It is better to limit the recession of inferior oblique to about 10 mm as this produces the new insertion to the lateral border of inferior rectus muscle.*
- *In superior oblique, larger recessions (12-15 mm) can be performed by passing under superior rectus.*
- Larger degrees of vertical squints can be corrected by combined recession and resection of obliques.
- *Recession of only one oblique muscle without corresponding shortening of antagonist give only 50% effect, since the oblique muscles provide only 1/3 of elevation or depression of globe.*

Suggested Readings

1. Adlers physiology of eye, clinical application, 11th edition; 2011.
2. American Academy of Ophthalmology: Basic clinical course, section 8.
3. Becker-Shaffers diagnosis and therapy of glaucomas, 8th edition; 2009.
4. Bloomsbery English Dictionary.
5. Chhablani J, Rao PS, Venkata A, Rao HL, et al. Choroidal thickness profile in healthy subjects. Indian Journal of Ophthalmology. 2014.
6. Dada T, Sharma R. Scanning laser polarimetry in glaucoma. AJO. 2015;62(9).
7. Dada T. All India Ophthalmologic Society guidelines for medical management of primary open angle glaucoma.
8. Duke Elders practice of refraction, 10th edition; 2014.
9. Fedman JL, Gowers P. Textbook of Ophthalmology: Retina and Vitreous.
10. Glaucoma in clinical practice: Leydhecker
11. Gopal L. Transition to MIVS (Micro incisional vitrectomy surgery) AIOS CME series No. 13: 2015.
12. Greers ocular pathology.
13. Haldipukar SS, Shikari HT, Gokhale V. Wound construction in manual small incision cataract surgery: IJO. 2009;59.
14. Hamilton RC. Anatomy of eye and orbit.
15. Jaffe NS, Jaffe MS, Jaffe CF. Cataract surgery and its complications.
16. Jain MK. Medical management of ocular inflammations.
17. Jain SS, Shah M. Facts about silent thief glaucoma: IJCP.
18. Kalever V. Marginal corneal ulcer.
19. Leibowitz HM, Waring GO. Corneal disorders: clinical diagnosis and management. 2nd edition.
20. Narang P, Agarwall A. Clinical outcomes of Parsplicata anterior vitrectomy; Two years result. Indian Journal of Ophthalmology. 2015.
21. Nema HV, Nema N, Shetty PR, Shetty A. Recent advances in Ophthalmology 10.
22. Nema HV, Nema N. Recent advances in Ophthalmology. 2013;11(11).
23. Outcome of treatment of congenital NLD obstruction: IJO: December-January 2015.
24. Parsons' Diseases of Eye, 22nd edition; 2015.
25. Shield's Textbook of glaucoma, 6th edition; 2011.
26. Sing K, Khanna R. Step by step glaucoma surgery. AIOS CME series No. 14.
27. Snellen RS, Lamp MA. Clinical anatomy of eye.
28. Sood D. Advances in the management of primary adult glaucomas: AIOS CME series No. 10.
29. Sreedhar U. General principles of corneal surgery: Ophthalmology Today;12(1)2011.
30. Stellard's eye surgery, 7th edition.
31. Sugar HS. Surgical anatomy of glaucoma. Survey of Ophthalmology.
32. The anatomy of limbus: Eye (London); 1989.
33. Thoft S. 'The cornea', scientific foundation and clinical practices, 4th edition; 2005.
34. Viscocanalostomy: Indian J Ophthalmol. February 2013.
35. Wolff's anatomy of eye and orbit: Vol. 1 & 2.

Index

Page numbers followed by *f* refer to figure, and *t* refer to table

A

Abducent nerve 228
Adenoma, pituitary 169, 169*f*
Adie's pupil 91
Alkaptonuria 49
Allergy 228
Amacrine cells 129, 130
Amaurosis 225
Amenorrhea 171
Ampulla 201
Anisocoria, physiological 90
Annulus of Zinn 181, 224, 231
Anterior chamber 54*f*, 62, 64*f*
   angle of 63
   boundaries of 62, 62*f*
   dimensions of 63*f*
   measurements of 62, 63
Anterior ciliary vessels, foramina for 17
Anterior scleral foramen, external scleral margin of 16
Antiglaucoma surgeries 9, 56*f*
Applanation 71
Aqueous
   circulation of 89
   flare 68, 68*f*
   humor 67, 69
      channels 66*f*
      composition of 68
      functions of 69
      measurements 68
      nonprotein concentration of 69
      outflow of 75
      oxygen concentration of 69
Arachnoiditis, optochiasmatic 170
Arcus juvenilis 49*f*
Arcus senilis 48
Area of Martegiani 115
Area of sella 165
Areolar tissue
   subcutaneous 180, 191
   submuscular 174, 180
Argyll Robertson pupil 91
Artery, infraorbital 220
Ascorbate 69
Asteroid hyalosis 118
Axial proptosis 225
Axoplasmic transport 158

B

Basal lamina 28
   inner 98
   outer 98
Basement membrane 28
Baush and Lomb keratometer 38
Bayer's calculators 36
Berger's space 114, 115
Bicarbonate ions 69
Bipolar cells function 129
Bitot's spots 48, 49*f*
Blaskovics technique 190
Bleeding disorders 56
Blindness, ipsilateral 169*f*
Blood vessels 94
Blue limbal incision 57
Bone 211
   forming lacrimal fossa 202*f*
   frontal 211
   maxillary 211
   zygomatic 211
Bouquet of central cones 143
Bowman's layer 28
Bowman's membrane 28, 32, 46, 47
   functions of 28
   termination of 50, 51
Brain
   inferior surface of 162*f*
   sagittal section of 163*f*
Brow ptosis 174
Brow suspension 175
Bruch's membrane 97
   structure of 97*f*
   thickness of 98
Bulbar conjunctiva, attachments of 9
Buphthalmos 34, 35*f*

C

Cadaveric eye 21
Canal of Hannover 110
Canal of Schlemm 17, 47, 52, 55, 64-66
Canaliculus, punctum of 200*f*
Canthal angle 187
Canthal tendon, lateral 182-184, 218
Cantholysis, lateral 186, 195*f*
Capsular tension ring 118
Capsule of Tenon 9
Capsulotomy
    anterior 104, 104*f*, 105
    posterior 104, 105*f*
Carcinoma breast 214
Cardiovascular diseases 71
Carotid
    artery, internal 162, 227
    system
        external 218
        internal 218
Cataract
    extraction
        conventional extracapsular 57, 58*f*
        intracapsular 57, 58*f*
    hypermature 107
    intumescent 100
    surgery 9, 10, 31, 36, 56, 57*f*, 58*f*, 103, 104, 118
        techniques of 57
Catarrhal ulcer 48
Cavernous sinus 228
Cells, horizontal 129
Central nervous system, part of 152
Cerebrospinal fluid 155, 162, 203
Chalazion 193*f*
    surgery 193
Chemosis 225
Chiasma
    anterior angle of 168
    length of 161
    part of 169*f*
    posterior angle of 170
    superior part of 170
Chiasmal lesions 168, 171
Chiasmatic cistern 162
Chloride ions 68, 69
Cholinesterase inhibitors 21
Choriocapillaris, outer basal lamina of 98
Choroid 96
    dimensions of 96, 98
    functions of 98
    length of 96
    structure of 96, 97*f*
    thickness of 96
Choroidal detachment 55
Choroidal pigment 15
Ciliary arteries
    long posterior 19
    short posterior 19
Ciliary body 91, 95
    anterior face of 62
    capillaries of 69
    dimensions of 94, 95
    functions of 95
    pars plana of 119
    pars plicata of 119
    parts of 92*f*
    posteromedial surface of 81
    structure of 92, 92*f*
    surface marking of 95
    total length of 95
Ciliary epithelial cells 94
Ciliary epithelium 93, 94
Ciliary flush 15
Ciliary muscle 92
    contraction of 93
    tone 67
Ciliary nerves
    long 20
    short 20
Ciliary process, structure of 94*f*
Ciliary sulcus 82, 84
    average diameter of 82
Cloquet's canal 113-115, 118
Closed angle glaucoma 70
Coaxial microincision cataract surgery 57, 58*f*
Collagen
    diseases 15
    fibers 118
    vascular disorders, limbal manifestation of 48
Collarette, thickness of 89
Color-coded contour map 39
Computerized corneal topography 39
Cones, high density of 141
Congestion, circumcorneal 17
Conjunctiva 7, 9, 10, 10*f*, 32, 50, 190
    bulbar 8-10
    burns of 12
    dimensions of 12
    diseases of 46, 48

fornicial 8
lamina propria of 47
measurements of 6, 12
palpebral 186
portions of 7, 7f
squamous cell carcinoma of 49f
structure of 6, 6f
Conjunctival epithelium 11, 12f
Conjunctival flap 52
fornix-based 9, 9f, 54f
Conjunctival fornix 7, 182, 199f
Conjunctival impression cytology 11, 11f
Conjunctival sac 8
dimension of 8f
level of 12
Conjunctival scarring 12f
Conjunctivitis
phlyctenular 49f
vernal 49f
Connective tissues, condensation of 86
Contact lenses 31
Copper deposit 48
Cornea 2, 26, 32, 33, 35, 54, 62
abscess of 48
anterior
layer of 27
surface of 33f
Bowman's membrane of 47
central third of 36
curvature of 35, 41
dimensions of 26f
internal diameter of 17
layers of 27f, 32
measurements of 26, 44
posterior surface of 33f, 36
refractive index of 41
shape of 35
structure of 26, 27f
surface area of 32
thickness of 42f
topography of 39f
Corneal astigmatism
anterior 35
posterior 36
Corneal curvature
measurement of 37
normal variations of 35
Corneal decompensation 118
Corneal diameter 32, 34
enlarged 35f
horizontal 35f
measurement of 33

Corneal epithelium 27f
Corneal incision 56
Corneal injury 28
Corneal innervation 32
Corneal pachymetry 44
Corneal reflex, keratoscopic 38f
Corneal stroma 28f
subjacent fibers of 64
Corneal thickness 41, 42, 44, 72
measurement of 42
Corneal topographer 35
Corneal topographic zones 36, 37f
Corneal ulcers, marginal 48
Corneolimbal junction 50, 55, 79
Corneoscleral junction 17
Corneoscleral limbus 65
Corneoscleral meshwork 64
Corneoscleral tunnel incision, conventional square-shaped 60f
Corrugator supercilii 173
Cortex 102
anterior 105
peripheral 105
Cranial cavity 161
Cranial fossa 163, 163f
middle 163
Cranial nerves 152
Craniofacial anomalies 210
Craniofacial syndromes 187
Craniopharyngioma 168, 169
Cushing syndrome 171
Cyclocryotherapy 55
Cyclodestructive procedures 55, 95
Cysticercosis, intraocular 118
Cystoid
cicatrix 21
macular edema 144

D

Dacryocystectomy 185, 206
Dacryocystitis 203, 207f
acute 204f
chronic 204f
Dacryocystorhinostomy 185, 206, 208
Deep lamellar keratoplasty 29
Deep pretarsal aponeurosis 218
Demyelination 168
Depression 234
Descemet's membrane 29, 30f, 32, 46, 47, 55, 65

posterior surface of 30
termination of 29, 50, 51, 64
Diabetes mellitus 31, 71
Diabetic retinopathy, proliferative 118
Diaphragma sella 162
Dilator pupillae 86, 89
Diplopia 217, 222, 223
    horizontal 223
Dorsum sellae 164
Down syndrome 210
Draeger tonometer 72
Drainage angle, measurements of 67
Dry eye 12
Dua's layer 29, 30f, 32
Duane's retraction syndrome 214
Dysgerminomas 169
Dyskeratosis, benign 48
Dysplasia, fibrous 227
Dystrophies 37

E

Ectasias 37
Ectopic pinealomas 169
Ectropion correction surgeries 194
Edinger-Westphal nucleus 86
Egger's line 115
Ehlers-Danlos syndrome 15
Electronic indentation tonometry 74
Emmetropes 16
Emphysema, surgical 221
Endocrine dysfunction 171
Endophthalmitis 118
    postoperative 57
Endothelial cell
    density 31
    single layer of 85
Endothelium 30, 30f, 32
    basal lamina of 29
    specular micrograph of 31f
Enophthalmos 214, 215f, 222
    measurements 215f
Entropion lower lid, correction of 194f
Entropion surgery 194
Enucleation 227
Epiretinal membrane surgery 118
Episclera 15
Episcleritis 49f
Epithelial cells 101
    enlargement of 11
    separation of 11
    small 11

Epithelioma, intraepithelial 48
Epithelium 27, 32, 102
    anterior 87
        pigmented 94
    basal lamina of 28
    normal 11
    posterior 87
    primary function of 27
Erggellet's space 114
Ethmoid bone 211
Ethmoidal artery, anterior 223
Ethmoidal canals
    anterior 216, 225
    posterior 216, 225
Ethmoidal foramen, anterior 223
Everbush's technique 190
Exophthalmos 213
Extracellular space, small size of 101
Extraocular muscles
    dimensions of 235, 235f
    insertion of 16, 24, 236, 236f
    measurements of 229
    origins of 224
    tone of 70
Eye 56, 99
    anterior segment of 81
    aqueous drainage system of 64
    buphthalmic 35f
    drainage system of 197
    gross measurements of 1
    pain of 221
    swelling of 221
Eyeball 1
    anterior segment of 99
    center of 3
        rotation of 3, 3f, 236, 238, 239f
    diameter of 2
    dimensions of 2f
    equator of 2
    general
        dimensions 2
        measurements of 4
        structure of 1f
    lower displacement of 222
    nodal point of 3
    outer coat of 14
    parts of 85
    posterior segment of 112
    preserves shape of 24
    structure 1
    torsions of 238

Eyebrows 172, 172*f*, 173, 174
  dimensions of 172
  functions of 174
  hairs, loss of 174, 175*f*
  layers of 173, 173*f*
  measurements of 172
  structure of 173, 173*f*
Eyelids 1, 178
  colobomas, reconstructions of 195
  fibrous layer of 183, 183*f*
  functions of 195
  measurements of 178

F

Facial
  expression, muscles of 180*f*
  opening 209
Fasanella-Servat
  operation 190
  procedure, modification of 190
Fascia 202
  bulbi 9
  capsulopalpebral 184, 192
Fat, preaponeurotic pad of 181
Fetal nucleus 107
Fibers
  arrangement of 167, 167*f*
  bundles of 28*f*, 109
  temporal 157, 167
Fibrous tissue layer, subcutaneous 173
Fissure
  below ring transmit, part of 228
  transmits, intermediate portion of 228
Fontalis muscle 176*f*
Foramen, zygomatic 218
Foramina
  anterior group of 16
  middle group 17
  posterior 25
Fornices, extent of 8*f*
Fovea 128, 134, 135, 141, 151
  centralis 134
  depth of 143, 151
  diameter of 143
  dimensions of 143
  externa 143
  structure of 143*f*
  thickness of 143
  trochlearis 216
Foveal avascular zone 142*f*, 143
Foveal pit 143

Foveola 134, 141, 143, 151
Fracture 216, 224
  blowout 223
  floor 221*f*
  lateral wall 186219
  zygomatic 186
  zygomaticomaxillary complex 219
Friedenwald nomogram 23*f*
Frontal bone, orbital plate of 215
Frontalis 173
  muscle 176*f*
  sling, steps of 176
Frontoethmoidal suture 215
Frontozygomatic suture 218
Full thickness lid tear, repair of 194*f*

G

Galactorrhea 171
Ganglion cell 141
  layer 130, 132, 144, 145
    thickness of 130
GDx printout 150*f*
Giant retinal tear 118
Gland, pituitary 161, 164, 165
Glands of Krause 197, 199
Glands of Wolfring 197, 199
Glandulae lacrimalis 198
Glaucoma 19, 23*f*, 31, 70, 80, 138*f*, 146
  congenital 35*f*
  disease
    mild 71, 80
    moderate 71, 80
    severe 71, 80
  early diagnosis of 75
  evaluation of 42, 150
  filtering bleb 48
  genetic predisposition 70
  infantile 21
  pupillary block 83*f*
  relief of 83
  types of 70
Gliomas 168
Globe, support ligament of 218
Glucose 69
Goblet cell 6, 10, 10*f*, 11, 12*f*
  density 10, 11
  loss of 11, 12*f*
Goldmann tonometer 44, 72
Goldmann/Zeiss four mirror contact
    lens 146
Golgi apparatus 30

Gonioscopy 29
Gout, conjunctival episcleritis of 49
Granuloma 193*f*
   removal of 193*f*

H

Haller's layer 97
Heidelberg retina tomograph 147
   equipment 149*f*
   printout 149*f*
Hemianopia 169*f*, 170
   binasal 171
   bitemporal 171
   contralateral 168
   inferior altitudinal 170*f*
Hemianopic reaction 91
Hemidesmosome formation 28
Hemorrhage 55, 224
   subconjunctival 221
Henle's fiber layer 129, 143, 144
Horner's muscle 202
Horner's syndrome 214
Hruby lens 146
Hyaloid membrane
   anterior 113
   posterior 113, 118
Hyaloideocapsular ligament 115, 118
Hydrodilineation 106
Hydrodissection 105
Hydroprocedures 106, 106*f*
Hypermature shrunken lens 101*f*
Hypermaturity 101
Hypermetropia 16, 21
Hypertelorism 210
Hypertension, ocular 80
Hypoesthesia 219
   infraorbital 222
Hypoglobus 222
Hypophysis cerebri 164
Hypotelorism 210
Hypothalamus, activity of 70
Hypothyroidism 174
Hypotony, ocular 80

I

Incision
   chord length of 57, 58*f*
   depth of 60
   length of 61
   size of 123
   vertical 79

Inferior ophthalmic vein, tributaries of 229
Inferior orbital fissure
   boundaries of 229*f*
   dimensions of 229*f*
Inferior rectus muscle, dimensions of 232*f*
Infertility 171
Inflammations 168, 224, 228
Infraorbital nerve, injury of 222
Internal carotid artery, aneurysm of 228
Internal limiting membrane 131, 132, 144
Internal maxillary artery, sphenopalatine branch of 229
Intraocular foreign body, removal of 118
Intraocular lens 36
   implantation 103
Intraocular pressure 21, 22, 22*t*, 33, 34, 65, 69, 70, 72, 73, 80
   baseline 71, 80
   measurement of 44, 70
   normal 70
Intraocular tumors 118
Ipsilateral temporal retina 160
Iridectomy, peripheral 54*f*, 83*f*
Iridocyclitis, acute 87*f*
Iris 85
   anterior surface of 62
   diameter of 87, 88*f*
   dimensions of 89
   epithelium 87*f*
   functions of 88
   layers of 85, 86*f*
   muscles of 86*f*
   posterior surface of 81
   root of 89
   structure of 85, 86*f*
   thickness of 88, 88*f*
Iritis 91
Iron deposit 48

J

Jacod's triad 225
Juxtacanalicular trabecular meshwork tissue 55

K

Kasener compares 51
Kayser-Fleischer ring 48, 49*f*
Keratinzation 12
Keratitis 225

marginal 49*f*
phlyctenular 49*f*
Keratoconus 31, 40*f*
Keratocytes 29
Keratoglobus 34
Keratometer 35
Keratometric mires 38*f*
Keratometry 37
Keratoplasty 31
    lamellar 29
    penetrating 31
Keratoscope 35
Keratoscopy 38
Knee of Willebrand 168
Kuhnt Szymanowski procedure, modified 194

L

Lacrimal apparatus 1, 197
    measurements of 197
Lacrimal bone 203, 211, 222
    small portion of 204
Lacrimal canaliculi 197, 200
Lacrimal crest, anterior 223
Lacrimal fascia 202
Lacrimal fistula 204*f*
Lacrimal fossa 202, 207*f*, 223
    dimensions of 203, 203*f*
Lacrimal gland 197, 198
    accessory 197, 199
    normal 199*f*
    orbital portion of 198*f*
Lacrimal nerve 227
Lacrimal papilla 186
Lacrimal passages 197, 200, 205
    dimensions of 200*f*, 201*f*
    surface marking of 205*f*
Lacrimal puncta 197, 200
Lacrimal sac 198, 201, 202
    disorders 203
    surgeries 206*f*
        measurements 206
Lactate 68, 69
Lamina cribrosa 19, 154
Lamina fusca 15, 96
Lamina papyracea 222
Large volume camp surgeries 56
Laser iridotomy 83*f*
LASIK 32
Lateral rectus, check ligament of 218
Lateral wall, bones of 218

Layer of Henle 143
Lens 81, 109, 118
    anterior surface of 100
    capsule 103, 103*f*, 110
    colobomatous 100
    congenital anomaly of 100
    cortex 105
    diameter of 99
    dimensions of 99, 107
    dioptric power of 101
    epithelium 105
    equatorial diameter of 93
    fibers, regular arrangement of 101
    functions of 102
    intumescent 101*f*, 107
    measurements of 99
    normal 99*f*
        diameter of 100*f*
        thickness of 100
        width of 100
    posterior
        curvature of 93
        surface of 116*f*
    power of 101
    pump system of 101
    radius of curvature of 100
    refractive index of 101
    sagittal thickness of 93
    structure of 102, 102*f*
    surgical anatomy of 102, 106*f*
    suspensory ligament of 109
    thickness of 100
    weight of 101
    zonule diaphragm 99
Lenticonus 101
Leprosy 174, 175*f*
Levator
    action
        assessment of 189*f*
        measurement of 188
    aponeurosis, lateral horn of 218
    muscle, dimensions of 182*f*
    muscular portion of 182
    palpebrae superioris 188, 190
        check ligament of 218
        muscle 181, 195
        portion of 7
    resection 182, 190
Lid
    ecchymosis of 221
    edema 225, 228

emphysema of 223
free margin of 186
tear, full thickness 193
Ligament of Lockwood 218
Ligament of Weiger 83
Ligament of Whitnall 181, 188
Limbal border
　anterior 50
　posterior 50
Limbal incision 56, 57
Limbal line 50
Limbal stroma 79
Limbic keratitis, superior 48
Limbus 20, 46f, 56, 145
　deep pigmentation of 49
　dimensions of 49, 50f, 51, 51f
　functions of 47
　importance of 47
　landmarks of 49, 50f, 52
　limits of 46
　measurements of 46
　pannus, superior 48
　structure of 47, 47f
　surgical anatomy of 51, 51f
　zones of 50, 51f, 52f
Lower conjunctival fornix, inferior suspensory ligament of 192
Lower lid
　breadth of 185f
　coloboma, reconstruction of 195f
　gross measurements of 191, 191f
　length of 185f
　measurements of 191
　movement 192
　retraction 193
　structure of 191, 192f
　tarsal plate of 184, 192, 196
Lymphatics 223
Lymphoma 118

M

Macula 116, 135, 141, 151
　portions of 142f
Macular area 134
Macular fibers 157, 158
Macular hole surgery 118
Macular pucker 118
Macular region 132
Macular star 144, 144f
Madarosis 174
Makay-Marg tonometer 72

Marcus Gunn pupil 91
Marfan's syndrome 114
Marginal reflex distance 189, 190f
Maxilla
　frontal process of 222
　orbital plate of 220
Maxillary antrum 204
Medial canthal tendon 183, 184
　posterior limb of 182
Medial canthus
　distance of 187f
　rounding of 223
Medial palpebral ligament 185, 202, 203
Medial rectus 16, 122, 235, 236
　muscle 230
Medial wall 222f
　bones of 222
　fracture 223
　injury 223
Megalocornea 33
　corneal diameter variation of 34f
　simple 34
Megalophthalmos, megalocornea of 34
Meibomian glands 180
Melanocytes 86
Meningioma 168, 169, 227, 228
Meningitis 170
Microcornea 33
　corneal diameter variation of 34f
Microincision cataract surgery 57, 58f
Microphakia 100
Microspherophakia 101, 101f
Middle cranial fossa
　floor of 164
　lateral borders of 164
Minimally invasive vitreous surgeries 123, 124f
Miosis 91
Mittendorf's dots 115
Moll's glands 180
Moraxella lacunata 48
Morgagnian cataract 100
Morphine 91
Mucin spots 11
Muller's cells 128-130
Muller's fibers 144
Muller's muscle 7, 182, 183, 188, 195
　dimensions of 182f
Mullerectomy 190
Muscle
　extraocular 15, 119f

layer 173
plane 239f
superior oblique 232
Mydriasis 89, 91
Mydriatics 90
Myopia 21, 90, 115

N

Nanophthalmos 21
Nasal fibers 157, 158, 167
Nasal nerve, internal 223
Nasal quadrant 95
   superior 41
Nasal retina 132
   contralateral 160
Nasal retinal
   fibers 160f
   quadrant, inferior 167
Nasal vortex vein
   inferior 17
   superior 17
Nasociliary nerve 228
   anterior ethmoidal branch of 223
Nasolacrimal canal 220, 225
Nasolacrimal duct 198, 203
   obstruction, congenital 205
Nerve
   fiber index 150
   fiber layer 130, 132, 144, 153
      abnormal 147f
      normal 147f
   frontal 227
   infraorbital 220, 229
   loop of Axenfeld 17
   supratrochlear 216
   zygomatic 229
   zygomaticofacial 219
   zygomaticotemporal 218
Neurilemma sheath 153
Neuroretinal rim 136
Nomogram 22
Noncontact tonometer 72
Non-keratinized stratified epithelium 6
Nonprotein nitrogen 69
Normal retina, color of 133
Nuclear layer
   inner 129, 131, 144
   outer 129, 131, 143
Nucleus 102, 106
   embryonic 107

O

Oblique muscle, inferior 220, 234
Ochronosis 49
Oculomotor nerve
   inferior division of 228
   irritation of 91
   paralysis 90
   superior division of 228
Oncotic pressure 118
Open angle glaucoma 70
   primary 65
Open sky vitrectomy 120, 120f
Ophthalmic artery
   aneurysm of 227
   recurrent branch of 228
Ophthalmic vein
   inferior 228
   superior 228
Ophthalmoplegia 228
Ophthalmoscope 133
Ophthalmoscopy 146
Optic atrophy
   consecutive 138, 139f
   postneuritic 139, 140f
   primary 138, 139f
Optic axis 3f, 4, 4f, 236, 237f
Optic canal 223, 225, 226f
   diameter of 226
   enlargement of 227
Optic chiasma 155, 160f-163f, 164, 165, 167, 167f, 168
   central part of 169
   dimensions of 161, 161f
   measurements of 160
   portions of 161f
   position of 161
Optic disk 116, 134, 135, 137f, 138, 151, 154f
   color variations of 138
   drusen 140f
   measurements of 135
   melanocytoma of 141f
   near 98
Optic foraminae 164
Optic nerve 20f, 152-154, 155f, 213
   chiasmal junction 168, 169f
   contralateral 167
   dimensions of 153f
   diseases of 90, 91
   distal portion of 156f

fiber 156, 159, 160, 167
    extent of 152*f*
    layer 147
functions of 158
gliomas 227
head 70, 147
intracanalicular portion of 155
intracranial portion of 160
intraocular portion of 154*f*
measurements of 152, 159
portions of 153*f*
proximal portion of 156, 157, 157*f*
retrolaminar layer of 154
sheath meningioma 227
Optic neuritis 225
Optic neuropathy, anterior ischemic 140*f*
Optic papilla 153
Optical canal 156*f*
    dimensions of 226*f*
Optical coherence tomography 43, 138, 147
Optical pachymetry 42
Optical system, different parts of 24
Ora serrata 19*f*, 119*f*, 135, 145, 151
    approximate distance of 5*f*, 20*f*
    distance of 145
    near 98
Orbicularis oculi 173, 180, 202
    muscle 180*f*
        orbital portion of 192
Orbit 1, 209, 209*f*
    base of 209
    blowout fracture of 214
    bones of 211*f*
    communications of 225
    configuration of 213, 213*f*
    depth of 209
    dimensions of 209, 210*f*
    emphysema of 223
    eyeball relationship 213
    floor of 219, 220*f*
    lateral wall of 186, 217, 221*f*
    measurements of 209
    medial wall of 222
    roof of 215, 216*f*
    thinnest part of 222
    walls of 211, 212*f*, 215
Orbital apex 223, 224*f*
    syndrome 224, 225
Orbital axis 236, 237, 238*f*
Orbital cavity 213
Orbital cellulitis 214
Orbital conjunctiva 7
Orbital fissure
    inferior 225, 228, 229*f*
    superior 224, 225, 227, 227*f*, 228
Orbital floor
    bones of 220
    fracture 221
    injury 221*f*
Orbital hemorrhage 221
Orbital index 210
Orbital lobe 197, 198
Orbital margins 211
    bones of 212*f*
    inferior 212
    lateral 211
Orbital periostitis 224
Orbital plane 236
Orbital plate 222
Orbital roof 216
    bones of 215
    fracture 217
Orbital septum 7, 181, 183, 184, 202
Orbital tissues, fibrous contraction of 214
Orbital tubercle, lateral 218
Orbital wall
    destruction of 214
    injury
        lateral 217*f*, 219*f*
        medial 223*f*
    posterior extremities of 223
Orbscan 40, 43
Organs, edge of 48

P

Pachymeter 42, 43*f*
Paget's disease 227
Pain, neuralgic 225
Palatine bone 211
    orbital process of 220
Pallid disk edema 139, 140*f*
Palpebral fissure 186
    dimensions of 186*f*
    width of 189
Palpebral ligament 183, 184, 186
Palpebral lobe 197, 198
Palpebral muscle, inferior 184
Pansinusitis 228
Papery white disk 139*f*
Papilledema 139*f*
Parafovea 134, 141, 143, 151
Paralysis, pupillary 91
Paranasal air sinuses 221

Pars orbicularis 110
Pars plana 91, 95, 96, 110, 119*f*
　incision 55, 56
　surgeries 55, 56*f*
　surgical procedures 95
　vitrectomy 120, 121, 121*f*, 122*f*, 124*f*
　　incisions 122
Pars plicata 94, 96
　distance of 119*f*
　vitrectomy 120, 124
Patellar fossa 115
　edge of 111
Pellucid marginal degeneration 48
Pemphigus 12
Pentacam 40f, 43
Pericapsular membrane 102
Perifovea 134, 141, 143, 151
Periorbital tissues, communications of 221
Periostitis 228
Perkin's tonometer 72
Petit's canal 114
Phacoemulsification 57, 58*f*
Phlyctenular disease 48
Pigment cells 86
Pilocarpine 65
Pinguecula 48
Pit, floor of 143
Plasma 69
Plexiform layer
　inner 130, 132, 144
　outer 129, 131, 143
Pneumatic tonometer 72
Posterior chamber 81
　boundaries of 81*f*
　dimensions of 84
　measurements of 81
　parts of 81, 82*f*
　volume of 84
Posterior ciliary arteries, foramina for 19
Pre-Descemet's dystrophies 29
Procerus muscle 174
Proptosis 213, 214*f*, 217, 221, 228
　measurement 214*f*
Protein 69
Provocative test 21
Pseudoexfoliation syndrome 103
Pterygium 48, 49*f*
Pterygopalatine ganglion, orbital branch of 229
Ptosis 217, 225, 228
　correction of 175*f*, 176, 190

　measurements of 189
　mild congenital 191
　moderate 190*f*, 191
　severe 190*f*
　surgery 175
Pupil 89
　size 89, 90*f*
　　enlargement of 89
Pupillary diameter 90
Pupillary reactions 90
Pupillary zone width 89

Q

Quadrantanopia, superior 168

R

Raised intracranial tension 227
Recesses of Khunt 82
Recti muscle 119
　insertions 232
Recti, vertical 239*f*
Rectus
　inferior 16, 122, 235, 236
　lateral 16, 122, 235, 236
　muscle
　　inferior 231
　　lateral 230, 230*f*
　　superior 7, 230
Red swollen disk 139*f*
Refractive index 41, 107, 118
Refractive power 41
Refractive surgeries 42
Reticulum cell sarcoma 118
Retina 126, 134*f*
　anterior 133, 134, 151
　blood vessels of 116
　central 133, 134
　diameter of 151
　diseases of 90
　extent of 132, 132*f*, 146*f*
　general
　　features of 132
　　structure of 127
　histological structure of 127*f*
　histopathology of 147
　layer-by-layer structure of 126*f*
　measurements of 126, 151
　normal 133*f*, 148*f*
　peripheral 133-135, 145, 151
　posterior 133, 134, 151
　shape of 132

surface
    area of 151
        marking of 146*f*
    thickness of 126*f*, 132, 133*f*, 151
    topography of 133
    width of 151
Retinal detachment
    primary 118
    surgeries 9
Retinal layers, measurement of 131
Retinal nerve fiber layer 146, 150
    damage of 75
Retinal pigment epithelium 126, 127, 131, 142
    functions of 127
Retinal quadrant, superonasal 168
Retinal vein occlusion 118
Retinal vessels, central 155*f*
Retinopathy of prematurity 118
Rheumatoid arthritis 49*f*
Ring ulcer 48
Road traffic accidents 217

S

Sac
    lowermost portion of 202
    massage 205, 206*f*
    tumors of 203
    upper portion of 202
Sattler's layer 97
Scanning laser
    ophthalmoscopy 75
    polarimetry 147, 149
Scar tissue 28
Schiotz tonometry, calibration of 22, 73*f*
Schlemm's canal 52, 54, 64, 65
Schwalbe's line 29, 47, 50, 51
Schwann cell sheath 32
Sclera 8, 9, 14, 15, 20
    dimensions of 14*f*
    diseases of 48
    dorsal surface of 20*f*
    functions of 24
    measurements of 14, 24
    peripheral 49
    radius of curvature of 2
    small anterior portion of 62
    structure of 15
    surface of 19*f*
    temporal 16
    thickness of 15
    weak areas of 20, 21*f*

Scleral apertures 16
Scleral canal 136
Scleral coat, coronal diameter of 14
Scleral dimensions 14
Scleral flap
    lamellar 54*f*
    thickness of 54*f*
Scleral foramen, posterior 19
Scleral foramina 16*f*, 25
Scleral incision 56, 58
Scleral indentation 9
Scleral margin, internal 17
Scleral pocket incision 58
Scleral rigidity 20
    calculation of 23*f*
Scleral spur 52, 65
Scleral stroma 15
Scleral surface, posterior 153
Scleral tunnel 58
    corneal valve incision 60*f*
    incision 80
        architecture of 59
        classical 58
        conventional 59
    limits of 60
Scleritis 21
Sclerolimbal junction 50, 52
Sclerotic carotid arteries 170
Sclerotomy, posterior 56
Scotoma, central bitemporal hemianopic 168
Sella
    depth of 165
    diameter of 165
    dimensions of 165*f*
    measurements of 165
    portions of 164*f*
    turcica 162, 164, 165
    volume of 165
Shwalbe ring 64
Sickle cell retinopathy 118
Silvery striated appearance 146
Skin 173, 179, 191, 202
    of eyelids, tuberculosis of 174
Small incision cataract surgery 57, 58*f*, 61*f*
Sodium ions 69
Specular microscope 30*f*
Sphenoid
    body of 222
    bone 211
        primary tumor of 228
    greater wing of 218

lesser wing of 216
wing meningioma 224
Sphenoidal air sinus 162
Sphincter pupillae 86, 89
Squamous cell carcinoma 48, 49f
Squint
   concomitant 239
   horizontal 239
   paralytic 240
   surgical correction of 239
   vertical 241
Stab incision 123, 123f
Staphylococcal toxin 48, 49f
Steatoblepharon 193
Stereophotography 147
Steven Johnson syndrome 12
Strabismus surgery 15
Stroma 28, 32, 86, 93, 97
   functions of 29
Substantia propria 28
Sulcus chiasmaticus 164
Superficial scleral flap 52
Superior oblique muscle, dimensions of 233f
Superior ophthalmic vein, occlusion of 228
Superior orbital fissure, medial end of 223
Superior quadrantanopia, contralateral 169f
Superior rectus muscle
   dimensions of 231f
   sheath, expansion of 218
Suprachoroidal lamina 96
Suture
   double-armed 175f
   zygomaticofrontal 215, 216
   zygomaticosphenoid 218
Sympathetic system, palsy of 91
Synechia, posterior 87f
Systemic disorders 70

T

Tarsal conjunctiva 7, 192
Tarsal muscle, inferior 192
Tarsal plate 176f, 183
   dimensions of 185f
   surgical importance of 193
Tears, functions of 199
Telecanthus 187
Temporal vortex vein, inferior 17
Tenon's capsule 9, 10, 15, 47, 50

Tenon's fascia 9, 52
Tension glaucoma
   low 80
   normal 80
Terrien's marginal degeneration 48
Tonic pupil of Adie 91
Tonography 75
   technique of 76
Tonometers 71, 72
Tonometry 70, 71
Tonopen 72
Topography 37
Tournay's reaction 90
Trabecular meshwork 52, 64
Trabecular tissue block 54f
Trabeculectomy 52
   ostium 54f
   steps 54f
Trabeculotomy 54
Trachoma 12
Trachomatous pannus 49f
Transscleral laser cyclophotocoagulation 55, 95
Traquair junctional scotoma 168, 169f
Trauma 169, 187, 228
Traumatic telecanthus 223
Trochlear
   fossa 216
   injury 223
   nerve 228
Tuber cinereum 162
Tuberculum musculare 216
Tuberculum sellae 164
Tumors 168, 170, 224
Tunnel incision 123
   internal corneal lip of 60
Turbinate bone, inferior 204

U

Ultrasonic pachymetry 43
Upper eyelid, structure of 181f
Upper lid
   breadth of 178f
   elevation 188
   excursion 188
   gross measurements of 178
   length of 178f
   margin 189
   structure of 178, 179f
   tarsal plate of 184f, 196

Urea 69
Uveal meshwork 64
Uveal tract 85
   general dimensions of 85*f*
   measurements of 85
   parts of 85*f*
Uveitis 115
   anterior 17
Uveoscleral outflow 67, 92
Uveoscleral pathway 67

V

Vasculitis 118
Vein, infraorbital 220
Vernal disease 48
Videokeratography 39
Viscocanalostomy 54
Viscosity 118
Vision
   considerable loss of 225
   contralateral hemified of 160
Visual acuity 142
Visual axis 3, 4*f*, 236, 236*f*-238*f*
   opacification 104
Visual field defects 168
Visual impulses, conduction of 158
Visual loss 217
Vitrectomy 55, 118, 119*f*
   measurements 118
   surgeries, microincisional 123
   types of 120
Vitreous 112, 114*f*, 117*f*
   anterior surface of 81
   base 116, 118
      posterior 116
      region 132
   core 113
   cortex 113, 118
   dimensions of 118
   face, anterior 114
   functions of 117
   hemorrhage, nonresolving 118
   humor
      measurements of 112
      transparency of 117
   incarceration 118
   membranes 118
   opacities 118
   parameters 117
   primary 113
   prolapse 118
   secondary 113
   structure of 112, 112*f*
   surface, posterior 115
   surgical removal of 118
   tertiary 113
   topography 114
Vortex veins 17
   approximate distance of 18*f*
   positions of 18

W

Waardenburg syndrome 187
Walkers field loss 169
Weigers ligament 111
Wheelers operation, modified 194
White limbal incision 57
Whitnall's ligament 218
Whitnall's tubercle 218
Wieger's ligament 114

X

X-ray skull 221*f*

Y

Yellow swollen disk 139

Z

Zonular bundles 110, 110*f*
   anterior 110, 111
   posterior 110, 111
Zonular fibers, posterior group of 95, 96
Zonular fibrils, length of 110
Zonular fork 110
Zonular lamella 102
Zonular plexus 110
Zonules 81, 109, 109*f*, 115
   dimensions of 109
   extent of 109, 111
   functions of 111
   hyaloid 111
   insertion of 109
   loosening of 93
   measurements of 109
   of Zinn, measurements of 109
   parts of 110
   posterior limbs of 110
   resistance of 110
Zygoma 218
Zygomatic bone, orbital surface of 218, 220